HIGH-PROTEIN, LOW-CARB COOKBOOK

Published by: Medialusion Books
San Diego, CA
First Edition: 2025

DISCLAIMER AND TERMS OF USE

The information contained in this book is for educational and informational purposes only and is not intended as health or medical advice. Always consult a physician or other qualified health provider regarding any questions you may have about a medical condition or health objectives.

The author is not a medical doctor, registered dietitian, or licensed healthcare professional. The recipes, meal plans, and nutritional information provided in this book reflect the author's research and personal experience and are not intended to diagnose, treat, cure, or prevent any disease or health condition.

Before beginning any new dietary regimen, including a high-protein, low-carb diet, you should consult with your physician or healthcare provider, especially if you:

- Have any pre-existing medical conditions (including but not limited to diabetes, kidney disease, heart disease, or eating disorders)
- Are pregnant, nursing, or planning to become pregnant Are taking any medications or supplements
- Are under 18 years of age

Individual results may vary. The testimonials and examples provided in this book represent the author's personal experience and are not guarantees of results for all readers.

The nutritional information provided for each recipe is calculated to the best of the author's ability using standard nutritional databases and should be considered approximate. Actual nutritional content may vary based on specific brands, preparation methods, and ingredient substitutions. If you have specific dietary requirements or restrictions, please verify nutritional information independently.

The author and publisher disclaim any liability arising directly or indirectly from the use of this book. By continuing to read and use the recipes and information in this book, you acknowledge that you have read this disclaimer and agree to its terms.

ALLERGEN NOTICE

Recipes in this book may contain common allergens including dairy, eggs, nuts, soy, and shellfish. Please review ingredient lists carefully if you have food allergies or sensitivities. The author and publisher are not responsible for adverse reactions to foods consumed or items handled as a result of following the recipes in this book.

FOOD SAFETY

Proper food handling, preparation, and storage are essential to prevent foodborne illness. Follow USDA food safety guidelines for minimum internal cooking temperatures, storage times, and safe food handling practices. When in doubt, throw it out.

TABLE OF CONTENTS

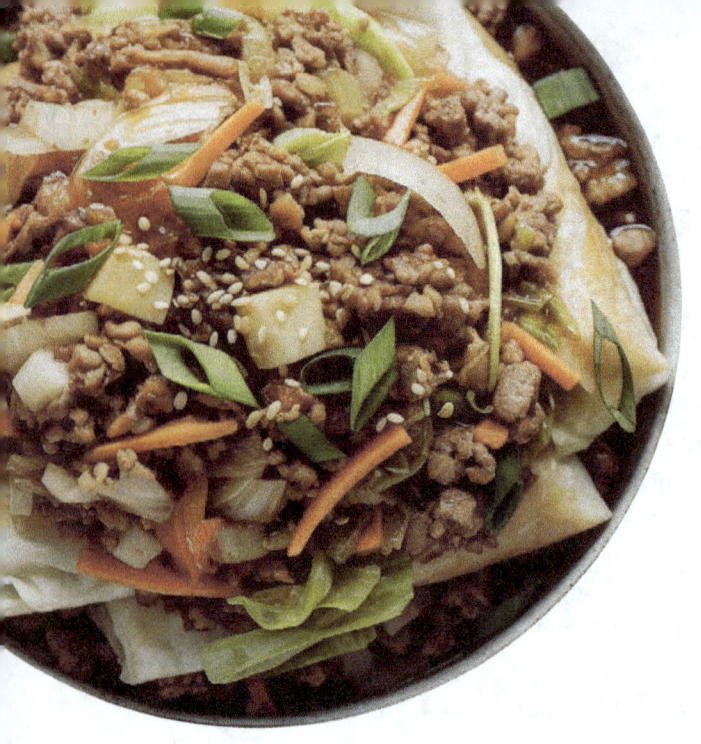

INTRODUCTION

I'm not a doctor or nutritionist. I'm a home cook who discovered that eating more protein and fewer carbs changed everything—my energy, my hunger between meals, and how I felt in my body.

This book isn't about achieving some perfect physique or following a trend. It's about feeling good, having energy for what matters, and simplifying food in a way that works with real life. After writing cookbooks on renal health, gut wellness, and food preservation, I've learned that sustainable eating isn't about perfection—it's about finding what nourishes you while fitting into your actual life.

These recipes come from my own kitchen, tested on family and friends who are brutally honest. They're not complicated restaurant creations. They're Tuesday night dinners when I'm tired, Sunday meal prep to survive the week, and comfort foods without the crash.

Before we get to the recipes, here's what you need to know about why this works and how to do it safely. Then I'll get out of your way and let you cook.

Important:
If you have health conditions, take medications, or have concerns, consult a healthcare provider before changing your diet significantly.

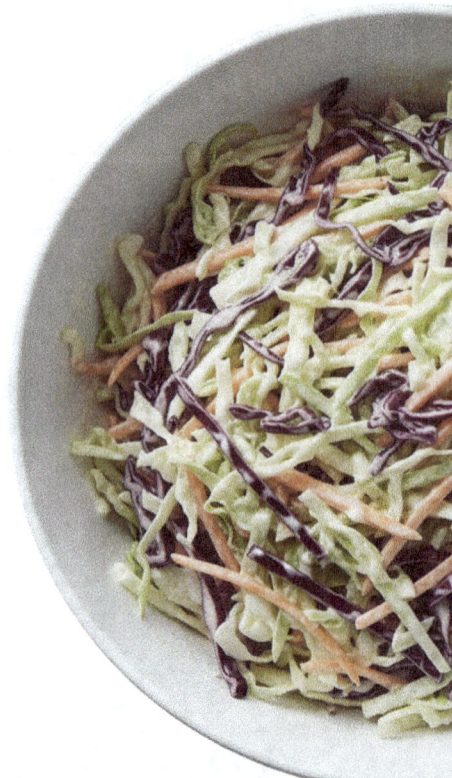

WHY THIS WORKS (THE SHORT VERSION)

The Carbohydrate Problem

When you eat carbs—especially refined ones like bread, pasta, and sugar—your blood sugar spikes, insulin floods your system, and a few hours later you crash and crave more carbs. This cycle promotes fat storage and makes it nearly impossible to feel satisfied.

The Protein Solution

Protein does the opposite:
- Keeps you full for hours
- Stabilizes blood sugar
- Preserves muscle mass
- Burns more calories during digestion

The Combination Effect

High protein + low carbs shifts your body from burning sugar to burning fat. You feel satisfied, energized, and free from constant hunger and cravings. Research consistently shows this approach outperforms low-fat diets for weight loss and metabolic health.

This Works Well For People Who:
- Crash between meals
- Feel hungry soon after eating carbs
- Struggle with sugar cravings
- Want to lose fat while keeping muscle
- Feel foggy or unfocused after meals
- Need a sustainable approach that actually works

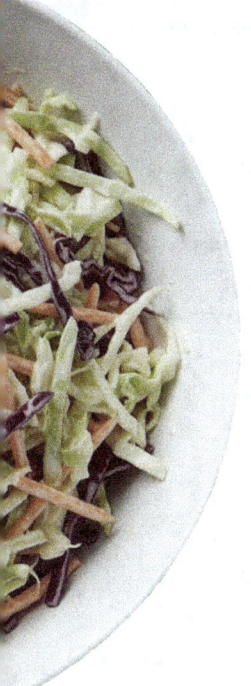

This May Not Be Right For:
- Endurance athletes training at very high volumes
- People with certain kidney conditions (check with your doctor)
- Pregnant or nursing women
- Anyone who feels better with more moderate carb restriction

The recipes give you a foundation you can adjust based on how your body responds.

THE BASICS

How Much Protein?
Simple calculation:
- **General health:** Your weight in pounds × 0.6-0.8 = daily protein grams
- **Weight loss/muscle building:** Your weight in pounds × 0.8-1.0 = daily protein grams
- **Very active:** Your weight in pounds × 1.0-1.2 = daily protein grams

Example: 150 lbs × 0.8 = 120g protein per day
Each recipe provides 25-40g protein per serving. Three meals gets you there.

Understanding Net Carbs
Net Carbs = Total Carbs - Fiber - Sugar Alcohols
Fiber and sugar alcohols don't raise blood sugar, so we subtract them.

Daily targets:
- **Strict low-carb (ketogenic):** 20-30g net carbs
- **Moderate low-carb:** 30-50g net carbs
- **Liberal low-carb:** 50-100g net carbs

Most recipes have under 10g net carbs per serving.

What to Eat
- **Proteins (eat freely):** Beef, pork, chicken, turkey, fish, seafood, eggs, cheese, Greek yogurt, cottage cheese.
- **Fats (essential for satisfaction):** Butter, olive oil, avocado oil, coconut oil, avocados, nuts, seeds, heavy cream, cheese.
- **Low-carb vegetables (eat generously):** Leafy greens, broccoli, cauliflower, zucchini, asparagus, green beans, peppers, mushrooms, tomatoes, cucumbers.
- **Seasonings:** All herbs and spices, salt, pepper, hot sauce, mustard, mayo, vinegar, lemon/lime juice

What to Avoid
- **Skip these:** Bread, pasta, rice, grains, beans, potatoes, corn, most fruits (except berries in small amounts), sugar, honey, processed foods, sugary drinks.
- **Watch for hidden carbs in:** Low-fat products, condiments, deli meats, "keto" products, restaurant meals.

YOUR KITCHEN SETUP

Essential Proteins to Stock

Fresh/Frozen: Eggs, chicken thighs, ground beef, ground turkey, bacon, frozen shrimp Pantry: Canned tuna, salmon, sardines.

Budget tip: Eggs, chicken thighs, and canned fish are your cheapest proteins. Buy meat on sale and freeze it.

Fats & Staples

Butter, olive oil, avocado oil, mayo, cauliflower rice, zucchini, almond flour, Parmesan, heavy cream.

Key Seasonings

Salt, pepper, garlic powder, onion powder, paprika, cumin, chili powder, Italian seasoning, fresh garlic, lemons/limes, Dijon mustard, hot sauce, soy sauce.

Weekly Shopping Template

Proteins (pick 2-3): Eggs, chicken, ground beef/turkey, fish, bacon.

Vegetables (pick 4-5): Greens, broccoli/cauliflower, zucchini, peppers, avocados.

Dairy: Butter, cream, cheese, yogurt.

MEAL PREP SHORTCUT

2-Hour Sunday Routine:

Hour 1	Hour 2
• Roast 3-4 lbs chicken thighs (hands-off) • Prep vegetables: wash lettuce, chop peppers/cucumbers • Hard-boil a dozen eggs	• Brown 2 lbs ground beef with taco seasoning • Cook bacon in the oven • Make cauliflower rice • Portion everything into containers

This gives you: Ready-to-eat proteins and components for 4-5 days of effortless meals.

USING THIS BOOK

Every recipe shows:

   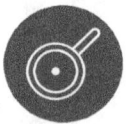

Quick
(30 min or less)   Budget-Friendly   Make-Ahead   One-Pan

- Macros: Calories, Protein, Fat, Net Carbs per serving
- Simple instructions, practical tips, money-saving ideas

Plan 5 dinners per week, not 7. Leave room for leftovers and life happening.
Keep breakfast simple. Eggs, yogurt, or leftover dinner.

WHAT TO EXPECT

Days 1-3   Slight adjustment as your body adapts. Drink water, get enough salt, eat enough fat.

Days 4-7   Energy stabilizes. Hunger between meals decreases.

Week 2   Cravings for sugar and carbs diminish significantly.

Week 3+:   Measurable results—better sleep, stable moods, mental clarity, and often weight loss.

IMPORTANT NOTES

This is not medical advice. I'm sharing what worked for me. Everyone is different. Work with your healthcare provider if you have medical conditions or take medications.

You don't have to be perfect. Even following this 80% of the time will likely improve how you feel compared to a high-carb diet.

Listen to your body. Some people need slightly more carbs (50-75g daily). Use these recipes as a framework, not rigid rules.

NOW, LET'S COOK

The recipes are organized by how you'll actually use them: quick weeknight dinners, make-ahead meals, budget-friendly options, and satisfying comfort foods.

Every recipe keeps protein high (25-40g per serving) and net carbs low (under 10g per serving). Every recipe is something I actually cook regularly. Every recipe is designed for real life.

Choose a few that appeal to you, make your shopping list, and start with what feels manageable. Find your favorites, master those, and build from there.

Your body will thank you.

SCIENTIFIC REFERENCES

The information in this introduction is based on peer-reviewed research from journals including the American Journal of Clinical Nutrition, New England Journal of Medicine, Journal of the American College of Nutrition, and Nutrition & Metabolism. For specific studies and a complete reference list, visit [your website] or search PubMed for terms like "low-carbohydrate diet weight loss" and "protein satiety.

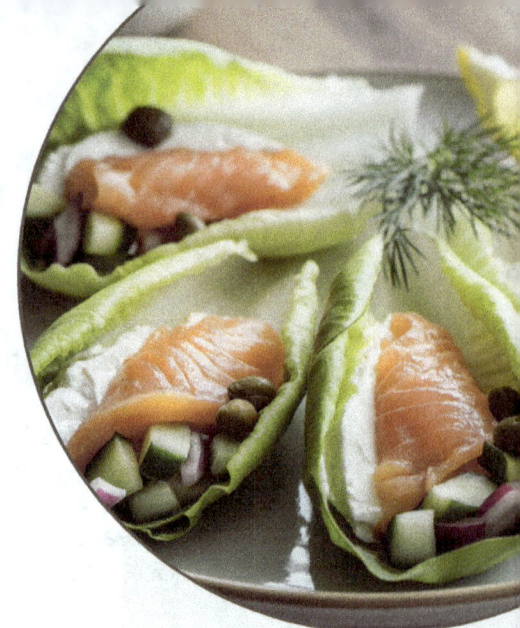

The first meal of the day sets the tone for everything that follows. When you start with a high-protein, low-carb breakfast, you'll notice something remarkable: you're not starving by 10 AM. That mid-morning crash and the desperate hunt for snacks simply disappears.

For years, I started my day with toast, cereal, or oatmeal, believing I was eating a "healthy" breakfast. By late morning, I'd be ravenous and reaching for whatever was convenient, which was rarely what I actually wanted to be eating. When I switched to protein-forward breakfasts, everything changed. My energy stayed stable, my focus sharpened, and I could easily make it to lunch without snacking.

The recipes in this chapter are designed for real mornings in real kitchens. Most take less than 10 minutes of active cooking time. Several can be made ahead on Sunday and reheated throughout the week. None require you to be a morning person or a skilled cook.

You'll notice I rely heavily on eggs. That's not an accident. Eggs are the most affordable, versatile, and nutritionally complete protein you can buy. A single large egg provides about 6 grams of high-quality protein, healthy fats, and virtually zero carbs for roughly 25 cents. When you're cooking for one or feeding a family, eggs are your best friend.

But this chapter isn't only eggs. You'll find options using breakfast sausage, bacon, smoked salmon, and Greek yogurt. You'll learn how to make egg-free breakfast bowls, protein-packed smoothies, and make-ahead egg muffins that travel well.

Breakfast Strategy Tips:
For rushed mornings: Make-ahead egg muffins, hard-boiled eggs with avocado, or Greek yogurt with nuts take less than 60 seconds to grab and go.

For leisurely mornings: Try the omelets or breakfast scrambles when you have 10-15 minutes to enjoy cooking.

For meal prep Sunday: The egg muffins and breakfast sausage patties can be made in bulk, refrigerated for 4 days or frozen for up to 2 months.

For budget-conscious cooks: Eggs, eggs, and more eggs. When they go on sale, I buy 5 dozen and hard-boil half of them immediately.

Now, let's make breakfast something you actually look forward to.

CHAPTER 1: BREAKFAST & BRUNCH

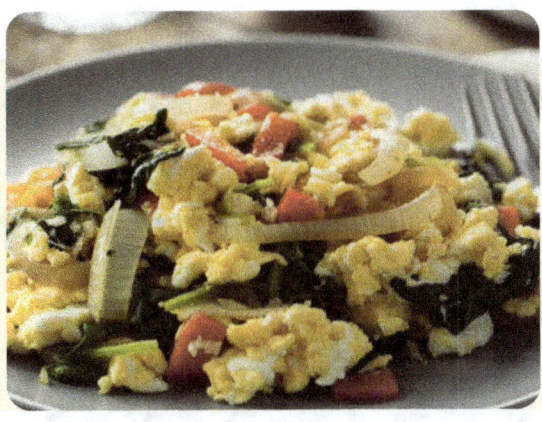

Classic Scrambled Eggs (Three Ways)

Quick   Budget-Friendly

 Serves: 1

 Prep Time: 2 min

 Cook Time: 5 min

Total: 7 min

MACROS PER SERVING:

Calories: 340 | Protein: 24g | Fat: 26g | Net Carbs: 2g

Ingredients:

- 3 large eggs
- 1 tablespoon butter
- 2 tablespoons heavy cream
- Salt and pepper to taste

Instructions:

1. Crack eggs into a bowl. Add heavy cream, salt, and pepper. Whisk with a fork until completely combined and slightly frothy.
2. Heat butter in a non-stick skillet over medium-low heat. Don't rush this. Medium-low is the key to creamy scrambled eggs.
3. Pour egg mixture into the skillet once butter is melted and foamy but not browning.
4. Let eggs sit undisturbed for 30 seconds, then gently push them from the edges toward the center with a spatula.
5. Continue cooking, stirring gently every 30 seconds, until eggs are just set but still glossy. They should look slightly underdone when you remove them from heat (they'll continue cooking from residual heat).

Variations:

Cheesy Scrambled Eggs (Add: ¼ cup shredded cheddar cheese in the last 30 seconds of cooking)
- **Macros per serving:** Calories: 440 | Protein: 31g | Fat: 34g | Net Carbs: 2g

Veggie Scrambled Eggs (Add: ¼ cup diced bell peppers and 2 tablespoons diced onion, cooked in butter before adding eggs + ½ cup spinach stirred in at the end)
- **Macros per serving:** Calories: 370 | Protein: 26g | Fat: 27g | Net Carbs: 4g

Tips:

Storage: Best eaten fresh, but you can refrigerate cooked eggs for up to 2 days. Reheat gently in the microwave for 30-45 seconds.

Budget hack: When eggs go on sale for under $2/dozen, stock up. They last 3-4 weeks in the refrigerator.

Make it travel-friendly: Scramble eggs, let cool completely, and store in a small container. Eat cold or reheat at work.

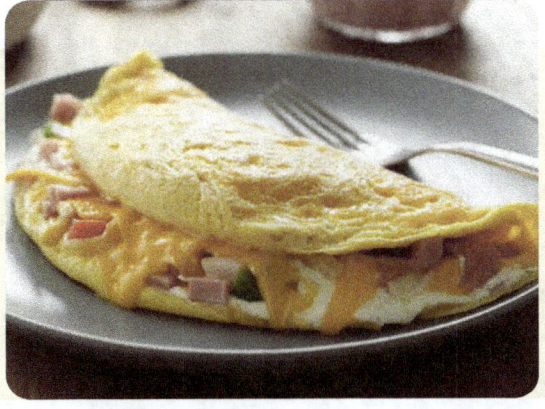

Denver Omelet

Quick

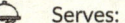 Serves: 1

 Prep Time: 5 min

 Cook Time: 8 min

 Total: 13 min

MACROS PER SERVING:

Calories: 420 | Protein: 32g | Fat: 29g | Net Carbs: 5g

Ingredients:

- 3 large eggs
- 2 tablespoons heavy cream
- 1 tablespoon butter
- ¼ cup diced ham
- 3 tablespoons diced bell pepper (any color)
- 2 tablespoons diced onion
- ¼ cup shredded cheddar cheese
- Salt and pepper to taste

Instructions:

1. Crack eggs into a bowl, add heavy cream, salt, and pepper. Whisk until well combined. Set aside.
2. Heat butter in an 8-inch non-stick skillet over medium heat. Add bell pepper and onion. Cook for 3-4 minutes until softened.
3. Add diced ham and cook for 1 minute more until heated through.
4. Pour egg mixture over the vegetables and ham. Tilt the pan to spread eggs evenly across the bottom.
5. Let eggs cook undisturbed for 2 minutes until edges begin to set.
6. Use a spatula to gently lift the edges, tilting the pan to let uncooked egg flow underneath. Continue until top is just slightly wet.
7. Sprinkle cheese over one half of the omelet. Fold the other half over the cheese using your spatula.
8. Cook for 1 more minute, then slide onto a plate.

Tips:

Make it easier: Skip the fold. Just add cheese on top of the eggs in step 7 and serve it open-faced.

Prep ahead: Dice all vegetables on Sunday and store in a container. In the morning, you'll only need 2-3 minutes of prep.

Substitutions: No ham? Use cooked bacon, sausage, or just make it with vegetables and extra cheese.

Storage: Omelets are best fresh, but leftovers can be refrigerated for 1 day and reheated gently in the microwave.

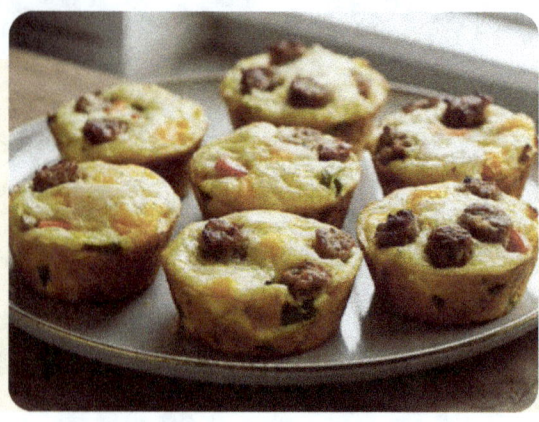

Sausage & Cheese Egg Muffins

Quick   Budget-Friendly   Make-Ahead

Serves: 6 (2 muffins per serving)

Prep Time: 10 min

Cook Time: 20 min

Total: 30 min

MACROS PER SERVING (2 muffins):

Calories: 285 | Protein: 22g | Fat: 20g |
Net Carbs: 2g

Ingredients:

- 12 large eggs
- ¼ cup heavy cream
- ½ pound breakfast sausage (bulk or removed from casings)
- 1 cup shredded cheddar cheese
- ¼ cup diced bell pepper
- 2 tablespoons diced onion
- ½ teaspoon salt
- ¼ teaspoon black pepper
- ¼ teaspoon garlic powder
- Cooking spray

Instructions:

1. Preheat oven to 350°F. Spray a 12-cup muffin tin generously with cooking spray.
2. Heat a skillet over medium-high heat. Add sausage and cook, breaking it into small crumbles, until browned and cooked through (about 5-6 minutes). Drain excess fat if needed.
3. Add bell pepper and onion to the skillet with sausage. Cook for 2 minutes until slightly softened. Remove from heat.
4. In a large bowl, whisk together eggs, heavy cream, salt, pepper, and garlic powder until well combined.
5. Divide the sausage mixture evenly among the 12 muffin cups (about 1 heaping tablespoon per cup).
6. Divide the shredded cheese evenly among the muffin cups.
7. Pour egg mixture into each muffin cup, filling about three-quarters full. Stir each cup gently with a fork to distribute ingredients.
8. Bake for 18-20 minutes until eggs are set in the center and tops are lightly golden.
9. Let cool in the pan for 5 minutes, then run a butter knife around the edges and pop them out.

Tips:

Storage: Refrigerate in an airtight container for up to 4 days, or freeze for up to 2 months. Freeze them on a baking sheet first, then transfer to a freezer bag to prevent sticking.

Reheating: From refrigerator, microwave 2 muffins for 45-60 seconds. From frozen, microwave for 90 seconds to 2 minutes.

Budget win: Make a double batch when sausage is on sale. Freeze half for quick breakfasts later.

Variations: Swap sausage for bacon, ham, or go vegetarian with extra vegetables and cheese. Add spinach, mushrooms, or sun-dried tomatoes.

Meal prep strategy: Make these every Sunday. Grab 2 on your way out the door for a complete 285-calorie, 22g protein breakfast.

  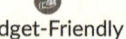

Bacon & Avocado Plate

Quick   Budget-Friendly

Serves: 1

Prep Time: 2 min

Cook Time: 10 min

Total: 12 min

MACROS PER SERVING:

Calories: 465 | Protein: 28g | Fat: 38g |
Net Carbs: 3g

Ingredients:

- 4 strips bacon
- 2 large eggs
- ½ medium avocado
- Salt and pepper to taste
- Optional: hot sauce

Instructions:

1. Cook bacon in a skillet over medium heat until crispy (about 8-10 minutes), flipping once halfway through. Transfer to a paper towel-lined plate.
2. Pour out all but 1 tablespoon of bacon grease from the skillet (save the rest for cooking other meals).
3. Crack eggs into the skillet with remaining bacon grease. Cook to your preference: 3 minutes for sunny-side up with runny yolk, 4 minutes for medium, 5 minutes for fully cooked yolk.
4. While eggs cook, slice avocado and arrange on a plate. Season with salt and pepper.
5. Add eggs and bacon to the plate. Serve with hot sauce if desired.

Tips:

Oven bacon: For easier cleanup, bake bacon at 400°F for 15-18 minutes on a foil-lined baking sheet. Perfect for making larger batches.

Save that grease: Store leftover bacon fat in a jar in the refrigerator. Use it to cook eggs, sauté vegetables, or add flavor to ground beef.

Make it portable: Hard-boil the eggs instead, pack with bacon and avocado in a container. Sprinkle avocado with lemon juice to prevent browning.

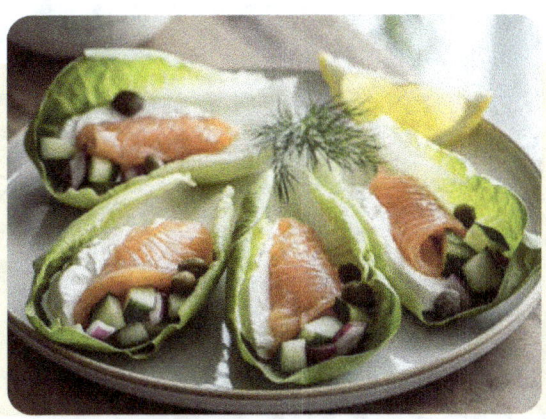

Smoked Salmon Cream Cheese Roll-Ups

Quick

Serves: 1

Prep Time: 5 min

Cook Time: 0 min

Total: 5 min

MACROS PER SERVING:

Calories: 380 | Protein: 28g | Fat: 28g | Net Carbs: 4g

Ingredients:

- 4 oz smoked salmon
- 2 oz cream cheese, softened
- 4 large lettuce leaves (butter lettuce or romaine work best)
- 2 tablespoons diced cucumber
- 1 tablespoon diced red onion
- 1 teaspoon capers (optional)
- Fresh dill for garnish (optional)
- Lemon wedge

Instructions:

1. Lay lettuce leaves flat on a cutting board or plate.
2. Spread cream cheese evenly across each lettuce leaf (about ½ oz per leaf).
3. Divide smoked salmon among the 4 leaves, laying it flat on top of the cream cheese.
4. Sprinkle cucumber, red onion, and capers (if using) over the salmon.
5. Roll each lettuce leaf tightly like a burrito or leave open-faced if you prefer.

Tips:

Budget hack: Buy a whole side of smoked salmon when it's on sale (often around holidays). Slice and freeze in 4 oz portions.

Make it heartier: Add 2 hard-boiled eggs to this meal for an extra 12g protein and more staying power.

Substitute: No smoked salmon? Use canned salmon mixed with a bit of mayo, or even tuna. You'll save money and still hit your protein target.

Prep ahead: Assemble these the night before without the lettuce. In the morning, spread the salmon mixture onto fresh lettuce leaves.

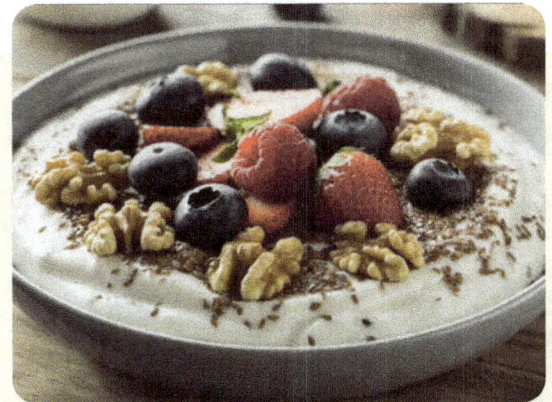

Greek Yogurt Protein Bowl

Quick Budget-Friendly

Serves: 1

Prep Time: 3 min

Cook Time: 0 min

Total: 3 min

MACROS PER SERVING:

Calories: 385 | Protein: 28g | Fat: 24g | Net Carbs: 9g

Ingredients:

- 1 cup plain Greek yogurt (full-fat)
- 2 tablespoons chopped walnuts or almonds
- 2 tablespoons ground flaxseed
- ¼ cup fresh berries (blueberries, raspberries, or strawberries)
- Optional: ½ teaspoon vanilla extract
- Optional: 5-6 drops liquid stevia or 1 teaspoon erythritol

Instructions:

1. Scoop Greek yogurt into a bowl.
2. If using vanilla extract or sweetener, stir it into the yogurt.
3. Top with nuts, ground flaxseed, and berries.
4. Mix everything together or eat it layered. Both ways work.

Tips:

Buy it right: Look for "plain Greek yogurt" with only milk and live cultures in the ingredients. Avoid varieties with added sugar or thickeners.

Full-fat vs. low-fat: Full-fat Greek yogurt keeps you fuller longer and has fewer carbs than low-fat versions (which often add sugar to compensate for taste).

Make it travel-ready: Layer ingredients in a mason jar. Pack nuts separately if you won't eat it for several hours (they'll get soggy).

Budget win: Buy large tubs of Greek yogurt instead of individual cups. You'll save 40-50% per serving.

Boost protein: Add 1 scoop of unflavored protein powder for an extra 20-25g protein. Macros become: Calories: 485 | Protein: 50g | Fat: 25g | Net Carbs: 10g

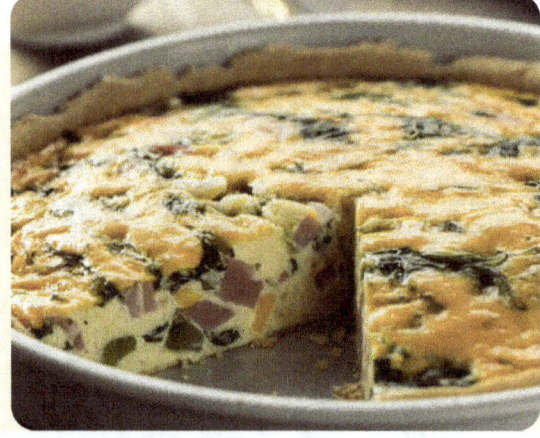

Breakfast Burrito Bowl

 Quick   One-Pan

 Serves: 1

Prep Time: 5 min

Cook Time: 10 min

 Total: 15 min

MACROS PER SERVING:

Calories: 520 | Protein: 35g | Fat: 38g | Net Carbs: 7g

Ingredients:

- 3 large eggs
- ¼ pound ground beef or turkey (about 4 oz)
- 2 tablespoons diced onion
- 2 tablespoons diced bell pepper
- 1 tablespoon butter
- ¼ cup shredded cheddar cheese
- ¼ medium avocado, diced
- 2 tablespoons salsa
- 1 tablespoon sour cream
- ½ teaspoon cumin
- ¼ teaspoon chili powder
- Salt and pepper to taste
- Optional: hot sauce, cilantro

Instructions:

1. Heat a large skillet over medium-high heat. Add ground meat, breaking it up with a spatula. Season with cumin, chili powder, salt, and pepper.
2. Cook meat for 4-5 minutes until browned. Add onion and bell pepper. Cook for 2 more minutes until vegetables soften.
3. Push meat mixture to one side of the skillet. Add butter to the empty side.
4. Crack eggs into the buttered side and scramble them, cooking for 2-3 minutes until just set.
5. Transfer everything to a bowl. Top with shredded cheese (the heat will melt it), diced avocado, salsa, and sour cream.
6. Add hot sauce and cilantro if using.

Tips:

Meal prep version: Cook the meat mixture in bulk on Sunday. In the morning, reheat 4 oz of meat while you scramble your eggs. Total morning time: 5 minutes.

Budget saver: Ground beef and turkey regularly go on sale. Buy 5 pounds, portion into 4 oz servings, and freeze.

No tortilla needed: This bowl is so satisfying, you won't miss the tortilla. But if you want one, look for low-carb tortillas with 3-5g net carbs.

Variations: Swap ground meat for chorizo, use pepper jack cheese for extra kick, or add jalapeños if you like it spicy.

Ham & Cheese Crustless Quiche

 Make-Ahead

 Serves: 6

Prep Time: 10 min

Cook Time: 35 min

Total: 45 min

MACROS PER SERVING:

Calories: 290 | Protein: 24g | Fat: 20g | Net Carbs: 3g

Ingredients:

- 10 large eggs
- ½ cup heavy cream
- 1 cup diced ham
- 1½ cups shredded cheddar cheese, divided
- ½ cup diced onion
- ½ cup diced bell pepper
- 1 cup fresh spinach, chopped
- ½ teaspoon salt
- ¼ teaspoon black pepper
- ¼ teaspoon garlic powder
- Cooking spray

Instructions:

1. Preheat oven to 375°F. Spray a 9-inch pie dish or similar baking dish with cooking spray.
2. In a large bowl, whisk together eggs, heavy cream, salt, pepper, and garlic powder until well combined.
3. Add ham, 1 cup of the shredded cheese, onion, bell pepper, and spinach to the egg mixture. Stir to combine.
4. Pour mixture into the prepared baking dish. Sprinkle the remaining ½ cup cheese on top.
5. Bake for 30-35 minutes until the center is set and the top is lightly golden. A knife inserted in the center should come out clean.

Tips:

Storage: Refrigerate for up to 4 days. Reheat individual slices in the microwave for 60-90 seconds.

Freeze it: Wrap individual slices in plastic wrap, then place in a freezer bag. Freeze for up to 2 months. Reheat from frozen for 2-3 minutes in the microwave.

Variations: Endless possibilities here. Try bacon and Swiss, sausage and pepper jack, or go vegetarian with mushrooms, tomatoes, and feta.

Make it Sunday, eat all week: This is my go-to make-ahead breakfast. Cut it into portions Sunday night, and you have breakfast ready for 6 days.

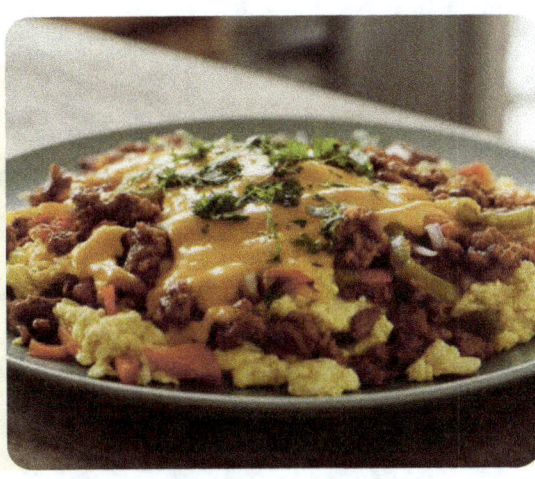

Chorizo & Pepper Scramble

Quick   One-Pan

 Serves: 1

 Prep Time: 3 min

 Cook Time: 8 min

 Total: 11 min

MACROS PER SERVING:

Calories: 475 | Protein: 32g | Fat: 36g | Net Carbs: 5g

Ingredients:

- 3 large eggs
- 2 oz fresh Mexican chorizo (removed from casing)
- ¼ cup diced bell pepper
- 2 tablespoons diced onion
- ¼ cup shredded pepper jack cheese
- 1 tablespoon chopped cilantro (optional)
- Salt to taste

Instructions:

1. Heat a non-stick skillet over medium-high heat. Add chorizo, breaking it into small pieces with a spatula.
2. Cook chorizo for 3-4 minutes until browned and cooked through.
3. Add bell pepper and onion to the skillet. Cook for 2 minutes until softened.
4. While vegetables cook, crack eggs into a bowl and whisk with a fork. Add a pinch of salt.
5. Pour eggs into the skillet with the chorizo and vegetables. Let sit for 30 seconds, then gently scramble until eggs are just set, about 2 minutes.
6. Remove from heat and sprinkle with pepper jack cheese. The heat from the eggs will melt it.

Tips:

Spice level: Mexican chorizo is typically spicy. If you prefer milder, use regular breakfast sausage and add ¼ teaspoon chili powder.

Drain or don't: Chorizo releases a lot of fat. If there's excessive grease in the pan after cooking the meat, drain most of it before adding vegetables.

Make it a bowl: Serve over a handful of fresh spinach or shredded lettuce for extra volume without extra carbs.

Batch option: Cook a pound of chorizo at once, divide into 2 oz portions, and refrigerate or freeze. Breakfast becomes a 5-minute affair.

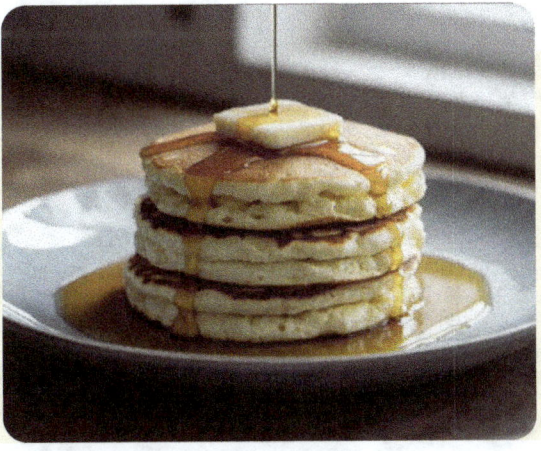

Cottage Cheese Pancakes

Quick

 Serves: 1
(makes 3 small pancakes)

 Prep Time: 5 min

 Cook Time: 8 min

 Total: 13 min

MACROS PER SERVING:

Calories: 320 | Protein: 28g | Fat: 18g | Net Carbs: 8g

Ingredients:

- ½ cup cottage cheese (full-fat)
- 2 large eggs
- ¼ cup almond flour
- ½ teaspoon vanilla extract
- ¼ teaspoon cinnamon
- Pinch of salt
- ½ teaspoon baking powder
- 1 tablespoon butter for cooking
- Optional: sugar-free syrup, butter for topping

Instructions:

1. Add cottage cheese, eggs, almond flour, vanilla extract, cinnamon, salt, and baking powder to a blender or food processor. Blend until smooth, about 30 seconds.
2. Let batter rest for 2-3 minutes. It will be thicker than regular pancake batter.
3. Heat butter in a non-stick skillet over medium-low heat. Don't use high heat or the pancakes will burn before cooking through.
4. Pour about ⅓ of the batter into the skillet to form one pancake. These stay small (about 4 inches across) because they're delicate.
5. Cook for 3 minutes until bubbles form on the surface and edges look set. Flip carefully.
6. Cook for 2 more minutes on the second side. Transfer to a plate.
7. Repeat with remaining batter, making 2 more pancakes.
8. Serve with a pat of butter and sugar-free syrup if desired.

Tips:

Texture note: These won't be fluffy like regular pancakes. They're denser and more custard-like, but very satisfying.

No blender? Mash the cottage cheese with a fork until mostly smooth, then whisk in the other ingredients. You'll have some lumps, but that's okay.

Make ahead: These reheat well. Make a double batch, refrigerate for up to 3 days, and reheat in a toaster or microwave.

Toppings: Try them with a dollop of Greek yogurt and berries, or spread with almond butter for extra protein and healthy fats.

Protein Coffee Smoothie

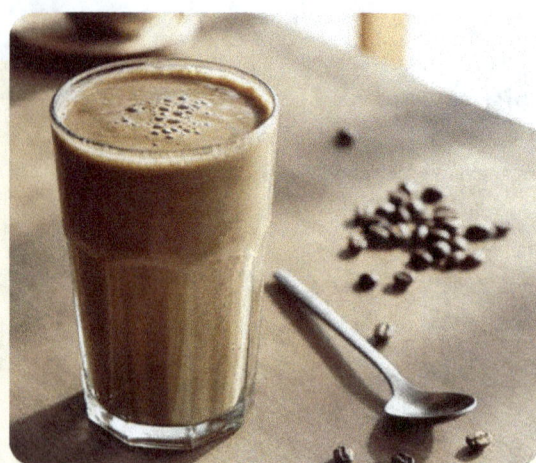

Quick

 Serves: 1

 Prep Time: 3 min

 Cook Time: 0 min

Total: 3 min

MACROS PER SERVING:
Calories: 285 | Protein: 30g | Fat: 15g | Net Carbs: 5g

Ingredients:

- 1 cup cold brewed coffee (or cooled regular coffee)
- 1 scoop vanilla or chocolate protein powder (about 25g protein)
- 2 tablespoons heavy cream
- 1 tablespoon almond butter
- ½ cup ice
- Optional: 5-6 drops liquid stevia or 1 teaspoon erythritol
- Optional: 1 tablespoon unsweetened cocoa powder for extra chocolate flavor

Instructions:

1. Add all ingredients to a blender.
2. Blend on high for 30-45 seconds until smooth and frothy.
3. Pour into a glass or travel cup.
4. Drink immediately or refrigerate for up to 24 hours (shake before drinking if separated).

Tips:

Cold brew is key: Room temperature or warm coffee will melt your ice and make this watery. Use cold brew or refrigerate your coffee after brewing.

Protein powder choice: Use whatever protein powder you prefer. Whey, casein, or plant-based all work. Check that it has at least 20g protein per scoop.

Make it ahead: Blend everything except ice the night before. Store in the refrigerator. In the morning, add ice and blend for 20 seconds.

Budget version: Skip the almond butter and add an extra tablespoon of heavy cream. You'll save about $0.50 per serving.

Not a coffee person? Replace coffee with unsweetened almond milk and add ½ teaspoon instant espresso powder for a hint of coffee flavor without the full intensity.

Spinach & Feta Egg Cups

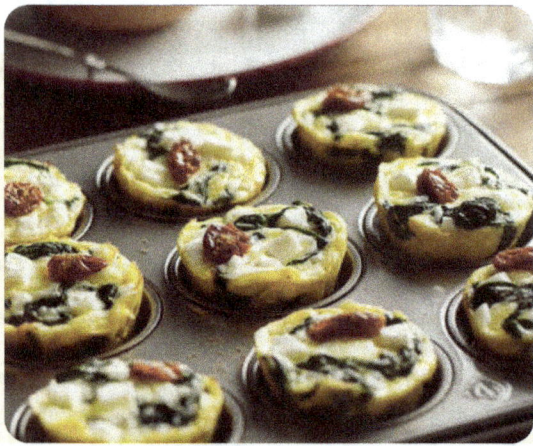

 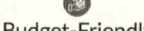
Make-Ahead   Budget-Friendly

 Serves: 6 (2 cups per serving)

 Prep Time: 10 min

 Cook Time: 20 min

Total: 30 min

MACROS PER SERVING (2 cups):
Calories: 220 | Protein: 16g | Fat: 16g | Net Carbs: 2g

Ingredients:

- 12 large eggs
- ¼ cup heavy cream
- 2 cups fresh spinach, chopped
- ¾ cup crumbled feta cheese
- 2 tablespoons diced sun-dried tomatoes (packed in oil, drained)
- 2 cloves garlic, minced
- ½ teaspoon dried oregano
- ½ teaspoon salt
- ¼ teaspoon black pepper
- Cooking spray

Instructions:

1. Preheat oven to 350°F. Spray a 12-cup muffin tin generously with cooking spray.
2. In a large bowl, whisk together eggs, heavy cream, salt, pepper, and oregano until well combined.
3. Add chopped spinach, feta cheese, sun-dried tomatoes, and minced garlic to the egg mixture. Stir to distribute evenly.
4. Divide mixture evenly among the 12 muffin cups, filling each about three-quarters full. You can use a ladle or large spoon for this.
5. Bake for 18-20 minutes until eggs are set in the center and tops are lightly golden.

Tips:

Storage: Keep in an airtight container in the refrigerator for up to 4 days, or freeze for up to 2 months.

Reheating: From fridge, microwave 2 cups for 45-60 seconds. From frozen, microwave for 90 seconds to 2 minutes.

Prep the spinach: You can use frozen spinach instead of fresh. Thaw it completely and squeeze out all excess water before adding to the eggs.

Budget hack: When feta is on sale, buy extra and freeze it. It crumbles easily even when frozen.

Mediterranean breakfast: Serve these with sliced cucumber, tomatoes, and olives for a complete meal.

Breakfast Sausage Patties (Homemade)

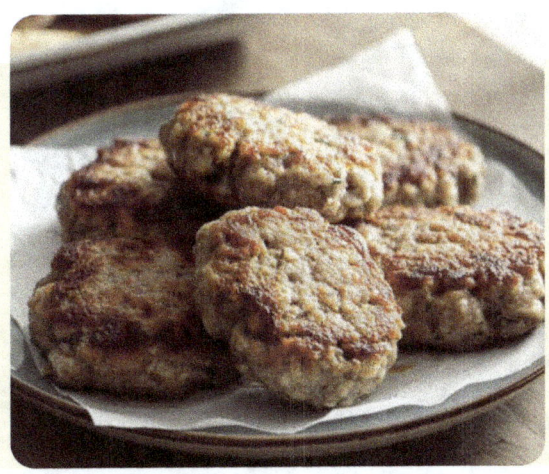

Make-Ahead   Budget-Friendly

🍽 Serves: 8 (2 patties per serving)

❄ Prep Time: 10 min

🍲 Cook Time: 10 min

⏲ Total: 20 min

MACROS PER SERVING (2 patties):
Calories: 260 | Protein: 18g | Fat: 20g |
Net Carbs: 1g

Ingredients:

- 2 pounds ground pork
- 2 teaspoons dried sage
- 1 teaspoon salt
- 1 teaspoon black pepper
- ½ teaspoon garlic powder
- ½ teaspoon onion powder
- ½ teaspoon dried thyme
- ¼ teaspoon red pepper flakes (optional, for a kick)
- ¼ teaspoon ground fennel (optional, for Italian-style sausage)

Instructions:

1. Add all ingredients to a large bowl.
2. Mix thoroughly with your hands until seasonings are evenly distributed. Don't overmix or the meat will get tough.
3. Divide mixture into 16 equal portions (about 2 oz each). Roll each into a ball, then flatten into a patty about ½ inch thick.
4. Heat a large skillet over medium heat. No oil needed (the pork has enough fat).
5. Working in batches, cook patties for 4-5 minutes per side until browned and cooked through to an internal temperature of 160°F.
6. Transfer cooked patties to a paper towel-lined plate to drain excess grease.

Tips:

Storage: Refrigerate cooked patties for up to 4 days, or freeze for up to 3 months. Place parchment paper between patties before freezing to prevent sticking.

Reheating: Microwave 2 patties for 45-60 seconds from refrigerated, or 90 seconds from frozen.

Why homemade? Store-bought breakfast sausage often contains added sugar, fillers, and preservatives. Making your own costs less and you control exactly what goes in.

Batch cooking: Make a triple batch when pork goes on sale. Freeze in portions for quick protein all month.

Serving suggestions: Pair with scrambled eggs, or break up a patty and add to a breakfast scramble or omelet.

Keto "Oatmeal"

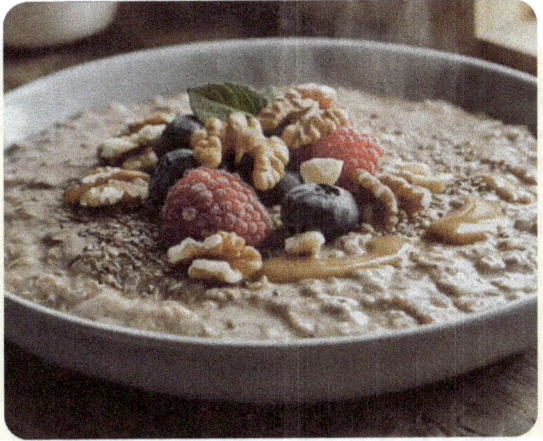

Quick   Budget-Friendly

🍽 Serves: 1

❄ Prep Time: 2 min

🍲 Cook Time: 3 min

⏲ Total: 5 min

MACROS PER SERVING:
Calories: 420 | Protein: 18g | Fat: 34g |
Net Carbs: 6g

Ingredients:

- 3 tablespoons hemp hearts (hemp seeds)
- 2 tablespoons ground flax
- 1 tablespoon almond flour
- 1 tablespoon chia seeds
- ¾ cup unsweetened almond milk
- 2 tablespoons heavy cream
- ½ teaspoon vanilla extract
- ½ teaspoon cinnamon
- Pinch of salt
- Optional: 5-6 drops liquid stevia or 1 teaspoon erythritol
- Optional toppings: 1 tablespoon chopped walnuts, 2 tablespoons berries, 1 tablespoon almond butter

Instructions:

1. Add hemp hearts, ground flax, almond flour, and chia seeds to a small pot or microwave-safe bowl.
2. Add almond milk, heavy cream, vanilla extract, cinnamon, salt, and sweetener (if using). Stir well to combine.
3. **Stovetop method:** Heat over medium-low heat, stirring frequently, for 3-4 minutes until mixture thickens to oatmeal consistency.
4. **Microwave method:** Microwave on high for 90 seconds. Stir, then microwave for another 60 seconds. Let sit for 1 minute to thicken.

Tips:

Texture adjustment: This gets very thick as it cools. If you like it thinner, add more almond milk. If you prefer it thicker, use less liquid or add more chia seeds.

Flavor variations: Try cocoa powder and a few sugar-free chocolate chips for chocolate "oatmeal." Or add pumpkin pie spice and 2 tablespoons pumpkin puree for fall flavor.

Make ahead: Mix dry ingredients in batches and store in small containers or bags. In the morning, just add liquid and heat.

Budget note: Hemp hearts are pricey but worth it for the complete protein profile (10g per 3 tablespoons). Buy in bulk online to save money.

Not like real oatmeal: Manage your expectations. This won't taste exactly like oats, but it's warm, satisfying, and keeps you full for hours.

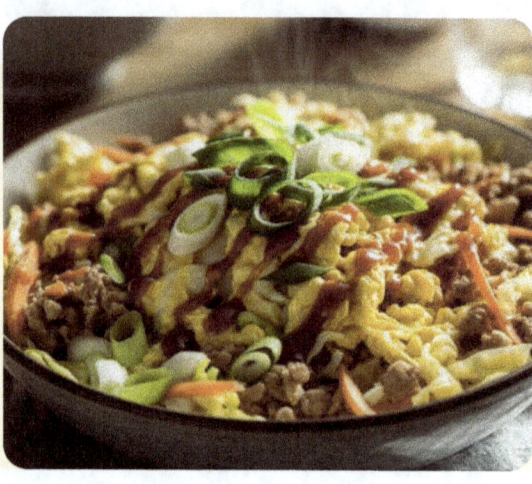

Egg Roll in a Bowl (Breakfast Version)

  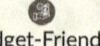

Quick   One-Pan   Budget-Friendly

 Serves: 2

 Prep Time: 5 min

 Cook Time: 12 min

Total: 17 min

MACROS PER SERVING:

Calories: 420 | Protein: 28g |
Fat: 30g | Net Carbs: 6g

Ingredients:

- ½ pound ground pork or turkey
- 3 cups shredded cabbage (about ½ small cabbage or use coleslaw mix)
- 1 cup shredded carrots (or use coleslaw mix)
- 4 large eggs
- 2 tablespoons soy sauce (or coconut aminos)
- 1 tablespoon sesame oil
- 2 cloves garlic, minced
- 1 teaspoon fresh ginger, grated (or ½ teaspoon ground ginger)
- 2 green onions, sliced
- Salt and pepper to taste
- Optional: sriracha or hot sauce for serving

Instructions:

1. Heat sesame oil in a large skillet or wok over medium-high heat.
2. Add ground pork and cook, breaking it into crumbles, for 4-5 minutes until browned and cooked through.
3. Add garlic and ginger to the skillet. Cook for 30 seconds until fragrant.
4. Add cabbage and carrots. Stir-fry for 3-4 minutes until cabbage wilts and vegetables soften.
5. Push everything to one side of the skillet. Crack eggs into the empty side.
6. Scramble the eggs for 2-3 minutes until just cooked, then mix them into the cabbage and meat.
7. Add soy sauce and stir everything together. Cook for 1 more minute.
8. Divide between two bowls and top with sliced green onions.
9. Serve with sriracha or hot sauce if desired.

Tips:

Time saver: Buy pre-shredded coleslaw mix. It's cabbage and carrots already mixed and ready to go.

Meal prep: This reheats beautifully. Make a double batch and refrigerate portions for up to 4 days.

Budget win: Ground pork is often cheaper than ground beef or turkey. Stock up when it's on sale.

Make it spicier: Add ¼ teaspoon red pepper flakes when cooking the meat, or top with more sriracha.

Add crunch: Top with sesame seeds or crushed pork rinds for texture contrast.

CHAPTER 1 SUMMARY

You now have 15 high-protein, low-carb breakfast options that range from 2-minute assembly to 30-minute meal prep projects. Here's how to think about using them:

For the busiest mornings (under 5 minutes):
- Greek Yogurt Protein Bowl
- Bacon & Avocado Plate (with pre-cooked bacon)
- Smoked Salmon Roll-Ups
- Hard-boiled eggs from your meal prep

For typical weekday mornings (5-15 minutes):
- Any of the scrambled egg variations
- Denver Omelet
- Breakfast Burrito Bowl
- Chorizo & Pepper Scramble
- Egg Roll in a Bowl

For Sunday meal prep (make once, eat all week):
- Sausage & Cheese Egg Muffins
- Ham & Cheese Crustless Quiche
- Spinach & Feta Egg Cups
- Breakfast Sausage Patties

For weekend leisurely cooking:
- Cottage Cheese Pancakes
- Any of the omelets or scrambles
- Trying new variations of the recipes

My Personal Weekly Breakfast Rotation:
I keep it simple during the week. Here's what a typical week looks like for me:

- **Monday-Friday:** Grab 2 egg muffins from the fridge (made Sunday) or scramble 3 eggs with whatever vegetables I have on hand. Total time: 2-7 minutes depending on whether I'm reheating or cooking fresh.
- **Saturday:** I take my time and make an omelet or try a new recipe variation.
- **Sunday:** After I make my egg muffins for the week, I usually have some of the mixture left. I cook it as a mini frittata and eat it while I'm doing the rest of my meal prep.

Budget Breakfast Strategy:
If you're watching your spending, focus on eggs, eggs, and more eggs. A dozen costs $2-4 depending on your location and provides 72 grams of protein. That's about 3-4 cents per gram of protein, making eggs the most affordable protein source available.

When you see good sales:
- Bacon under $4/pound: buy 3-5 pounds, freeze in portions
- Sausage under $2/pound: buy 5 pounds, make patties, freeze
- Eggs under $2/dozen: buy 5 dozen, hard-boil half

Protein Timing for Breakfast:
Research shows that eating 25-30 grams of protein at breakfast helps control appetite throughout the day. Every recipe in this chapter meets or exceeds that target. If you're used to carb-heavy breakfasts (cereal, toast, pastries), you'll notice a dramatic difference in how long you stay satisfied.

What About Coffee?
I didn't include it in these recipes because most people have their coffee routine dialed in. But if you're used to sweetened coffee drinks, that's an easy place to eliminate unnecessary carbs. Black coffee has zero carbs. Coffee with heavy cream has 1-2g net carbs per cup. A Starbucks grande caramel macchiato has 33g of carbs.

If you need sweetness in your coffee, use liquid stevia, monk fruit sweetener, or erythritol. Skip the sugar and flavored syrups.

Common Breakfast Mistakes:
1. **Skipping breakfast entirely, then overeating at lunch.** If you're truly not hungry in the morning, that's fine. But if you're skipping because you're rushed, meal prep is your answer.
2. **Not eating enough protein.** A single egg and a piece of fruit isn't going to cut it. You need 25-30g minimum to feel satisfied until lunch.
3. **Relying on "low-carb" packaged breakfast foods.** Most bars and shakes are expensive and less satisfying than real food. Save your money and make egg muffins instead.
4. **Eating the same thing every single day.** Even if you love eggs, eat them 7 days straight and you'll burn out. Rotate through at least 3-4 breakfast options.

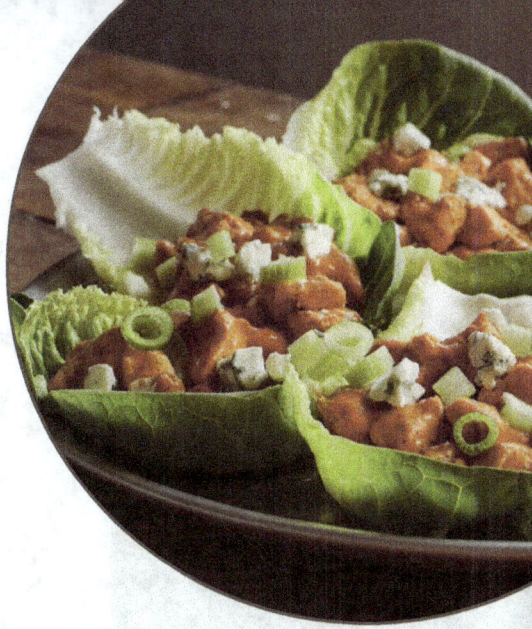

This is the chapter you'll use most. These are the recipes that answer the 5 PM question: "What's for dinner?" when you're tired, hungry, and have maybe 30 minutes before everyone needs to eat.

I'm not going to pretend you have the energy for complicated techniques or exotic ingredients on a Tuesday night. These recipes use straightforward methods, common ingredients, and deliver complete meals in 30 minutes or less. Most are one-pan affairs that won't leave you with a sink full of dishes.

Every recipe in this chapter provides at least 25 grams of protein per serving and keeps net carbs under 8 grams. You're getting complete, satisfying meals that support your goals without requiring a culinary degree or three hours of your evening.

The recipes are organized by protein type (chicken, beef, pork, fish) simply because that's how most people shop and plan. When chicken goes on sale, you'll know exactly where to find quick chicken recipes. When you defrost ground beef at lunch, you can flip to that section and pick your dinner.

Weeknight Dinner Strategy:

Monday through Friday, keep it simple. Pick from this chapter. Cook once, eat tonight. Some recipes deliberately make extra portions for tomorrow's lunch or another dinner later in the week.

Wednesday or Thursday, use leftovers. If you cooked Sunday or Monday and have extra protein, throw together a quick salad or vegetable side. Dinner in 10 minutes.

Friday, either go super simple or order takeout. You made it through the week. If you want to cook, great. If you want someone else to cook, also great. This isn't about perfection.

What you won't find in this chapter:
- Recipes requiring 15+ ingredients
- Techniques that need special equipment or skills
- Marinades that need 4+ hours (everything here uses quick marinades or none at all)
- Recipes that dirty every pan in your kitchen
- Foods that need to "rest" or "sit" for extended periods

What you will find:
- Dinner on the table in 30 minutes or less
- Recipes using ingredients you can find at any regular grocery store
- Methods so straightforward that even cooking-averse family members can help
- Meals that reheat well for lunch the next day
- Real food that actually tastes good
- Let's cook some dinner.

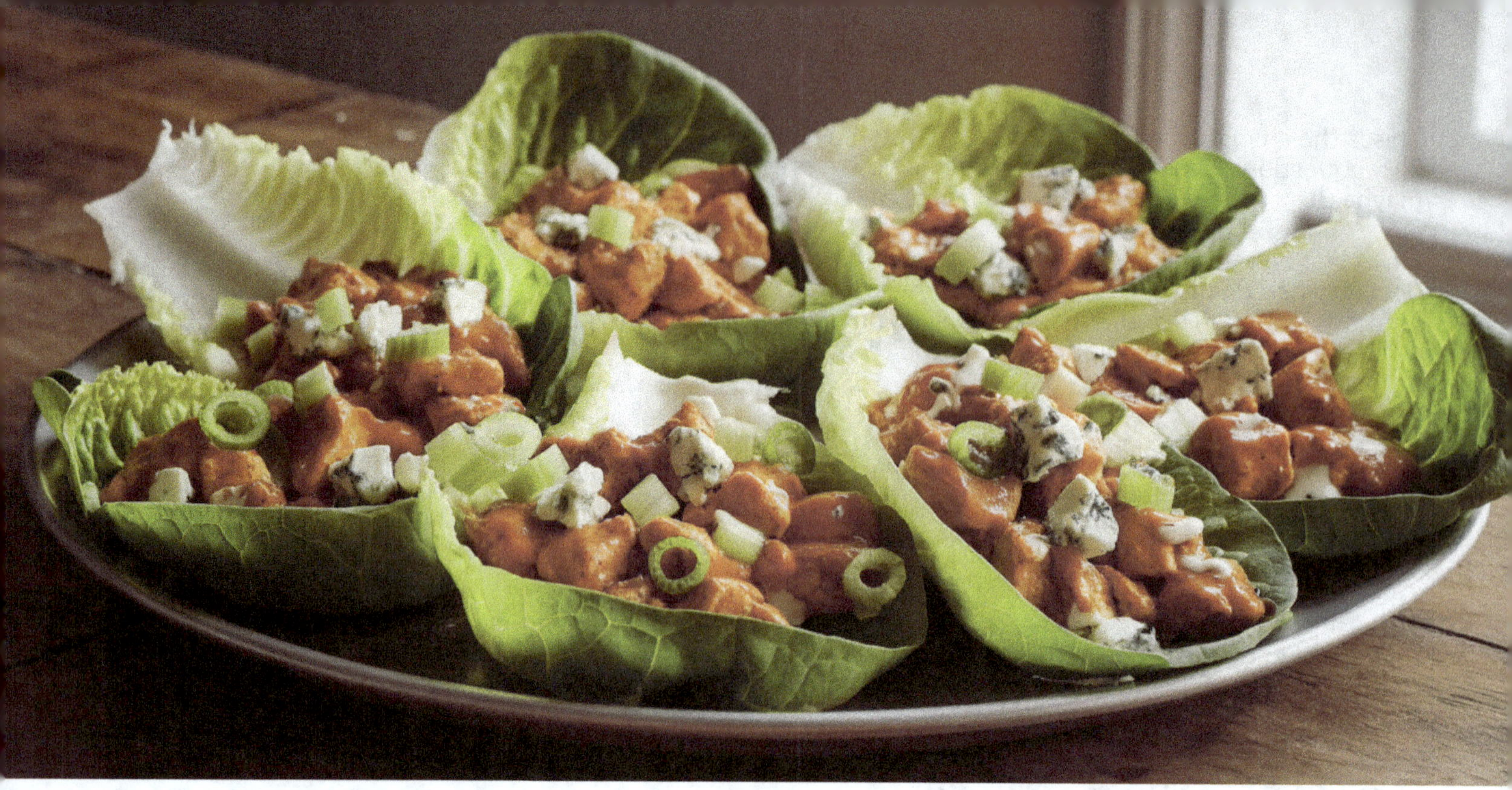

CHICKEN RECIPES

Chicken is the weeknight protein MVP. It's affordable, versatile, cooks quickly, and most people like it. I'll be honest: boneless, skinless chicken breasts are the most popular cut, but they're also the easiest to overcook into dry, flavorless hockey pucks.

That's why most of these recipes use chicken thighs. They're more forgiving, stay juicy even if you overcook them slightly, have more flavor, and cost less. But if you prefer chicken breasts, you can substitute them in any recipe. Just reduce cooking time by 2-3 minutes and use a meat thermometer to avoid overcooking (target 165°F internal temperature).

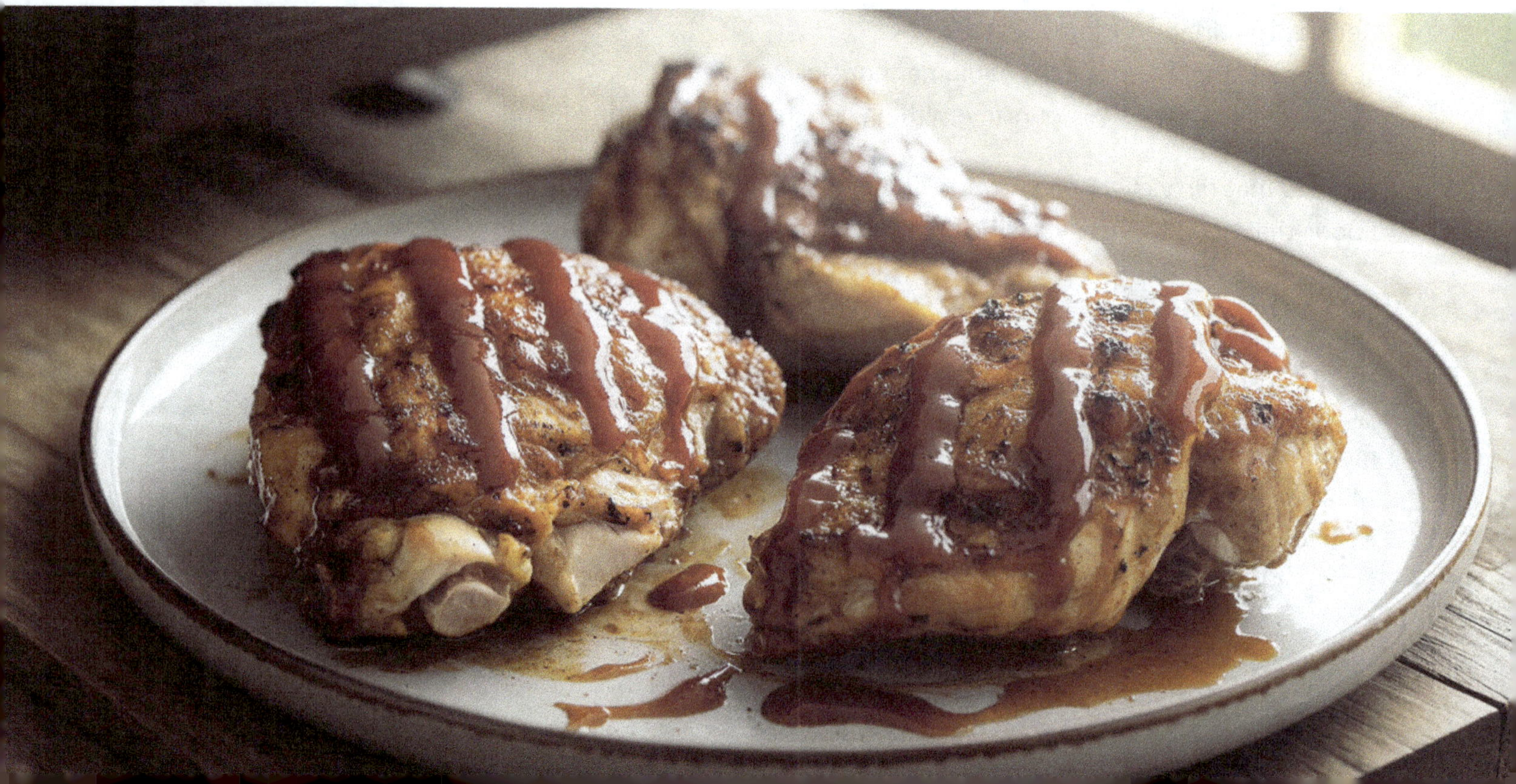

Garlic Butter Chicken Thighs

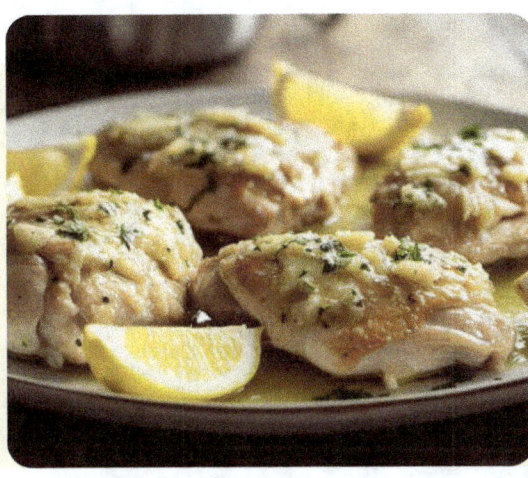

Quick   One-Pan   Budget-Friendly

 Serves: 4

 Prep Time: 5 min

 Cook Time: 20 min

 Total: 25 min

MACROS PER SERVING:

Calories: 420 | Protein: 38g |
Fat: 28g | Net Carbs: 2g

Ingredients:

- 8 boneless, skinless chicken thighs (about 2 pounds)
- 4 tablespoons butter, divided
- 6 cloves garlic, minced
- 1 teaspoon Italian seasoning
- ½ teaspoon paprika
- ½ teaspoon salt
- ¼ teaspoon black pepper
- 2 tablespoons fresh parsley, chopped (or 2 teaspoons dried)
- Optional: lemon wedges for serving

Instructions:

1. Pat chicken thighs dry with paper towels. Season both sides with salt, pepper, paprika, and Italian seasoning.
2. Heat 2 tablespoons butter in a large skillet over medium-high heat.
3. Add chicken thighs to the skillet. Cook for 6-7 minutes without moving them (this creates a good sear).
4. Flip chicken and cook for another 6-7 minutes until cooked through (internal temperature of 165°F). Transfer chicken to a plate.
5. Reduce heat to medium. Add remaining 2 tablespoons butter to the skillet.
6. Add minced garlic and cook for 1 minute, stirring constantly, until fragrant. Don't let it burn.
7. Return chicken to the skillet and spoon the garlic butter over it. Cook for 1 more minute.

Tips:

Don't skip the pat-dry step. Wet chicken won't sear properly. It'll steam instead, and you'll lose that delicious browned exterior.

Chicken breast substitute: Use 4 chicken breasts (about 6 oz each). Reduce cooking time to 5-6 minutes per side.

Make it a complete meal: Serve over cauliflower rice or with roasted broccoli. Both take about the same 20 minutes and can cook while you make the chicken.

Storage: Refrigerate for up to 4 days. Reheat gently in the microwave or in a skillet with a splash of water to prevent drying out.

Budget win: Chicken thighs regularly go on sale for $1.50-2.50/pound. Stock up and freeze in portions.

Sheet Pan Chicken & Broccoli

Quick   One-Pan   Budget-Friendly

 Serves: 4

 Prep Time: 10 min

 Cook Time: 20 min

 Total: 30 min

MACROS PER SERVING:

Calories: 385 | Protein: 36g |
Fat: 24g | Net Carbs: 5g

Ingredients:

- 2 pounds boneless, skinless chicken thighs, cut into 2-inch pieces
- 6 cups broccoli florets (about 2 heads)
- 3 tablespoons olive oil, divided
- 4 cloves garlic, minced
- 1 teaspoon paprika
- 1 teaspoon garlic powder
- 1 teaspoon onion powder
- ¾ teaspoon salt, divided
- ½ teaspoon black pepper, divided
- ¼ cup grated Parmesan cheese
- Optional: red pepper flakes for heat

Instructions:

1. Preheat oven to 425°F. Line a large baking sheet with parchment paper or spray with cooking spray.
2. In a large bowl, toss chicken pieces with 2 tablespoons olive oil, half the minced garlic, paprika, garlic powder, onion powder, ½ teaspoon salt, and ¼ teaspoon pepper.
3. Spread chicken in a single layer on one half of the baking sheet.
4. In the same bowl (no need to wash), toss broccoli with remaining 1 tablespoon olive oil, remaining garlic, remaining ¼ teaspoon salt, and remaining ¼ teaspoon pepper.
5. Spread broccoli on the other half of the baking sheet.
6. Roast for 18-20 minutes until chicken is cooked through (165°F internal temperature) and broccoli is tender with some crispy edges.
7. Remove from oven and sprinkle everything with Parmesan cheese. Let the residual heat melt the cheese for 1-2 minutes.

Tips:

Even cooking: Cut chicken into similar-sized pieces so they cook evenly. If some pieces are much smaller, they'll dry out.

Crispy broccoli: Make sure broccoli florets are completely dry before tossing with oil. Water prevents browning.

Make it spicy: Add ½ teaspoon red pepper flakes to the chicken seasoning, or sprinkle them on top before serving.

Meal prep friendly: This reheats exceptionally well. Make a double batch Sunday and eat it all week.

Swap the vegetable: Don't like broccoli? Use cauliflower, Brussels sprouts (halved), green beans, or asparagus. Same cooking time.

Chicken Parmesan (Almond Flour Breading)

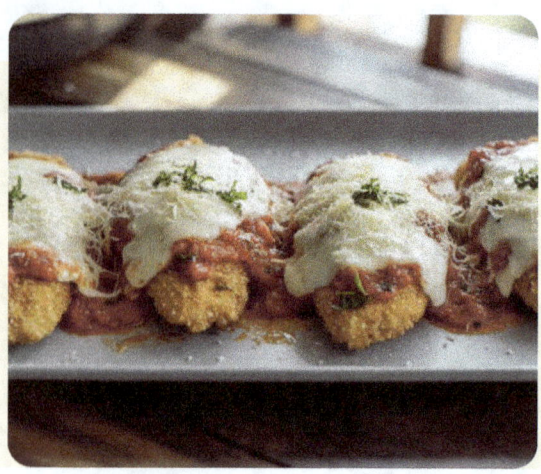

 Quick

 Serves: 4

 Prep Time: 10 min

 Cook Time: 20 min

 Total: 30 min

MACROS PER SERVING:

Calories: 445 | Protein: 42g | Fat: 26g | Net Carbs: 6g

Ingredients:

- 4 boneless, skinless chicken breasts (about 6 oz each), pounded to even thickness
- 1 cup almond flour
- ½ cup grated Parmesan cheese, divided
- 2 large eggs
- 1 teaspoon Italian seasoning
- ½ teaspoon garlic powder
- ½ teaspoon salt
- ¼ teaspoon black pepper
- 3 tablespoons olive oil for cooking
- 1 cup sugar-free marinara sauce (check label for 3-5g net carbs per ½ cup)
- 1 cup shredded mozzarella cheese
- Fresh basil for garnish (optional)

Instructions:

1. Preheat oven to 400°F.
2. Set up breading station: In a shallow bowl, mix almond flour, ¼ cup Parmesan cheese, Italian seasoning, garlic powder, salt, and pepper. In another shallow bowl, beat eggs.
3. Dip each chicken breast in egg, letting excess drip off, then dredge in almond flour mixture, pressing to adhere. Set breaded chicken on a plate.
4. Heat olive oil in a large oven-safe skillet over medium-high heat.
5. Add breaded chicken breasts and cook for 3-4 minutes per side until golden brown. They won't be cooked through yet.
6. Remove skillet from heat. Top each chicken breast with ¼ cup marinara sauce, then divide mozzarella cheese evenly among them. Sprinkle remaining ¼ cup Parmesan on top.
7. Transfer skillet to oven and bake for 10-12 minutes until cheese is melted and bubbly, and chicken reaches 165°F internal temperature.

Tips:

Pound it even: Use a meat mallet or heavy pan to pound chicken breasts to even thickness (about ¾ inch). This ensures even cooking.

No oven-safe skillet? After browning chicken in a regular skillet, transfer to a baking dish before adding sauce and cheese, then bake.

Make the sauce stick: Let browned chicken cool for 1 minute before adding sauce. This helps prevent sauce from sliding off.

Serve it with: Zucchini noodles, spaghetti squash, or a simple salad.

Storage: Refrigerate for up to 3 days. Reheat in the oven at 350°F for best texture (microwave makes the breading soggy).

Watch the marinara: Many store-bought marinara sauces are loaded with sugar. Check labels and choose one with 3-5g net carbs per ½ cup.

Lemon Herb Grilled Chicken

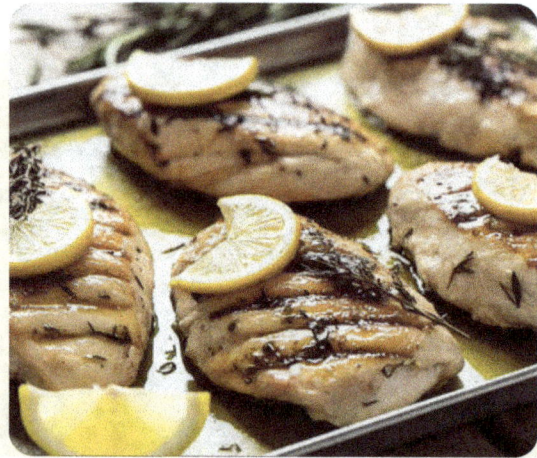

 Quick   Budget-Friendly

 Serves: 4

 Prep Time: 5 min

 Cook Time: 12 min

Total: 17 min

MACROS PER SERVING:

Calories: 295 | Protein: 38g | Fat: 14g | Net Carbs: 2g

Ingredients:

- 4 boneless, skinless chicken breasts (about 6 oz each)
- 3 tablespoons olive oil
- Juice of 1 lemon (about 3 tablespoons)
- Zest of 1 lemon
- 3 cloves garlic, minced
- 1 tablespoon fresh rosemary, chopped (or 1 teaspoon dried)
- 1 tablespoon fresh thyme, chopped (or 1 teaspoon dried)
- 1 teaspoon salt
- ½ teaspoon black pepper

Instructions:

1. In a small bowl, whisk together olive oil, lemon juice, lemon zest, garlic, rosemary, thyme, salt, and pepper.
2. Place chicken breasts in a shallow dish or large zip-top bag. Pour marinade over chicken and turn to coat. Let sit for 5-10 minutes while you preheat the grill (or you can marinate up to 2 hours if you have time).
3. Preheat grill or grill pan to medium-high heat (about 400°F). Oil the grates.
4. Remove chicken from marinade and shake off excess. Place on grill.
5. Cook for 5-6 minutes without moving, until you get good grill marks.
6. Flip and cook for another 5-6 minutes until internal temperature reaches 165°F.
7. Remove from grill and let rest for 3-5 minutes before slicing.

Tips:

No grill? No problem. Use a grill pan on the stovetop or bake at 425°F for 18-20 minutes.

Prevent sticking: Make sure grill is hot and grates are clean before adding chicken. Oil the grates just before cooking.

Don't press it: Resist the urge to press down on the chicken with your spatula. This squeezes out juices and makes it dry.

Batch cook it: Double the recipe. Use half for dinner tonight, slice the rest for salads, wraps, or quick protein additions throughout the week.

Storage: Refrigerate for up to 4 days. This chicken is great cold in salads or reheated gently.

Buffalo Chicken Lettuce Wraps

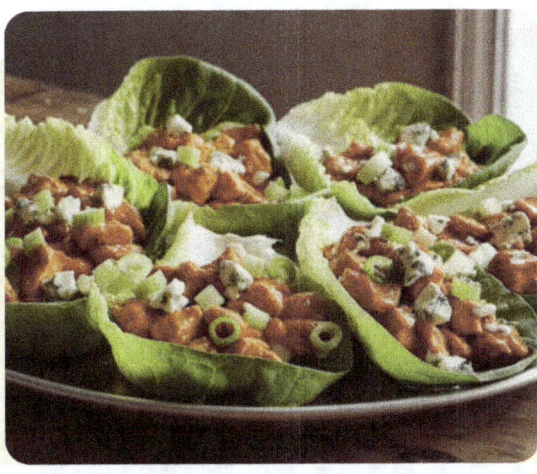

Quick   One-Pan

Serves: 4

Prep Time: 10 min

Cook Time: 12 min

Total: 22 min

MACROS PER SERVING:
Calories: 340 | Protein: 32g | Fat: 21g | Net Carbs: 4g

Ingredients:
- 1½ pounds boneless, skinless chicken breasts, diced into ½-inch pieces
- 3 tablespoons butter
- ½ cup Frank's RedHot sauce (or your favorite hot sauce)
- 1 teaspoon garlic powder
- ½ teaspoon salt
- 12 large lettuce leaves (butter lettuce, romaine, or iceberg)
- ½ cup blue cheese dressing (or ranch)
- 1 cup diced celery
- ½ cup crumbled blue cheese (optional)
- 2 green onions, sliced

Instructions:
1. Heat a large skillet over medium-high heat. Add diced chicken and season with garlic powder and salt.
2. Cook chicken for 8-10 minutes, stirring occasionally, until cooked through and lightly browned.
3. Reduce heat to low. Add butter and hot sauce to the chicken. Stir until butter melts and chicken is coated in buffalo sauce. Cook for 1-2 minutes more.
4. Remove from heat.
5. To assemble: Place a lettuce leaf on a plate. Add about ⅓ cup buffalo chicken. Top with a drizzle of blue cheese dressing, some diced celery, crumbled blue cheese (if using), and green onions.
6. Repeat with remaining lettuce leaves.

Tips:
Spice level: Frank's RedHot is medium heat. Want it milder? Use half hot sauce, half melted butter. Want it spicier? Add a dash of cayenne pepper.

Make it a bowl: Skip the lettuce wraps and serve buffalo chicken over shredded cabbage or cauliflower rice with all the toppings.

Meal prep: Cook the buffalo chicken in bulk. Store in the fridge for up to 4 days. Assemble fresh lettuce wraps each day.

Blue cheese alternative: If you don't like blue cheese, use ranch dressing and shredded cheddar instead.

Rotisserie shortcut: Use a store-bought rotisserie chicken. Shred the meat, toss with butter and hot sauce, and heat through. Dinner in 5 minutes.

Creamy Tuscan Chicken

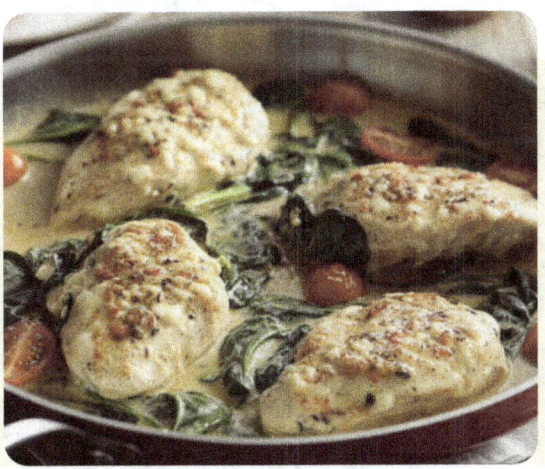

Quick   One-Pan

Serves: 4

Prep Time: 5 min

Cook Time: 20 min

Total: 25 min

MACROS PER SERVING:
Calories: 465 | Protein: 40g | Fat: 32g | Net Carbs: 5g

Ingredients:
- 4 boneless, skinless chicken breasts (about 6 oz each)
- 2 tablespoons olive oil
- 4 cloves garlic, minced
- 1 cup heavy cream
- ½ cup chicken broth
- ½ cup grated Parmesan cheese
- 1 cup cherry tomatoes, halved
- 2 cups fresh spinach
- 1 teaspoon Italian seasoning
- ½ teaspoon salt
- ¼ teaspoon black pepper
- ¼ teaspoon red pepper flakes (optional)

Instructions:
1. Season chicken breasts with salt, pepper, and Italian seasoning on both sides.
2. Heat olive oil in a large skillet over medium-high heat. Add chicken and cook for 5-6 minutes per side until golden and cooked through (165°F internal temperature). Transfer to a plate.
3. In the same skillet, add garlic and cook for 30 seconds until fragrant.
4. Add chicken broth and use a wooden spoon to scrape up any browned bits from the bottom of the pan.
5. Add heavy cream and Parmesan cheese. Stir until cheese melts and sauce is smooth.
6. Add cherry tomatoes and spinach. Cook for 2-3 minutes until spinach wilts and tomatoes soften slightly.
7. Return chicken to the skillet and spoon sauce over it. Add red pepper flakes if using.
8. Simmer for 2-3 minutes until sauce thickens slightly and chicken is heated through.

Tips:
Thin it out: If sauce gets too thick, add a splash more chicken broth.

Chicken thighs: These work great too. Use 8 boneless, skinless thighs and adjust cooking time to 6-7 minutes per side.

Sun-dried tomatoes: Swap cherry tomatoes for ½ cup chopped sun-dried tomatoes (packed in oil, drained). More intense flavor.

Serve it over: Zucchini noodles, cauliflower rice, or spaghetti squash. All soak up the creamy sauce beautifully.

Storage: Refrigerate for up to 3 days. The sauce may thicken in the fridge. Reheat gently with a splash of broth or cream.

Chicken Stir-Fry (Cauliflower Rice)

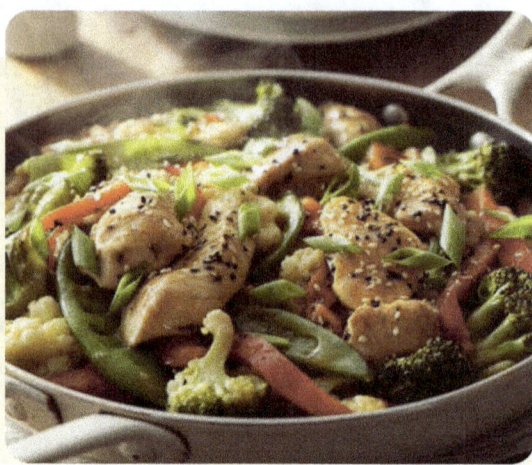

  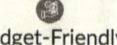
Quick   One-Pan   Budget-Friendly

 Serves: 4

 Prep Time: 10 min

 Cook Time: 15 min

 Total: 25 min

MACROS PER SERVING:
Calories: 295 | Protein: 32g | Fat: 13g | Net Carbs: 7g

Ingredients:
- 1½ pounds boneless, skinless chicken breasts or thighs, cut into 1-inch pieces
- 3 tablespoons sesame oil or avocado oil, divided
- 4 cups cauliflower rice (fresh or frozen)
- 2 cups broccoli florets
- 1 red bell pepper, sliced
- 1 cup snap peas
- 3 cloves garlic, minced
- 1 tablespoon fresh ginger, grated
- 3 tablespoons soy sauce (or coconut aminos)
- 1 tablespoon rice vinegar
- ½ teaspoon red pepper flakes (optional)
- 2 green onions, sliced
- 1 tablespoon sesame seeds

Instructions:
1. Heat 1 tablespoon oil in a large skillet or wok over high heat.
2. Add chicken pieces in a single layer. Cook without stirring for 3-4 minutes until browned on one side.
3. Flip and cook for another 3-4 minutes until cooked through. Transfer chicken to a plate.
4. Add remaining 2 tablespoons oil to the skillet. Add broccoli, bell pepper, and snap peas. Stir-fry for 3-4 minutes until vegetables are crisp-tender.
5. Push vegetables to the side. Add garlic and ginger to the center. Cook for 30 seconds until fragrant.
6. Add cauliflower rice. Stir-fry for 2-3 minutes until heated through and any excess moisture evaporates.
7. Return chicken to the skillet. Add soy sauce, rice vinegar, and red pepper flakes (if using). Toss everything together and cook for 1 minute more.
8. Remove from heat. Top with sliced green onions and sesame seeds.

Tips:
Frozen cauliflower rice: If using frozen, don't thaw it first. Just add it frozen and cook an extra minute or two.

High heat is key: Stir-fries need high heat to get that slightly charred, restaurant-quality flavor. Don't be afraid to crank up the burner.

Prep ahead: Cut all vegetables and chicken the night before. Store separately in the fridge. Cooking time becomes 10 minutes.

Make it saucier: Double the soy sauce and rice vinegar. Add 1 teaspoon of sesame oil for extra flavor.

Protein swap: Shrimp, beef, or pork all work great in this recipe. Just adjust cooking time as needed.

BBQ Chicken Thighs (Sugar-Free Sauce)

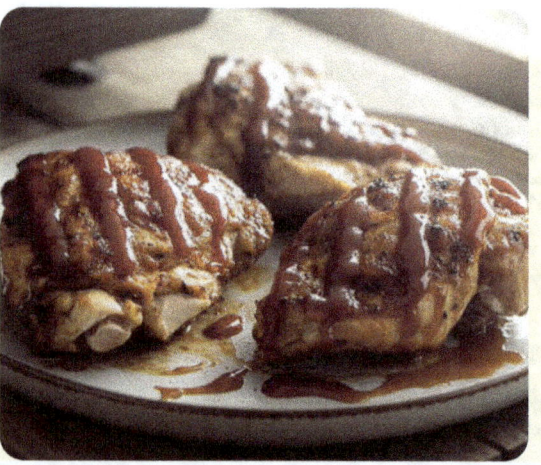

 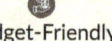
Quick   Budget-Friendly

 Serves: 4

 Prep Time: 5 min

 Cook Time: 25 min

 Total: 30 min

MACROS PER SERVING:
Calories: 410 | Protein: 36g | Fat: 26g | Net Carbs: 6g

Ingredients:
- 8 bone-in, skin-on chicken thighs (about 2½ pounds)
- 1 teaspoon salt
- ½ teaspoon black pepper
- ½ teaspoon garlic powder
- ½ teaspoon paprika
- ¾ cup sugar-free BBQ sauce (store-bought or homemade, see recipe below)

For Quick Sugar-Free BBQ Sauce (optional, if making your own):
- ¾ cup tomato sauce
- 2 tablespoons apple cider vinegar
- 2 tablespoons Worcestershire sauce
- 2 tablespoons erythritol or monk fruit sweetener
- 1 teaspoon liquid smoke
- 1 teaspoon garlic powder
- 1 teaspoon onion powder
- ½ teaspoon smoked paprika
- Salt to taste

Instructions:
1. Preheat oven to 425°F. Line a baking sheet with foil and place a wire rack on top (this helps chicken get crispy all around).
2. Pat chicken thighs dry with paper towels. Season both sides with salt, pepper, garlic powder, and paprika.
3. Place chicken thighs skin-side up on the wire rack.
4. Bake for 20 minutes.
5. Remove from oven and brush generously with BBQ sauce (about 2 tablespoons per thigh).
6. Return to oven and bake for 5 more minutes until sauce is caramelized and sticky.
7. **Optional BBQ Sauce Instructions:** Mix all sauce ingredients in a small saucepan. Simmer over medium-low heat for 10-15 minutes, stirring occasionally, until thickened. Store leftover sauce in the fridge for up to 2 weeks.

Tips:
Store-bought sauce: G Hughes, Primal Kitchen, and Lillie's Q all make good sugar-free BBQ sauces. Check that net carbs are under 2g per 2 tablespoons.

No wire rack? Place chicken directly on the foil-lined baking sheet. Flip halfway through cooking for even browning.

Grill it: These work great on the grill too. Cook over medium heat for 10 minutes per side, then brush with sauce and grill 2-3 more minutes.

Meal prep: Make a double batch. Shred leftover chicken and use it for quick BBQ chicken salads, lettuce wraps, or scrambles.

Bone-in vs. boneless: Bone-in chicken stays juicier and has more flavor. But boneless works too. Reduce cooking time to 15 minutes total.

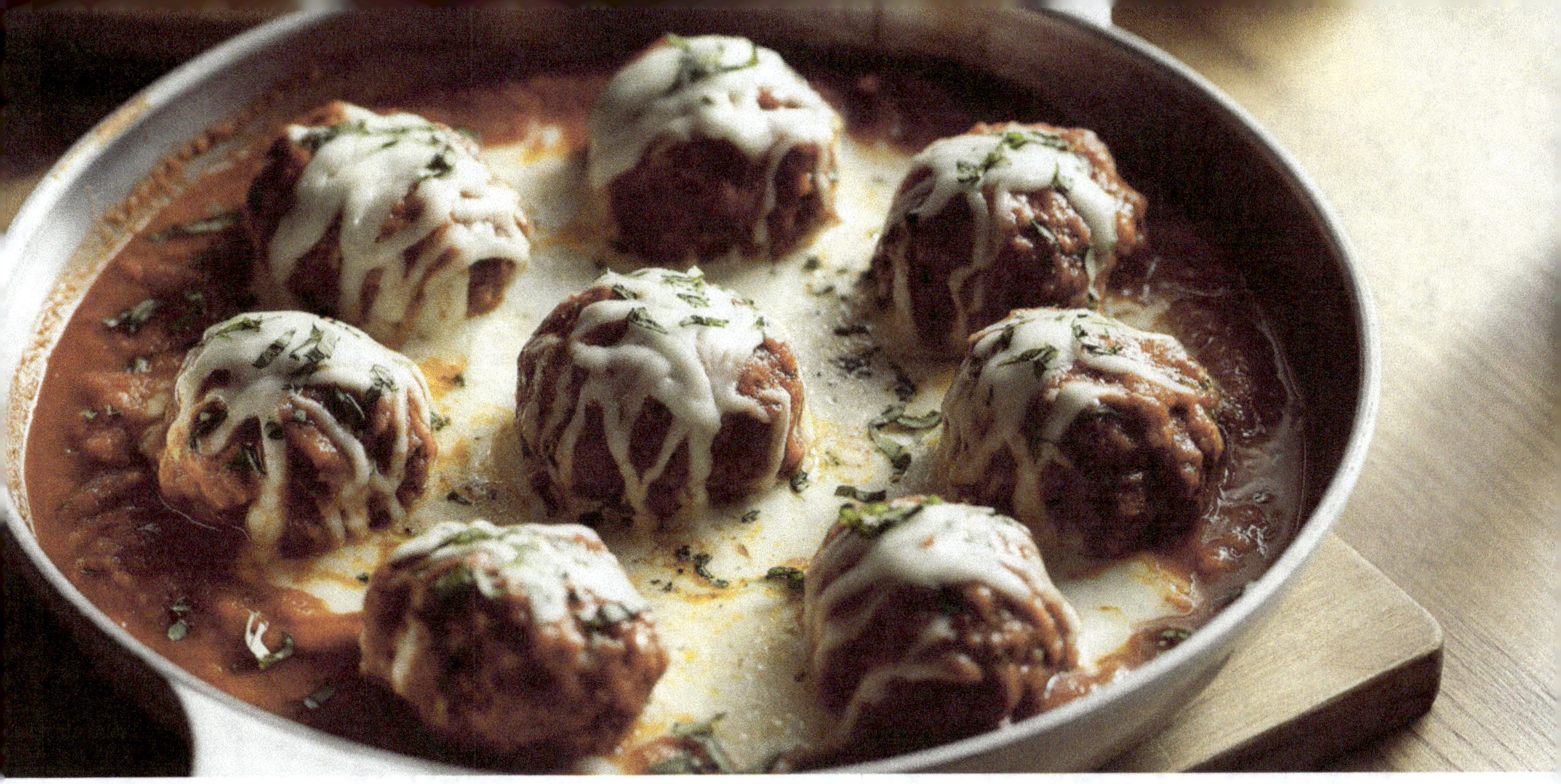

BEEF RECIPES

Beef gets a bad reputation in some diet circles, but when you choose the right cuts and cook them properly, it's one of the most satisfying and nutrient-dense proteins available. It's rich in iron, B vitamins, and provides complete protein with excellent bioavailability.

Ground beef is my weeknight hero. It's affordable, cooks quickly, and transforms into a dozen different meals. I buy 80/20 ground beef (not the super lean stuff) because the fat keeps it flavorful and juicy. Plus, when you're eating low-carb, you need those healthy fats for energy and satiety.

For steaks and whole cuts, I use a meat thermometer religiously. Overcooked beef is a tragedy. For reference: 130-135°F is medium-rare, 135-145°F is medium, 145-155°F is medium-well. I pull my steaks at 130°F and let them rest (they'll continue cooking and reach 135°F).

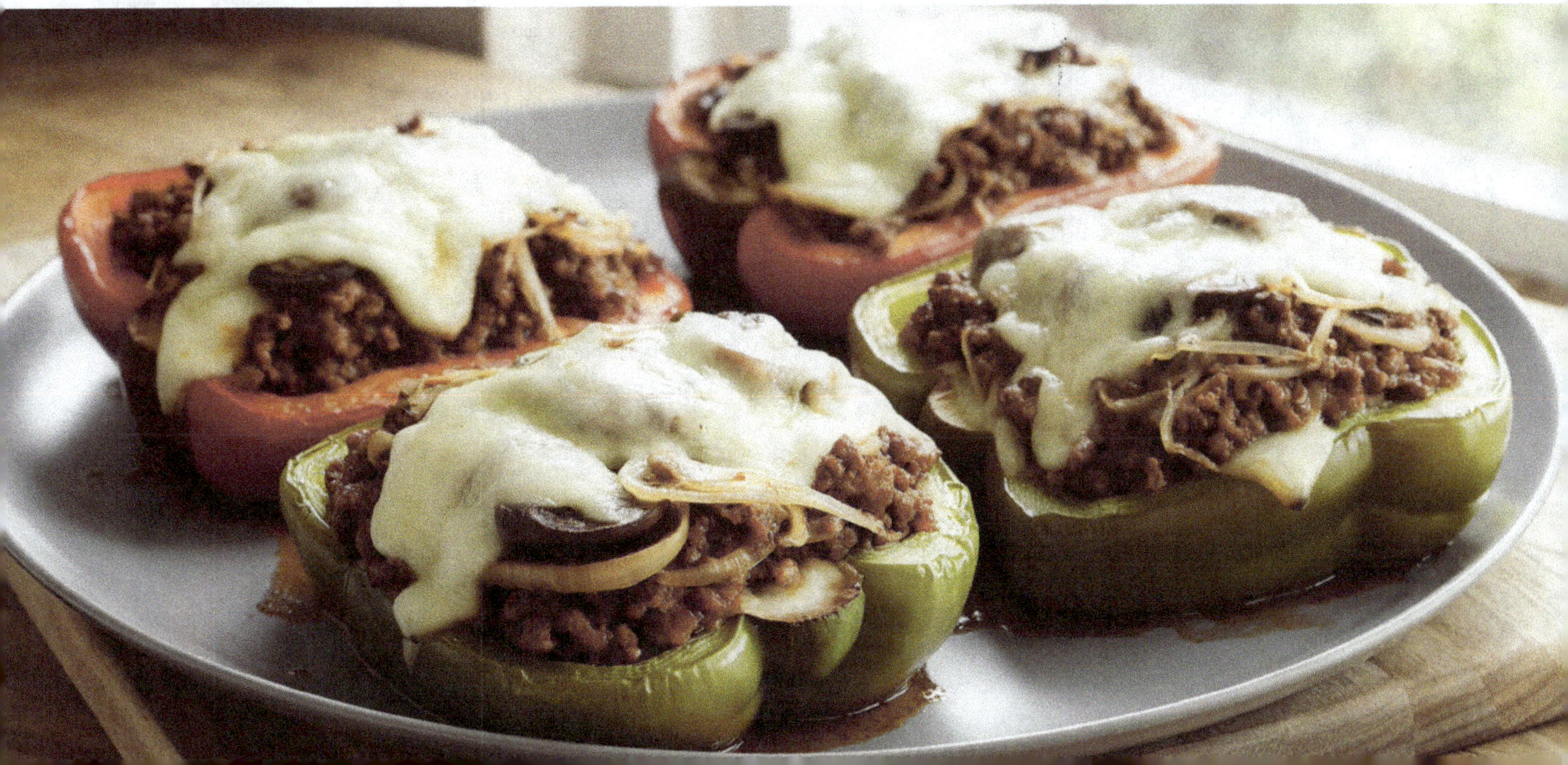

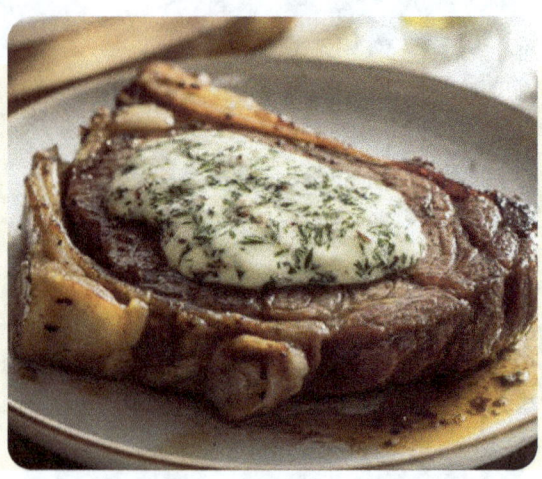

Pan-Seared Ribeye with Herb Butter

Quick

🍽 Serves: 2

✳ Prep Time: 5 min

⏲ Cook Time: 12 min

🍳 Total: 17 min

MACROS PER SERVING:
Calories: 580 | Protein: 42g | Fat: 44g | Net Carbs: 1g

Ingredients:
- 2 ribeye steaks (10-12 oz each, about 1 inch thick)
- 2 tablespoons avocado oil or other high-heat oil
- Salt and black pepper
- 4 tablespoons butter, softened
- 2 cloves garlic, minced
- 1 tablespoon fresh parsley, chopped
- 1 teaspoon fresh thyme, chopped (or ½ teaspoon dried)
- ½ teaspoon lemon zest

Instructions:
1. Remove steaks from refrigerator 20-30 minutes before cooking (room temperature steaks cook more evenly).
2. While steaks come to temperature, make herb butter: Mix softened butter with garlic, parsley, thyme, and lemon zest. Set aside.
3. Pat steaks completely dry with paper towels. Season generously with salt and pepper on both sides.
4. Heat oil in a large cast-iron or heavy skillet over high heat until it just begins to smoke.
5. Carefully place steaks in the hot skillet. Don't touch them. Let them sear for 4-5 minutes without moving.
6. Flip steaks and cook for another 3-4 minutes for medium-rare (130-135°F internal temperature), or adjust time for your preferred doneness.
7. Transfer steaks to a plate or cutting board. Top each with half the herb butter and let rest for 5 minutes (this allows juices to redistribute).
8. Slice against the grain if desired, or serve whole.

Tips:
Don't skip the rest: Those 5 minutes make a huge difference in juiciness. Cutting immediately causes all the juices to run out.

Cast iron is best: It retains heat better than other pans and creates an amazing crust. If you don't have one, use the heaviest skillet you own.

No fancy cuts needed: This method works with any steak. NY strip, sirloin, or even skirt steak. Just adjust cooking time based on thickness.

Make extra herb butter: Double the butter recipe and freeze half. Pull it out whenever you're cooking steak, chicken, or fish.

Serve it with: Roasted asparagus, sautéed mushrooms, or a simple salad. Keep the sides simple so the steak shines.

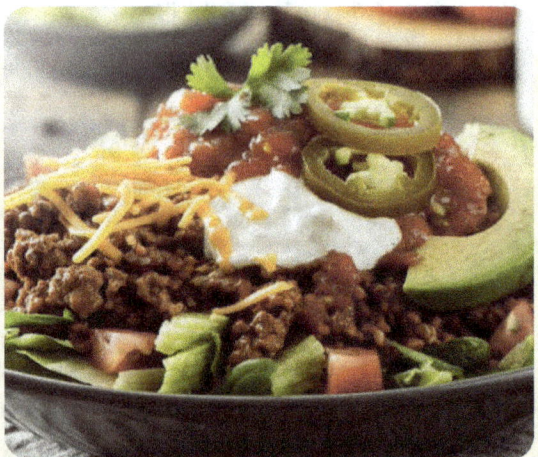

Ground Beef Taco Bowl

  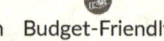
Quick   One-Pan   Budget-Friendly

 Serves: 4

 Prep Time: 5 min

 Cook Time: 15 min

 Total: 20 min

MACROS PER SERVING:
Calories: 445 | Protein: 32g | Fat: 30g | Net Carbs: 7g

Ingredients:
- 1½ pounds ground beef (80/20)
- 2 tablespoons taco seasoning (store-bought or homemade, see below)
- ¼ cup water
- 4 cups shredded lettuce
- 1 cup shredded cheddar cheese
- 1 cup diced tomatoes
- 1 cup diced avocado (about 1 large avocado)
- ½ cup sour cream
- ¼ cup salsa
- ¼ cup sliced jalapeños (optional)
- 2 tablespoons fresh cilantro, chopped

Homemade Taco Seasoning (makes about ⅓ cup):
- 2 tablespoons chili powder
- 1 tablespoon cumin
- 1 tablespoon paprika
- 2 teaspoons garlic powder
- 2 teaspoons onion powder
- 1 teaspoon oregano
- 1 teaspoon salt
- ½ teaspoon black pepper
- ½ teaspoon cayenne (optional, for heat)

Instructions:
1. Heat a large skillet over medium-high heat. Add ground beef and cook, breaking it up with a spatula, for 6-8 minutes until browned and cooked through.
2. Drain excess fat if there's more than 2 tablespoons in the pan (a little fat adds flavor).
3. Add taco seasoning and water to the beef. Stir well and cook for 2-3 minutes until water evaporates and beef is coated in seasoning.
4. While beef cooks, divide lettuce among 4 bowls.
5. Top each bowl with seasoned beef (about ½ cup per bowl), then add cheese, tomatoes, avocado, sour cream, salsa, jalapeños (if using), and cilantro.

Tips:
Taco seasoning: Store-bought packets work but often contain sugar and fillers. Make your own blend and store it in a jar. Use 2-3 tablespoons per pound of meat.

Meal prep: Cook a double batch of taco meat on Sunday. Use it for taco bowls, scrambles, stuffed peppers, or lettuce wraps throughout the week.

Budget hack: Ground beef goes on sale frequently. Buy 5 pounds when it's under $3/lb, portion into 1½ lb packages, and freeze.

Make it spicier: Add diced jalapeños to the meat while cooking, or use hot salsa.

Swap the protein: Ground turkey, chicken, or pork all work with these same seasonings.

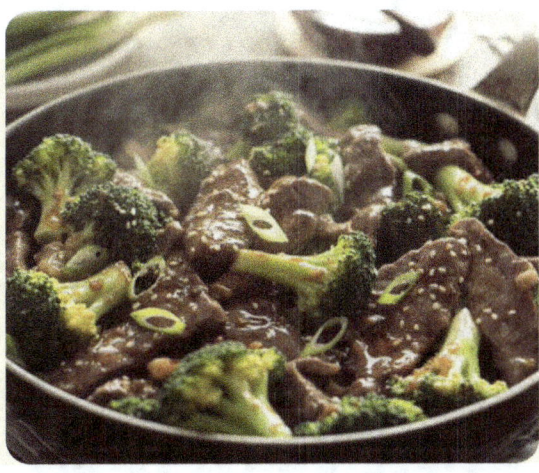

Beef & Broccoli Stir-Fry

Quick   One-Pan

 Serves: 4

 Prep Time: 10 min

Cook Time: 12 min

Total: 22 min

MACROS PER SERVING:

Calories: 380 | Protein: 34g | Fat: 22g | Net Carbs: 8g

Ingredients:

- 1½ pounds flank steak or sirloin, sliced thin against the grain
- 6 cups broccoli florets
- 3 tablespoons avocado oil, divided
- 4 cloves garlic, minced
- 1 tablespoon fresh ginger, grated
- ¼ cup soy sauce (or coconut aminos)
- 2 tablespoons rice vinegar
- 1 tablespoon sesame oil
- 1 teaspoon erythritol or 5-6 drops liquid stevia (optional, for slight sweetness)
- ¼ teaspoon red pepper flakes
- 1 tablespoon sesame seeds
- 2 green onions, sliced

Instructions:

1. In a small bowl, whisk together soy sauce, rice vinegar, sesame oil, sweetener (if using), and red pepper flakes. Set aside.
2. Heat 1 tablespoon avocado oil in a large skillet or wok over high heat.
3. Add beef slices in a single layer. Don't overcrowd the pan (work in batches if needed). Cook for 2-3 minutes without stirring until browned.
4. Flip and cook for another 1-2 minutes. Transfer beef to a plate. It's okay if it's slightly undercooked; it'll finish cooking later.
5. Add remaining 2 tablespoons oil to the skillet. Add broccoli and stir-fry for 3-4 minutes until bright green and crisp-tender.
6. Push broccoli to the sides. Add garlic and ginger to the center. Cook for 30 seconds until fragrant.
7. Return beef to the skillet along with any accumulated juices. Pour sauce over everything.
8. Toss everything together and cook for 1-2 minutes until sauce thickens slightly and coats the beef and broccoli.
9. Remove from heat. Top with sesame seeds and sliced green onions.

Tips:

Slice it thin: Partially freeze the beef for 20 minutes before slicing. This makes it easier to cut thin, even slices against the grain.

High heat matters: Like all stir-fries, high heat is essential. If your pan isn't hot enough, the beef will steam instead of sear.

Serve it over: Cauliflower rice if you want to make it more filling. Or just eat it as-is for a lighter meal.

Meal prep: This reheats well for up to 3 days. The broccoli will soften a bit but still tastes great.

Switch the vegetable: Snap peas, green beans, or bell peppers all work beautifully here.

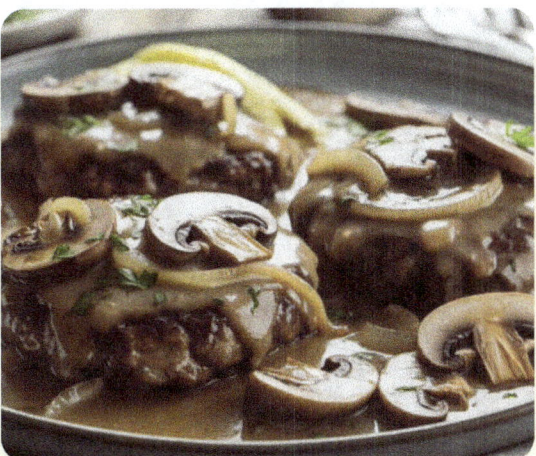

Salisbury Steak with Mushroom Gravy

 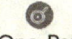 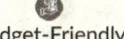
Quick   One-Pan   Budget-Friendly

 Serves: 4

 Prep Time: 10 min

Cook Time: 20 min

Total: 30 min

MACROS PER SERVING:

Calories: 465 | Protein: 36g | Fat: 32g | Net Carbs: 6g

Ingredients:

For the patties:
- 1½ pounds ground beef (80/20)
- 1 large egg
- ¼ cup almond flour
- 2 tablespoons onion, finely minced
- 2 cloves garlic, minced
- 1 teaspoon Worcestershire sauce
- ½ teaspoon salt
- ¼ teaspoon black pepper

For the gravy:
- 2 tablespoons butter

- 8 oz mushrooms, sliced
- 1 small onion, sliced
- 2 cloves garlic, minced
- 1½ cups beef broth
- ½ cup heavy cream
- 1 tablespoon Worcestershire sauce
- ½ teaspoon xanthan gum (optional, for thicker gravy)
- Salt and pepper to taste
- Fresh parsley for garnish

Instructions:

1. In a large bowl, combine ground beef, egg, almond flour, minced onion, garlic, Worcestershire sauce, salt, and pepper. Mix gently with your hands until just combined.
2. Form into 4 oval-shaped patties, about ¾ inch thick.
3. Heat a large skillet over medium-high heat. Add patties and cook for 4-5 minutes per side until browned and cooked through. Transfer to a plate.
4. In the same skillet, add butter. Once melted, add mushrooms and sliced onion. Cook for 5-6 minutes until softened and browned.
5. Add garlic and cook for 30 seconds.
6. Pour in beef broth and Worcestershire sauce. Use a wooden spoon to scrape up any browned bits from the bottom of the pan.
7. Bring to a simmer and cook for 3-4 minutes to reduce slightly.
8. Stir in heavy cream. If you want a thicker gravy, sprinkle xanthan gum over the sauce while whisking constantly (it thickens quickly, so add a little at a time).
9. Season with salt and pepper to taste.
10. Return patties to the skillet and spoon gravy over them. Simmer for 2-3 minutes until heated through.

Tips:

Don't overmix: When forming patties, mix just until combined. Overmixing makes them tough.

Make an indent: Press a small indent in the center of each patty with your thumb before cooking. This prevents them from puffing up in the middle.

No xanthan gum? Let the gravy simmer longer to reduce and thicken naturally, or skip thickening altogether. It'll be thinner but still delicious.

Serve it with: Mashed cauliflower, roasted green beans, or a simple salad.

Storage: Refrigerate for up to 3 days. Reheat gently on the stovetop with a splash of broth.

Philly Cheesesteak Stuffed Peppers

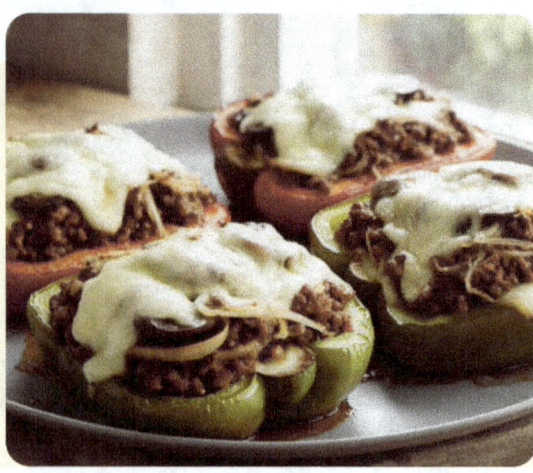

Quick   Budget-Friendly

Serves: 4

Prep Time: 10 min

Cook Time: 20 min

Total: 30 min

MACROS PER SERVING:

Calories: 420 | Protein: 32g | Fat: 26g | Net Carbs: 8g

Ingredients:

- 4 large bell peppers (any color)
- 1 pound ground beef (or thinly sliced ribeye/sirloin if you prefer)
- 1 tablespoon olive oil
- 1 medium onion, sliced
- 8 oz mushrooms, sliced
- 2 cloves garlic, minced
- 1 teaspoon Worcestershire sauce
- ½ teaspoon salt
- ¼ teaspoon black pepper
- 1½ cups shredded provolone cheese (or mozzarella)

Instructions:

1. Preheat oven to 400°F.
2. Cut bell peppers in half lengthwise. Remove seeds and membranes. Place cut-side up in a baking dish. Set aside.
3. Heat olive oil in a large skillet over medium-high heat. Add onion and mushrooms. Cook for 5-6 minutes until softened and starting to brown.
4. Add ground beef, breaking it up with a spatula. Cook for 5-6 minutes until browned and cooked through.
5. Add garlic, Worcestershire sauce, salt, and pepper. Cook for 1 minute more.
6. Divide the beef mixture evenly among the 8 pepper halves, filling each one.
7. Top each stuffed pepper with shredded cheese (about 3 tablespoons per pepper).
8. Bake for 12-15 minutes until peppers are tender and cheese is melted and bubbly.

Tips:

Tender peppers: If you prefer softer peppers, microwave the halves for 3-4 minutes before stuffing, then reduce baking time to 8-10 minutes.

Sliced steak version: For authentic Philly cheesesteak, use thinly sliced ribeye or sirloin instead of ground beef. Slice it super thin and cook it quickly in the skillet.

Cheese variety: Traditional cheesesteaks use provolone or Cheez Whiz (though that's not low-carb). Provolone, mozzarella, or even white American cheese all work.

Meal prep: These reheat beautifully. Make a double batch and refrigerate for up to 4 days.

Budget tip: Buy whole bell peppers rather than pre-cut. They're always cheaper.

Beef Cauliflower Fried Rice

 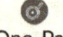 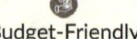
Quick   One-Pan   Budget-Friendly

Serves: 4

Prep Time: 10 min

Cook Time: 15 min

Total: 25 min

MACROS PER SERVING:

Calories: 380 | Protein: 30g | Fat: 24g | Net Carbs: 7g

Ingredients:

- 1 pound ground beef (80/20)
- 4 cups cauliflower rice (fresh or frozen)
- 3 tablespoons sesame oil or avocado oil, divided
- 3 large eggs, beaten
- 1 cup diced carrots (about 2 medium carrots)
- ½ cup frozen peas
- 3 cloves garlic, minced
- 1 tablespoon fresh ginger, grated
- 3 tablespoons soy sauce (or coconut aminos)
- 1 tablespoon rice vinegar
- 3 green onions, sliced
- 1 tablespoon sesame seeds

Instructions:

1. Heat 1 tablespoon oil in a large skillet or wok over high heat.
2. Add ground beef and cook, breaking it up, for 5-6 minutes until browned and cooked through. Transfer to a plate.
3. Add 1 tablespoon oil to the skillet. Pour in beaten eggs and scramble for 1-2 minutes until just cooked. Transfer to the plate with beef.
4. Add remaining 1 tablespoon oil to the skillet. Add carrots and peas. Stir-fry for 2-3 minutes.
5. Add garlic and ginger. Cook for 30 seconds until fragrant.
6. Add cauliflower rice. Stir-fry for 3-4 minutes until heated through and any excess moisture evaporates.
7. Return beef and eggs to the skillet. Add soy sauce and rice vinegar. Toss everything together and cook for 1-2 minutes.

Tips:

Frozen cauliflower rice: Use it frozen, don't thaw. It cooks perfectly from frozen and you avoid the extra moisture.

Get it crispy: The key to good fried rice (even cauliflower rice) is high heat and not stirring too much. Let it sit for 30 seconds at a time to get some browning.

Day-old trick: If making fresh cauliflower rice, pulse it in the food processor the day before and refrigerate overnight. This dries it out slightly and prevents mushiness.

Protein swaps: This works with ground turkey, chicken, pork, or shrimp. Just adjust cooking time.

Make it spicy: Add 1 teaspoon sriracha or sambal oelek with the soy sauce.

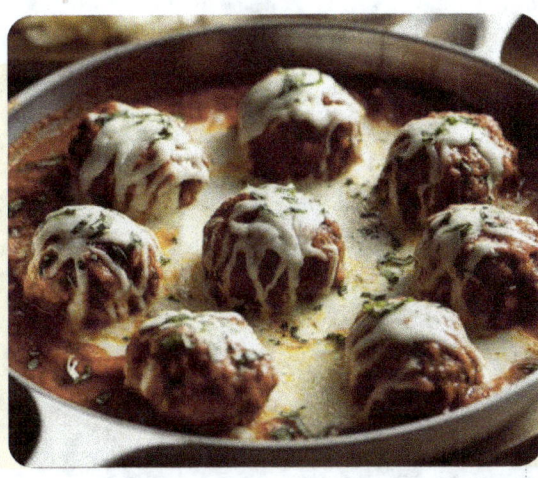

Meatballs in Marinara (No Pasta)

 Quick    Budget-Friendly

 Serves: 4 (5 meatballs per serving)

Prep Time: 10 min

Cook Time: 20 min

 Total: 30 min

MACROS PER SERVING:
Calories: 445 | Protein: 34g | Fat: 30g | Net Carbs: 7g

Ingredients:

For the meatballs:
- 1½ pounds ground beef (80/20)
- 1 large egg
- ½ cup grated Parmesan cheese
- ¼ cup almond flour
- 3 cloves garlic, minced
- 2 tablespoons fresh parsley, chopped (or 2 teaspoons dried)
- 1 teaspoon Italian seasoning
- ½ teaspoon salt
- ¼ teaspoon black pepper

For serving:
- 2 cups sugar-free marinara sauce
- ½ cup shredded mozzarella cheese
- Fresh basil for garnish

Instructions:

1. Preheat oven to 400°F. Line a baking sheet with parchment paper.
2. In a large bowl, combine ground beef, egg, Parmesan, almond flour, garlic, parsley, Italian seasoning, salt, and pepper. Mix gently with your hands until just combined.
3. Form into 20 meatballs (about 2 tablespoons of mixture each). Place on the prepared baking sheet.
4. Bake for 15-18 minutes until browned and cooked through (internal temperature of 160°F).
5. While meatballs bake, heat marinara sauce in a large skillet over medium heat.
6. Transfer cooked meatballs to the skillet with marinara. Spoon sauce over meatballs and simmer for 2-3 minutes.
7. Sprinkle mozzarella cheese over the top. Cover skillet and let sit for 1-2 minutes until cheese melts.

Tips:

Keep them moist: Don't overbake. Pull them at 160°F and they'll be juicy and tender.

Make them uniform: Use a cookie scoop or ice cream scoop to portion the meat. Uniform size means even cooking.

Serve it over: Zucchini noodles, spaghetti squash, or just eat them straight with the sauce. A side salad makes it a complete meal.

Freeze them: Make a triple batch. Freeze cooked meatballs on a baking sheet, then transfer to freezer bags. Thaw and reheat in marinara whenever you need a quick meal.

Ground turkey: Works great if you want a leaner option. Add 1 tablespoon olive oil to the mixture to keep them from drying out.

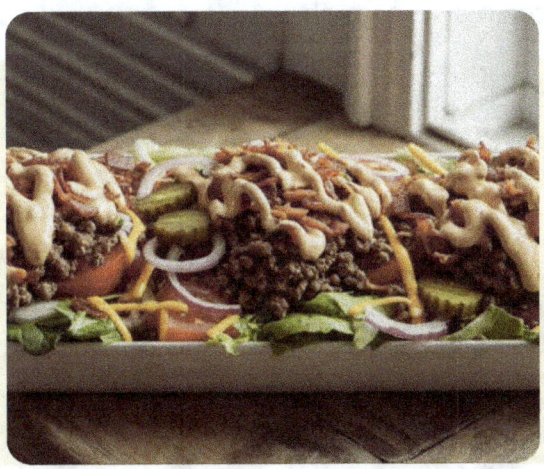

Bunless Bacon Burger Bowl

 Quick   One-Pan   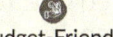 Budget-Friendly

Serves: 4

Prep Time: 5 min

 Cook Time: 15 min

 Total: 20 min

MACROS PER SERVING:
Calories: 520 | Protein: 36g | Fat: 38g | Net Carbs: 5g

Ingredients:

- 1½ pounds ground beef (80/20)
- 8 strips bacon
- 4 cups shredded lettuce (iceberg or romaine)
- 1 cup diced tomatoes
- ½ cup diced onion
- ½ cup diced pickles
- 1 cup shredded cheddar cheese
- ½ cup mayonnaise
- 2 tablespoons sugar-free ketchup (or regular ketchup if you don't mind 2-3g extra carbs)
- 1 tablespoon yellow mustard
- Salt and pepper to taste

Instructions:

1. Cook bacon in a large skillet over medium heat until crispy, about 8-10 minutes. Transfer to a paper towel-lined plate. Once cool, crumble or chop.
2. Pour out all but 1 tablespoon of bacon grease from the skillet.
3. Increase heat to medium-high. Add ground beef, season with salt and pepper, and cook for 6-8 minutes, breaking it up with a spatula, until browned and cooked through.
4. While beef cooks, divide shredded lettuce among 4 bowls.
5. In a small bowl, mix mayonnaise, ketchup, and mustard to make burger sauce.
6. Top each lettuce bowl with seasoned beef, crumbled bacon, tomatoes, onion, pickles, and shredded cheese.
7. Drizzle burger sauce over each bowl.

Tips:

Bacon in the oven: For easier cleanup, bake bacon at 400°F on a foil-lined baking sheet for 15-18 minutes. Less mess, more bacon capacity.

Secret sauce upgrade: Add 1 tablespoon diced pickles and ½ teaspoon garlic powder to the burger sauce. Now it tastes like Big Mac sauce.

Make it spicy: Use pepper jack cheese and add sliced jalapeños or a dash of hot sauce.

Meal prep: Cook the beef and bacon on Sunday. Store separately. Assemble fresh bowls each day.

Add avocado: Half an avocado per bowl adds healthy fats and makes it even more satisfying. Adds about 8g fat and 2g net carbs.

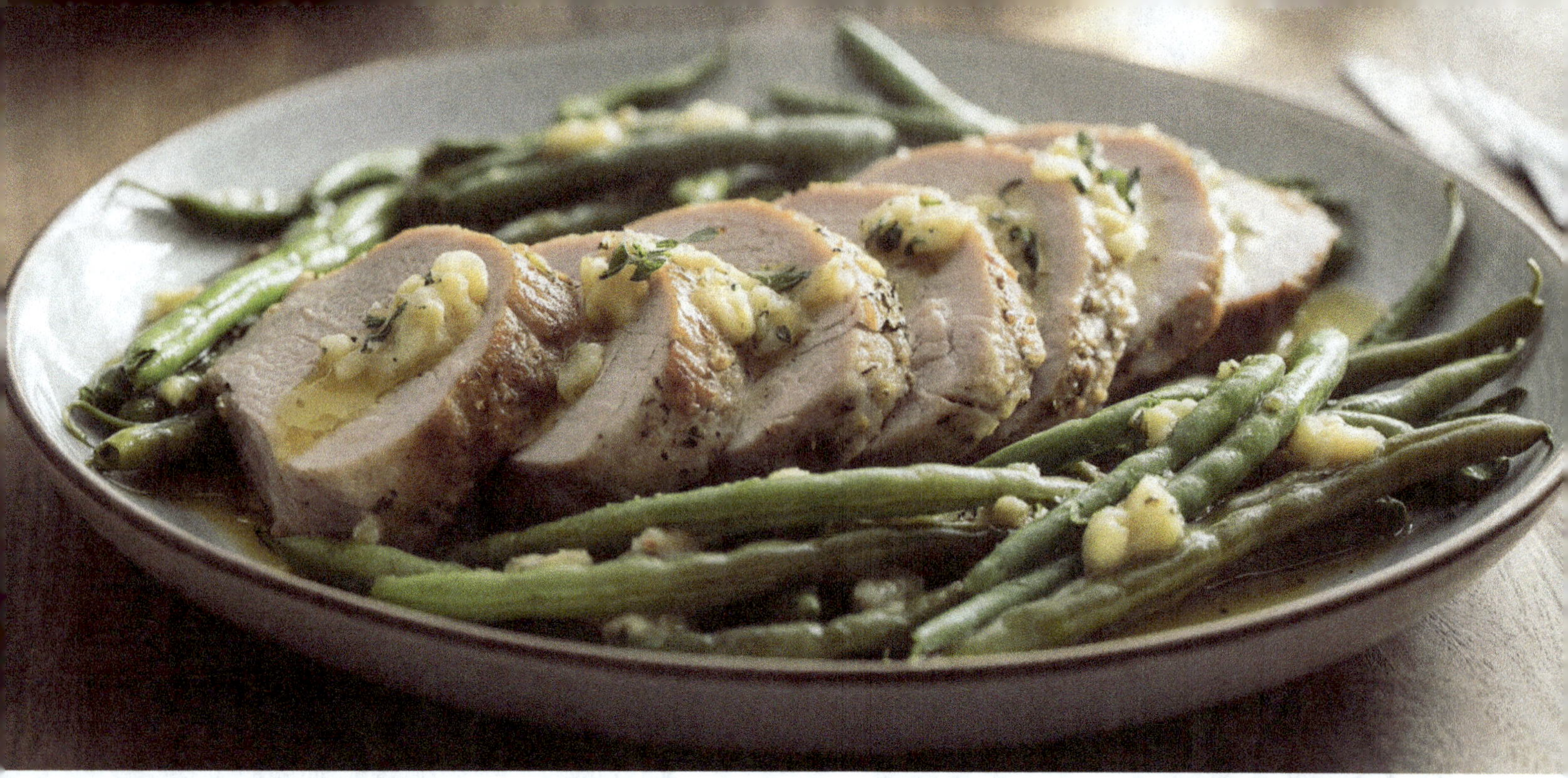

PORK RECIPES

Pork is an underrated weeknight protein. It's affordable, flavorful, and more forgiving than chicken (harder to overcook into sawdust). Plus, it pairs beautifully with both bold spices and simple seasonings.

Pork chops and tenderloin cook quickly, making them perfect for weeknights. Ground pork is incredibly versatile and often cheaper than ground beef. And let's be honest: bacon makes everything better.

One note on pork safety: The USDA lowered the recommended internal temperature for pork to 145°F (with a 3-minute rest) back in 2011. This means you can safely cook pork to medium, where it's still slightly pink and juicy. No more dry, gray pork chops.

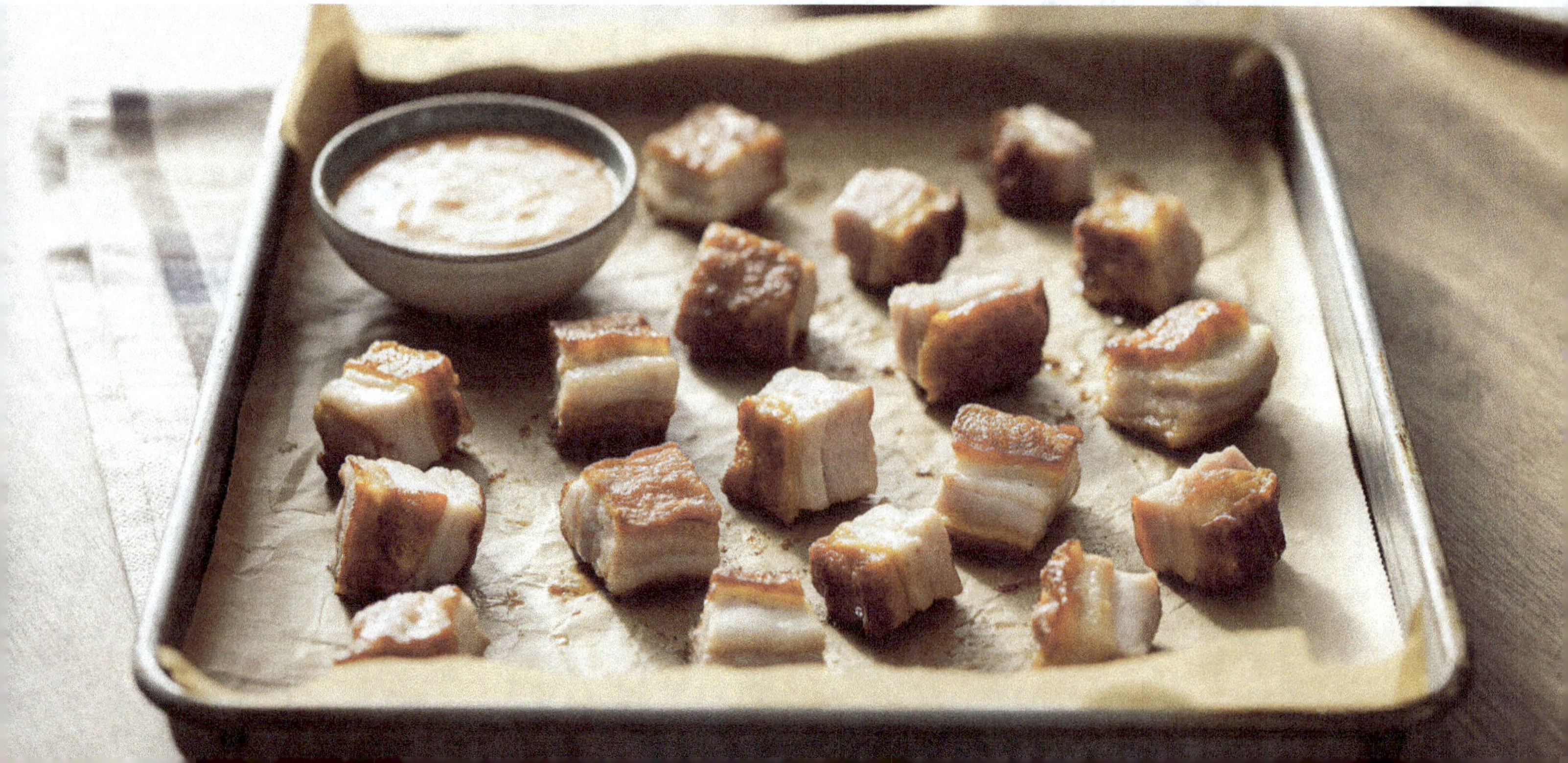

Pork Chops with Mustard Cream Sauce

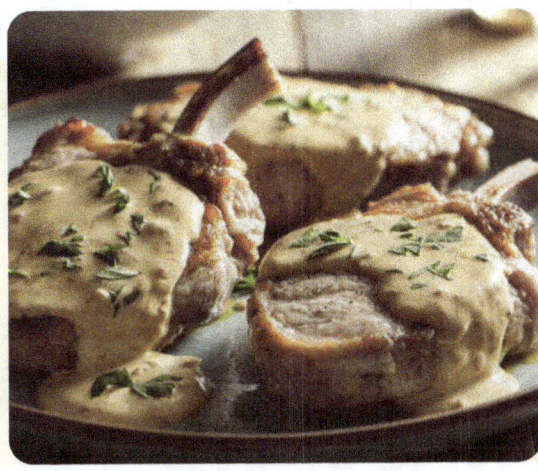

Quick   One-Pan

 Serves: 4

 Prep Time: 5 min

 Cook Time: 18 min

 Total: 23 min

MACROS PER SERVING:

Calories: 465 | Protein: 38g | Fat: 32g | Net Carbs: 3g

Ingredients:

- 4 boneless pork chops (about 6 oz each, ¾ inch thick)
- 2 tablespoons olive oil
- Salt and pepper
- 3 cloves garlic, minced
- ½ cup chicken broth
- ¾ cup heavy cream
- 3 tablespoons Dijon mustard
- 1 tablespoon whole grain mustard
- 1 teaspoon fresh thyme (or ½ teaspoon dried)
- Fresh parsley for garnish

Instructions:

1. Pat pork chops dry with paper towels. Season both sides generously with salt and pepper.
2. Heat olive oil in a large skillet over medium-high heat.
3. Add pork chops and cook for 4-5 minutes without moving them. Flip and cook for another 4-5 minutes until internal temperature reaches 145°F. Transfer to a plate.
4. Reduce heat to medium. Add garlic to the skillet and cook for 30 seconds until fragrant.
5. Add chicken broth and scrape up any browned bits from the bottom of the pan with a wooden spoon.
6. Add heavy cream, Dijon mustard, whole grain mustard, and thyme. Stir until smooth.
7. Simmer for 3-4 minutes until sauce thickens slightly.
8. Return pork chops to the skillet and spoon sauce over them. Cook for 1-2 minutes until heated through.

Tips:

Don't overcook: Pork chops dry out quickly when overcooked. Pull them at 145°F and let them rest. They'll be slightly pink in the center and perfectly juicy.

Even thickness: If your pork chops are uneven, pound the thick end with a meat mallet to create uniform thickness. This ensures even cooking.

Bone-in option: Bone-in pork chops work great too. Just add 2-3 minutes to the cooking time per side.

Serve it with: Roasted Brussels sprouts, sautéed green beans, or cauliflower mash. The sauce is so good you'll want something to soak it up.

Storage: Refrigerate for up to 3 days. Reheat gently to avoid drying out the meat.

Italian Sausage & Peppers

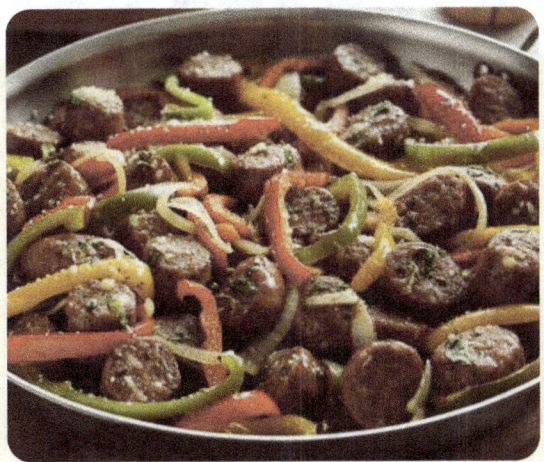

  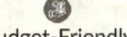
Quick   One-Pan   Budget-Friendly

 Serves: 4

 Prep Time: 8 min

 Cook Time: 20 min

 Total: 28 min

MACROS PER SERVING:

Calories: 420 | Protein: 28g | Fat: 30g | Net Carbs: 8g

Ingredients:

- 1½ pounds Italian sausage (mild or hot, links or bulk)
- 3 bell peppers (mix of colors), sliced into strips
- 1 large onion, sliced
- 3 cloves garlic, minced
- 1 tablespoon olive oil
- 1 teaspoon Italian seasoning
- ½ teaspoon salt
- ¼ teaspoon black pepper
- ¼ teaspoon red pepper flakes (optional)
- 2 tablespoons fresh basil, chopped (optional)
- Optional: grated Parmesan for serving

Instructions:

1. If using sausage links, cut each into 3-4 pieces. If using bulk sausage, form into 12-16 small patties.
2. Heat olive oil in a large skillet over medium-high heat.
3. Add sausage and cook for 8-10 minutes, turning occasionally, until browned on all sides and cooked through. Transfer to a plate.
4. In the same skillet, add bell peppers and onion. If the pan is dry, add another tablespoon of olive oil.
5. Cook for 6-7 minutes, stirring occasionally, until vegetables are softened and starting to caramelize.
6. Add garlic, Italian seasoning, salt, pepper, and red pepper flakes (if using). Cook for 1 minute.
7. Return sausage to the skillet. Toss everything together and cook for 2 more minutes.

Tips:

Bulk vs. links: Bulk sausage is often cheaper and cooks faster. Links have better presentation. Both work perfectly.

Sweet or hot: Use mild Italian sausage for family-friendly flavor, or hot Italian sausage if you like some kick.

Make it a complete meal: Serve over cauliflower rice or zucchini noodles. Or just eat it as-is with a side salad.

Meal prep gold: This reheats beautifully and actually tastes better the next day as flavors meld. Make a double batch.

Budget tip: Bell peppers are expensive. Buy them on sale and freeze sliced peppers for recipes like this. Or use just green peppers (the cheapest variety).

Pulled Pork Lettuce Wraps

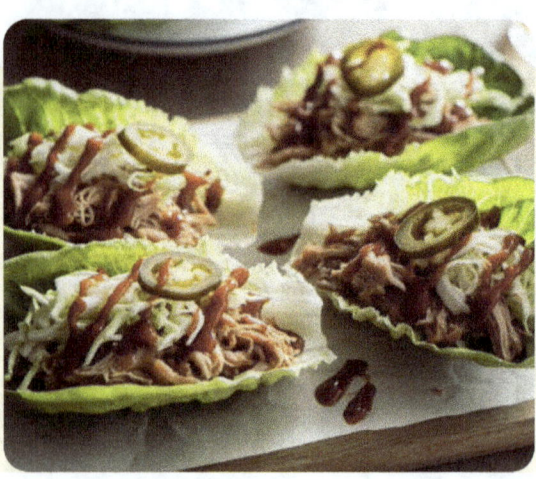

 Budget-Friendly   Make-Ahead

Serves: 8

Prep Time: 10 min

Cook Time: 4 hours (slow cooker)

Total: 4 hours 10 min

MACROS PER SERVING:
Calories: 380 | Protein: 32g | Fat: 24g | Net Carbs: 4g

Ingredients:

- 3 pounds pork shoulder (also called pork butt)
- 2 tablespoons olive oil
- 1 tablespoon chili powder
- 1 tablespoon paprika
- 1 tablespoon garlic powder
- 1 tablespoon onion powder
- 2 teaspoons cumin
- 1 teaspoon salt
- ½ teaspoon black pepper
- ½ cup chicken broth
- 3 tablespoons apple cider vinegar
- 2 tablespoons Worcestershire sauce

For serving:
- 16 large lettuce leaves (butter lettuce or romaine)
- 1 cup coleslaw mix
- ½ cup sugar-free BBQ sauce
- Optional: sliced jalapeños, diced onion, pickles

Instructions:

1. In a small bowl, mix chili powder, paprika, garlic powder, onion powder, cumin, salt, and pepper to make a rub.
2. Rub the pork shoulder all over with the spice mixture.
3. Heat olive oil in a large skillet over high heat. Sear the pork on all sides until browned, about 2-3 minutes per side.
4. Transfer pork to slow cooker. Add chicken broth, apple cider vinegar, and Worcestershire sauce.
5. Cover and cook on low for 7-8 hours or on high for 4-5 hours, until pork is very tender and easily shreds with a fork.
6. Remove pork from slow cooker. Shred with two forks, discarding any large pieces of fat.
7. Return shredded pork to the slow cooker and stir to coat with cooking liquid. Let sit for 5 minutes to absorb flavors.
8. To serve: Place about ⅓ cup pulled pork in a lettuce leaf. Top with coleslaw, a drizzle of BBQ sauce, and any optional toppings.

Tips:

Timing: This recipe takes 4+ hours, but it's completely hands-off. Perfect for Sunday meal prep while you're doing other things.

Instant Pot version: Sear pork in Instant Pot using sauté function, then pressure cook on high for 75 minutes with natural release. Total time: 2 hours.

Storage: Shredded pork keeps for up to 5 days in the fridge or 3 months in the freezer. Portion into containers for quick meals.

Beyond wraps: Use this pulled pork for breakfast scrambles, taco bowls, stuffed peppers, or just eat it plain with a side of vegetables.

Budget superstar: Pork shoulder is one of the cheapest cuts of meat (often $1.50-2.50/lb). One 3-pound roast feeds 8 people or gives you protein for a week.

Pork Tenderloin with Green Beans

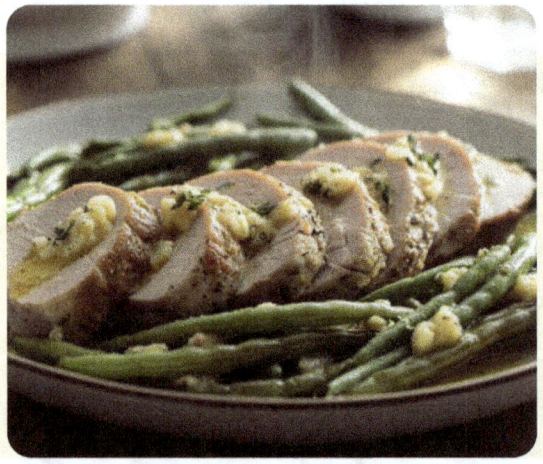

 Quick   One-Pan

Serves: 4

Prep Time: 8 min

Cook Time: 22 min

Total: 30 min

MACROS PER SERVING:
Calories: 320 | Protein: 36g | Fat: 16g | Net Carbs: 6g

Ingredients:

- 1½ pounds pork tenderloin
- 1 pound green beans, trimmed
- 3 tablespoons olive oil, divided
- 4 cloves garlic, minced
- 1 teaspoon paprika
- 1 teaspoon garlic powder
- 1 teaspoon dried thyme
- ¾ teaspoon salt, divided
- ½ teaspoon black pepper, divided
- 2 tablespoons butter
- 1 tablespoon lemon juice
- Optional: lemon wedges for serving

Instructions:

1. Preheat oven to 425°F.
2. Pat pork tenderloin dry. In a small bowl, mix paprika, garlic powder, thyme, ½ teaspoon salt, and ¼ teaspoon pepper. Rub all over the pork.
3. Heat 1 tablespoon olive oil in a large oven-safe skillet over high heat.
4. Sear pork for 2-3 minutes per side until browned all over. Transfer skillet to oven.
5. Roast for 12-15 minutes until internal temperature reaches 145°F. Remove from oven and transfer pork to a cutting board to rest.
6. While pork rests, add remaining 2 tablespoons olive oil to the same skillet over medium-high heat (careful, handle will be hot).
7. Add green beans, remaining ¼ teaspoon salt, and remaining ¼ teaspoon pepper. Sauté for 4-5 minutes until tender-crisp.
8. Add garlic and butter. Cook for 1 minute until garlic is fragrant.
9. Remove from heat and stir in lemon juice.
10. Slice pork into medallions and serve with green beans. Drizzle any accumulated juices from the cutting board over the pork.

Tips:

Let it rest: Don't skip the 5-minute rest. This allows juices to redistribute, keeping the pork moist.

Even cooking: Tuck the thin end of the tenderloin under itself and tie with kitchen twine if needed. This creates uniform thickness.

No oven-safe skillet? Sear the pork in a regular skillet, then transfer to a baking dish for roasting. Sauté green beans in the skillet while pork roasts.

Swap the vegetables: Asparagus, broccoli, or Brussels sprouts all work with the same cooking method.

Scaling: Pork tenderloin comes in various sizes (1-2 pounds). Adjust cooking time based on thickness, not weight. Use a thermometer.

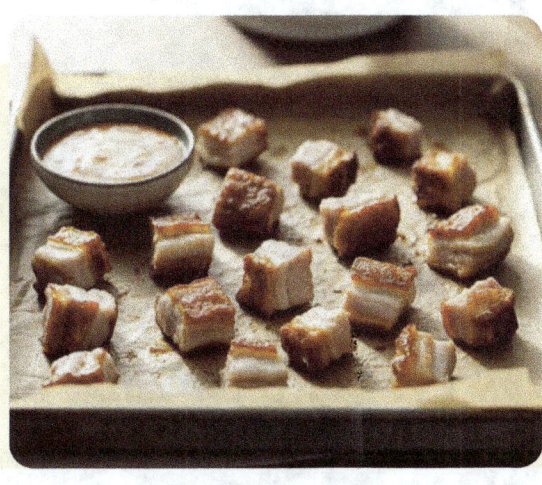

Crispy Pork Belly Bites

Quick

 Serves: 4

 Prep Time: 5 min

 Cook Time: 25 min

 Total: 30 min

MACROS PER SERVING:
Calories: 520 | Protein: 28g | Fat: 44g | Net Carbs: 1g

Ingredients:
- 2 pounds pork belly, cut into 1-inch cubes
- 2 teaspoons salt
- 1 teaspoon black pepper
- 1 teaspoon garlic powder
- ½ teaspoon smoked paprika
- ¼ teaspoon cayenne pepper (optional)

For the dipping sauce (optional):
- ¼ cup mayonnaise
- 1 tablespoon Dijon mustard
- 1 tablespoon sugar-free hot sauce
- ½ teaspoon garlic powder

Instructions:

1. Preheat oven to 425°F. Line a baking sheet with parchment paper or foil.
2. Pat pork belly cubes completely dry with paper towels (this is crucial for crispiness).
3. In a bowl, toss pork belly with salt, pepper, garlic powder, smoked paprika, and cayenne (if using).
4. Arrange pork belly pieces on the baking sheet in a single layer, not touching.
5. Roast for 25-30 minutes, flipping halfway through, until deeply golden and crispy on the outside.
6. While pork cooks, make dipping sauce by whisking together all sauce ingredients.
7. Let pork belly bites cool for 2-3 minutes before serving (they're extremely hot right out of the oven).
8. Serve with dipping sauce.

Tips:

Finding pork belly: Look in the fresh pork section or ask the butcher. Some stores sell it pre-sliced for Korean BBQ. If you can only find a slab, ask them to slice it for you.

Crispy secret: The drier the pork belly before cooking, the crispier it gets. Pat it dry thoroughly, then let it sit uncovered in the fridge for an hour if you have time.

Air fryer option: Cook at 400°F for 15-18 minutes, shaking the basket halfway through.

Save the fat: The rendered pork fat left on the baking sheet is liquid gold. Save it in a jar in the fridge and use it to cook eggs, vegetables, or anything else that needs fat.

Meal prep: These reheat well in a hot oven (425°F) for 5-7 minutes. Microwave makes them rubbery.

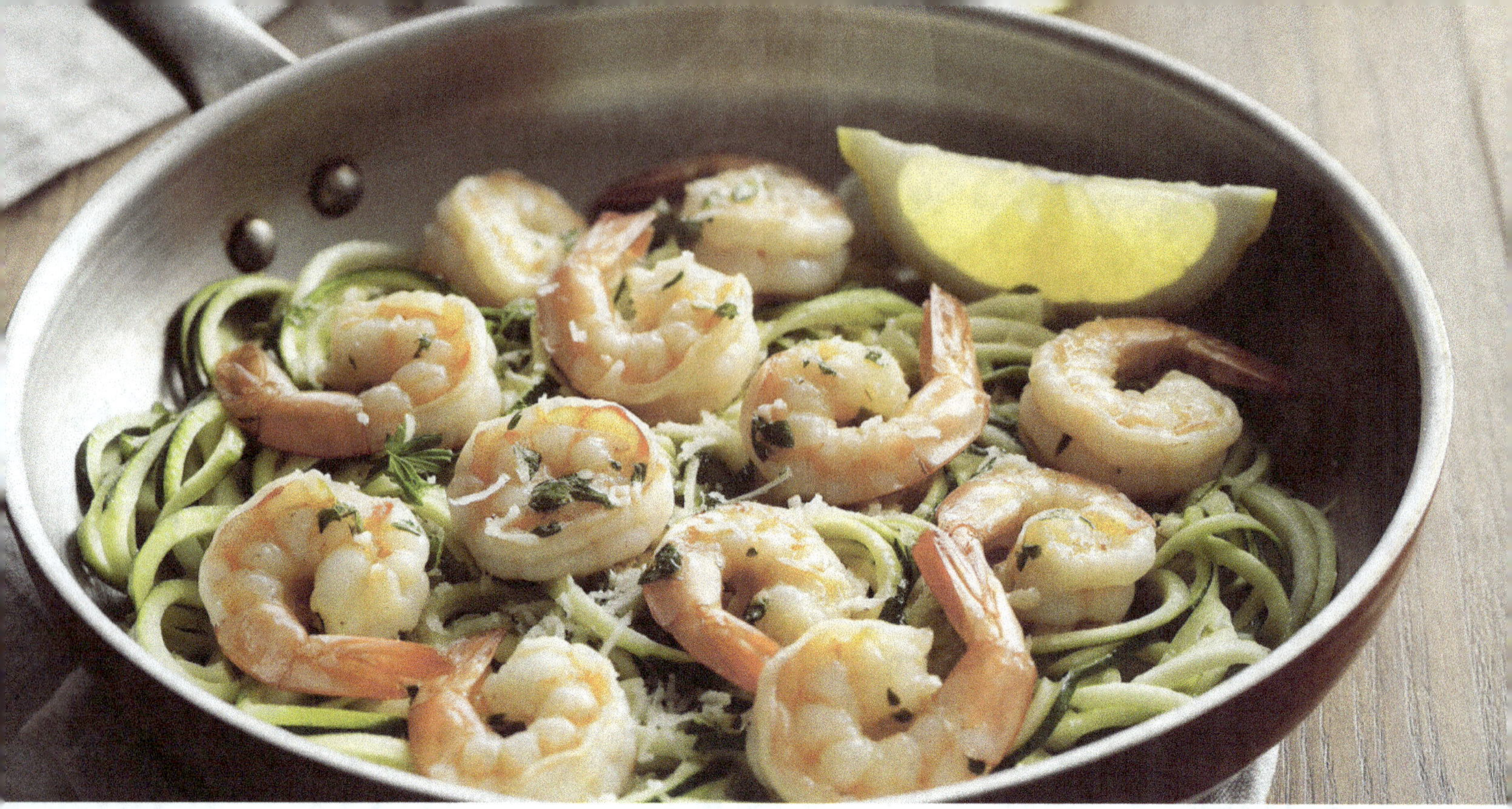

FISH & SEAFOOD RECIPES

Fish and seafood cook incredibly quickly, making them perfect for weeknights. They're also packed with omega-3 fatty acids and high-quality protein. The key is not to overcook them (most fish needs only 8-12 minutes total).

I know some people are intimidated by cooking fish, but these recipes are foolproof. If you can cook chicken, you can cook fish.

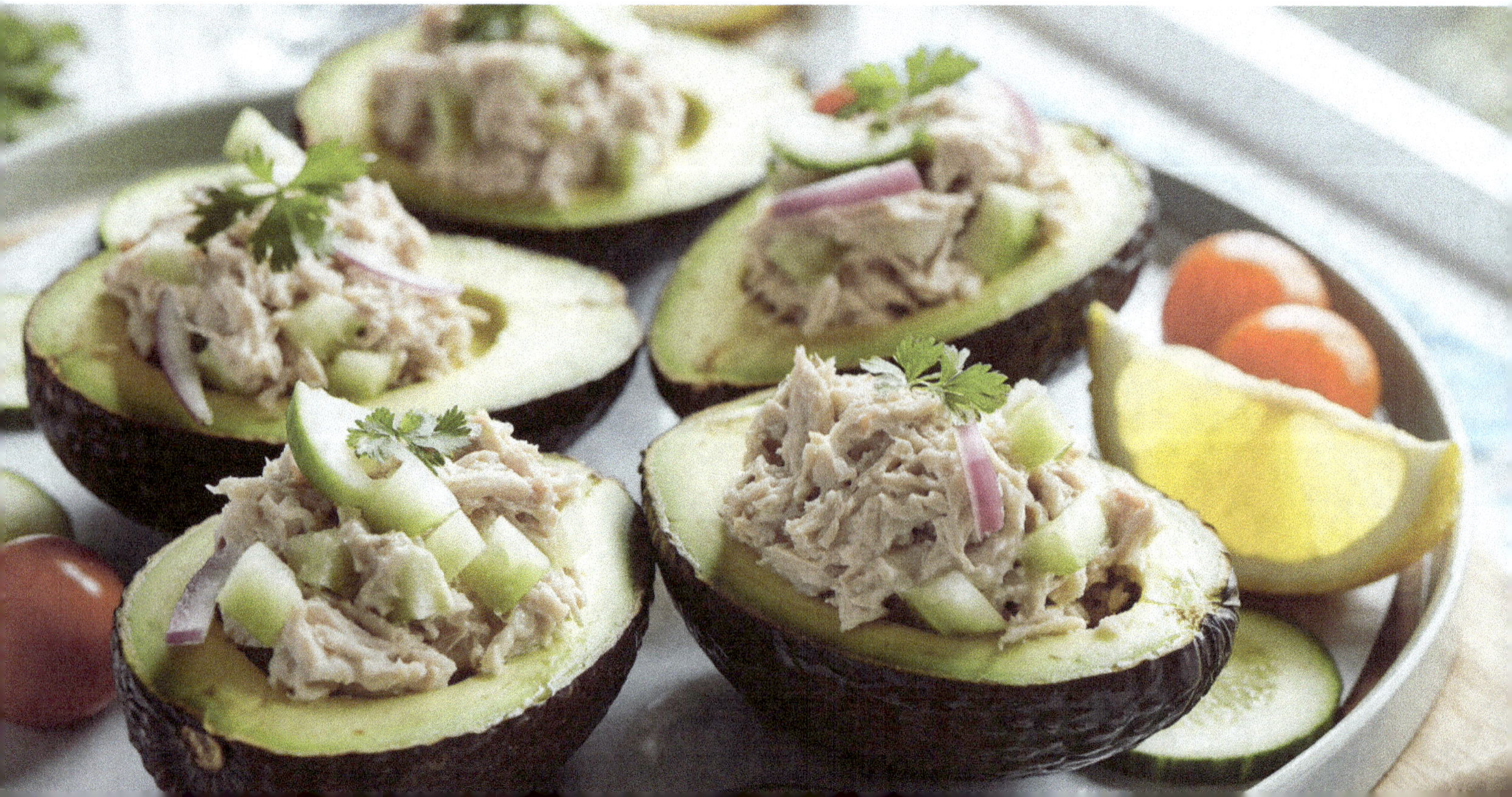

Lemon Garlic Butter Salmon

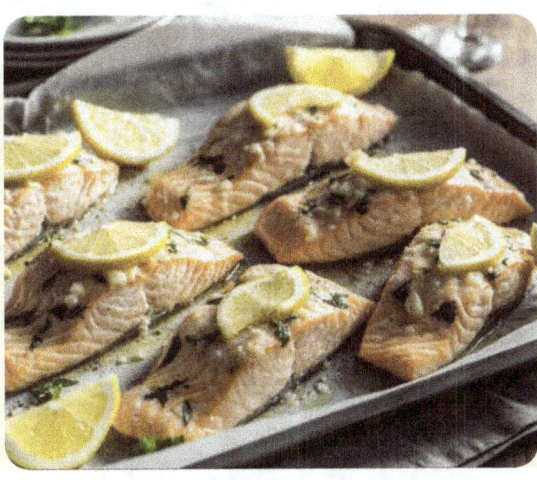

 Quick

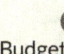 Budget-Friendly
(when salmon is on sale)

 Serves: 4

 Prep Time: 5 min

 Cook Time: 12 min

Total: 17 min

MACROS PER SERVING:
Calories: 420 | Protein: 34g | Fat: 30g | Net Carbs: 2g

Ingredients:
- 4 salmon fillets (6 oz each), skin-on or skinless
- 4 tablespoons butter, melted
- 4 cloves garlic, minced
- Juice of 1 lemon (about 3 tablespoons)
- Zest of 1 lemon
- 1 teaspoon dried oregano (or Italian seasoning)
- ½ teaspoon salt
- ¼ teaspoon black pepper
- 2 tablespoons fresh parsley, chopped
- Lemon wedges for serving

Instructions:
1. Preheat oven to 425°F. Line a baking sheet with parchment paper or foil.
2. Place salmon fillets on the prepared baking sheet, skin-side down if using skin-on.
3. In a small bowl, mix melted butter, garlic, lemon juice, lemon zest, oregano, salt, and pepper.
4. Brush the butter mixture generously over each salmon fillet.
5. Bake for 10-12 minutes until salmon is opaque and flakes easily with a fork. For thicker fillets, add 2-3 minutes.

Tips:
Don't overcook: Salmon continues cooking after you remove it from the oven. Pull it when it's just barely opaque in the center.

Skin-on or off: Both work. Skin-on helps the salmon hold together better. If you don't like eating the skin, just peel it off after cooking (it'll slide right off).

Wild vs. farmed: Wild salmon has fewer calories and more omega-3s, but it's pricier. Farmed salmon works fine for this recipe. Buy what fits your budget.

Frozen salmon: Totally fine to use. Thaw in the fridge overnight, then pat very dry before cooking.

Serve it with: Roasted asparagus, sautéed spinach, or a simple salad. Salmon is rich, so light sides balance it well.

Blackened Mahi-Mahi

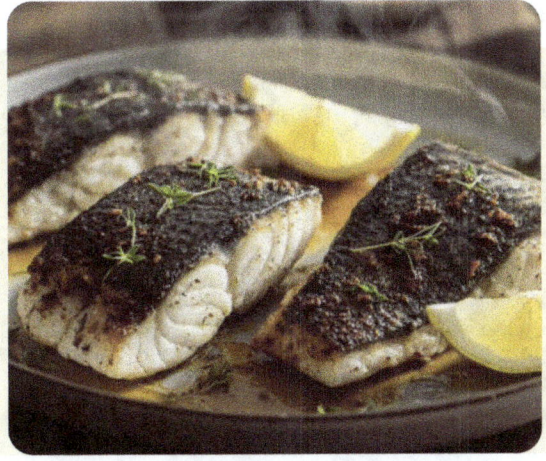

 Quick

 Serves: 4

 Prep Time: 5 min

 Cook Time: 10 min

Total: 15 min

MACROS PER SERVING:
Calories: 215 | Protein: 32g | Fat: 8g | Net Carbs: 2g

Ingredients:
- 4 mahi-mahi fillets (6 oz each)
- 2 tablespoons olive oil

Blackening spice:
- 1 tablespoon paprika
- 1 teaspoon garlic powder
- 1 teaspoon onion powder
- 1 teaspoon dried thyme
- ½ teaspoon cayenne pepper
- ½ teaspoon black pepper
- ½ teaspoon salt
- ¼ teaspoon oregano

Instructions:
1. In a small bowl, mix all blackening spice ingredients.
2. Pat fish fillets completely dry with paper towels.
3. Brush both sides of each fillet with olive oil.
4. Generously coat both sides of fish with blackening spice, pressing to adhere.
5. Heat a large cast-iron skillet or heavy pan over high heat until very hot (about 3 minutes).
6. Carefully place fish fillets in the hot skillet. Don't move them.
7. Cook for 4-5 minutes until the bottom is deeply charred and blackened.
8. Flip and cook for another 3-4 minutes until fish is opaque and flakes easily.

Tips:
Ventilation: Blackening creates smoke. Turn on your vent fan and open a window.

Cast iron is best: It gets hot enough to create that authentic blackened crust. Regular pans work but won't get the same char.

Spice level: This has some heat from the cayenne. Reduce to ¼ teaspoon for mild, or omit entirely for no heat.

Other fish: This method works with any firm white fish: cod, snapper, grouper, or even salmon.

Serve it with: Cauliflower rice, sautéed vegetables, or over a salad. The bold spices pair well with simple sides.

Garlic Shrimp Zoodles

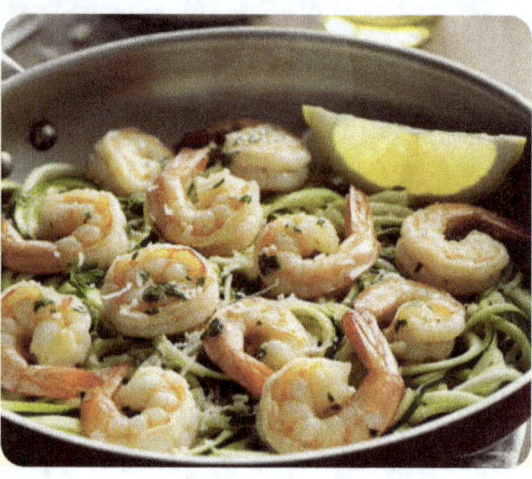

Quick   One-Pan

 Serves: 4

 Prep Time: 10 min

Cook Time: 8 min

Total: 18 min

MACROS PER SERVING:
Calories: 245 | Protein: 28g |
Fat: 12g | Net Carbs: 6g

Ingredients:
- 1½ pounds large shrimp, peeled and deveined
- 4 medium zucchini, spiralized into noodles (or 4 cups store-bought zoodles)
- 3 tablespoons olive oil, divided
- 6 cloves garlic, minced
- ¼ teaspoon red pepper flakes
- ½ teaspoon salt, divided
- ¼ teaspoon black pepper
- Juice of 1 lemon
- 2 tablespoons fresh parsley, chopped
- ¼ cup grated Parmesan cheese

Instructions:
1. Pat shrimp completely dry with paper towels. Season with ¼ teaspoon salt and pepper.
2. Heat 1 tablespoon olive oil in a large skillet over high heat.
3. Add shrimp in a single layer. Cook for 2 minutes without moving.
4. Flip and cook for another 1-2 minutes until pink and cooked through. Transfer to a plate.
5. Add remaining 2 tablespoons olive oil to the skillet. Reduce heat to medium-high.
6. Add garlic and red pepper flakes. Cook for 30 seconds until fragrant.
7. Add zucchini noodles and remaining ¼ teaspoon salt. Toss and cook for 2-3 minutes until just tender. Don't overcook or they'll get mushy and release too much water.
8. Return shrimp to the skillet. Add lemon juice and toss everything together.
9. Remove from heat. Top with parsley and Parmesan cheese.

Tips:
Drain the zoodles: Zucchini releases water when cooked. After spiralizing, pat zoodles dry with paper towels or let them sit in a colander for 15 minutes.

No spiralizer: Buy pre-spiralized zucchini noodles (most grocery stores sell them). Or use a vegetable peeler to make ribbons instead of noodles.

Frozen shrimp: Works great. Thaw under cold running water for 5 minutes, then pat very dry.

Make it creamier: Add 2-3 tablespoons of heavy cream or butter with the lemon juice.

Storage: Best eaten fresh. Zoodles get watery when reheated, but it's still edible for up to 2 days.

Tuna Avocado Boats

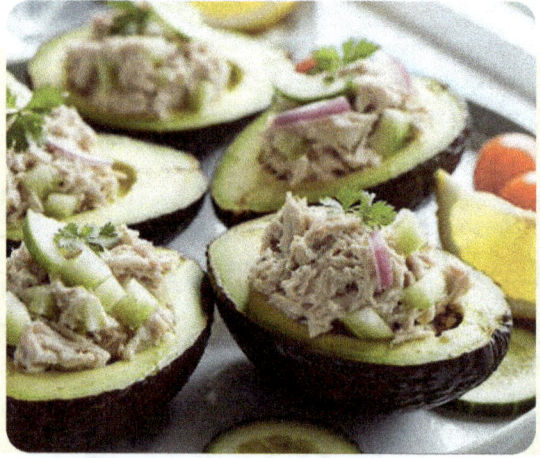

Quick   Budget-Friendly

 Serves: 2

 Prep Time: 10 min

 Cook Time: 0 min

Total: 10 min

MACROS PER SERVING:
Calories: 380 | Protein: 30g |
Fat: 26g | Net Carbs: 6g

Ingredients:
- 2 cans (5 oz each) tuna in water, drained
- 2 large avocados
- ¼ cup mayonnaise
- 2 tablespoons diced celery
- 2 tablespoons diced red onion
- 1 tablespoon lemon juice
- 1 teaspoon Dijon mustard
- ½ teaspoon garlic powder
- Salt and pepper to taste
- Optional: cherry tomatoes, cucumber slices, lettuce for serving

Instructions:
1. Cut avocados in half and remove pits. Scoop out about 1 tablespoon of flesh from each half to create a bigger cavity (eat this or add it to the tuna mixture).
2. In a bowl, combine drained tuna, mayonnaise, celery, red onion, lemon juice, Dijon mustard, and garlic powder. Mix well.
3. Season with salt and pepper to taste.
4. Divide tuna mixture among the 4 avocado halves, mounding it in the center.
5. Serve immediately, or cover and refrigerate for up to 2 hours before serving.

Tips:
Canned tuna types: Solid white albacore is more expensive but has a firmer texture. Chunk light tuna is cheaper and works fine.

Make it fancy: Add diced hard-boiled egg, capers, or fresh dill to the tuna mixture.

Meal prep: Mix the tuna salad and store separately from the avocados. Assemble just before eating to prevent the avocado from browning.

Not just boats: This tuna salad is great on its own, wrapped in lettuce, or stuffed into bell peppers or tomatoes.

Budget win: This entire meal costs about $3-4 per serving, depending on avocado prices. Canned tuna is one of the cheapest proteins available.

CHAPTER 2 SUMMARY

You now have 25 quick weeknight dinner recipes that take 30 minutes or less. Here's how to use them effectively:

Weekly Meal Planning Strategy:
Pick 4-5 recipes from this chapter each week. I know that sounds like a lot of variety, but remember:

- Two recipes will probably make leftovers for lunch
- You'll eat out or do leftovers one night
- You might repeat a favorite

My Actual Weekly Rotation:
I don't make 7 different recipes every week. That's exhausting. Here's what I actually do:

Monday: Make Recipe #1 (usually something easy like Ground Beef Taco Bowl)

Tuesday: Make Recipe #2 (something quick like Garlic Butter Chicken Thighs)

Wednesday: Eat leftovers from Monday or Tuesday

Thursday: Make Recipe #3 (often a one-pan meal like Sheet Pan Chicken & Broccoli)

Friday: Either very simple (like Tuna Avocado Boats) or order takeout

Weekend: Cook something that takes longer if I feel like it, or repeat a favorite from the week

Protein Shopping Strategy:
Buy what's on sale and plan around it:

- Chicken thighs under $2/lb? Make 2-3 chicken recipes this week.
- Ground beef on sale? Stock up and make beef recipes.
- Fish marked down for quick sale? Tonight's dinner is decided.

Batch Cooking for Efficiency:
Several of these recipes work well doubled:

- Cook 3 pounds of taco meat instead of 1.5
- Grill 8 pork chops instead of 4
- Make extra pulled pork (it freezes perfectly)

Store extras in portions. Future you will be grateful when dinner is just a reheat away.

Time-Saving Shortcuts I Actually Use:
- Pre-minced garlic from a jar (yes, fresh is better, but jarred is fast)
- Frozen vegetables (especially cauliflower rice, broccoli, green beans)
- Pre-shredded cheese (costs more, saves time)
- Rotisserie chicken when I'm too tired to cook (use in buffalo wraps, salads, or eat plain)

What Makes These Recipes Work:
Every recipe in this chapter follows these principles:

- **30 minutes or less** from start to finish
- **Simple ingredients** you can find anywhere
- **Minimal dishes** to wash
- **Macro-balanced** with protein as the star
- **Actually tastes good** (not just "healthy")

Common Mistakes to Avoid:

1. **Trying to make everything from scratch every night.** Some nights, simple is smart. Seasoned meat and steamed vegetables is a perfectly acceptable dinner.

2. **Not using a meat thermometer.** Guessing doneness leads to overcooked (dry) or undercooked (unsafe) meat. A $10 thermometer solves this forever.

3. **Cooking on too low heat.** Most proteins need medium-high to high heat to develop good flavor through browning. Low heat steams instead of sears.

4. **Forgetting to let meat rest.** Those 5 minutes matter. Resting allows juices to redistribute. Skip it and your cutting board becomes a puddle.

5. **Not salting enough.** Salt enhances flavor. Most home cooks don't use enough. Season generously.

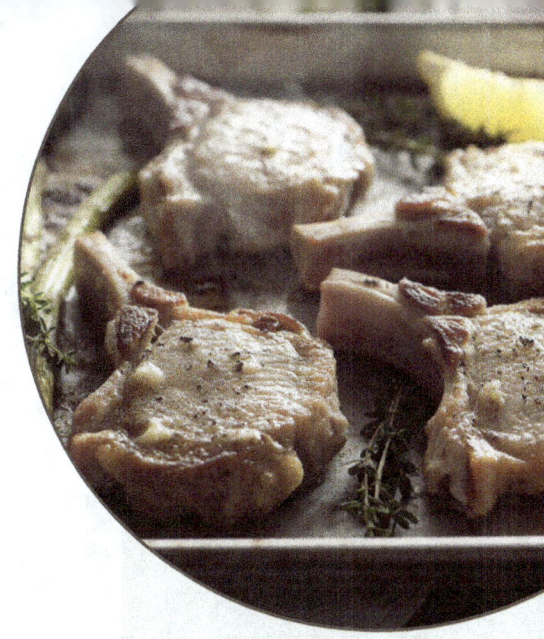

There are nights when even a 30-minute dinner feels like too much effort. That's what this chapter is about: complete, satisfying meals that dirty exactly one pan. No juggling multiple burners. No transferring ingredients between vessels. No pile of dishes mocking you after dinner.

These recipes use sheet pans, skillets, or baking dishes to cook your protein and vegetables together. Everything goes in, everything cooks, you eat, you wash one pan. That's it.

I'm not going to pretend these are gourmet restaurant meals. They're better than that. They're the meals you'll actually make on a Tuesday when you're exhausted. They're the recipes you'll return to week after week because they just work.

The Strategy Behind One-Pan Meals:

The key to successful one-pan cooking is choosing ingredients that cook in similar timeframes or layering ingredients so everything finishes together. Chicken thighs and broccoli both take about 20 minutes at 425°F. Sausage and peppers cook at the same rate in a skillet. When you pair proteins and vegetables strategically, one-pan cooking is effortless.

Most recipes in this chapter follow one of three methods:

Sheet Pan Method: Everything goes on a rimmed baking sheet and roasts together. Usually 20-25 minutes at 400-425°F. Minimal prep, maximum results.

Skillet Method: Start with protein, add vegetables as you go, everything stays in one pan. Often finished in the oven if needed.

Bake and Forget: Everything in a baking dish, into the oven, walk away for 30-40 minutes. Perfect for nights when you need to do other things while dinner cooks.

Tips for One-Pan Success:

1. **Cut everything the same size.** Uniform pieces cook evenly. If your chicken is in 2-inch chunks, cut your vegetables in similar sizes.

2. **Don't overcrowd the pan.** Everything needs space to roast, not steam. If things are touching everywhere, use a second pan or cook in batches.

3. **Use parchment paper or foil.** Makes cleanup even easier. Just throw it away.

4. **Flip halfway through** (for most recipes). This ensures even browning on all sides.

5. **Add delicate vegetables later.** Zucchini needs less time than Brussels sprouts. Add quick-cooking items partway through if needed.

6. **Let it rest.** Even sheet pan dinners benefit from 2-3 minutes of resting before serving.

What You Won't Find in This Chapter:

- Recipes requiring constant stirring or monitoring
- Meals that need multiple cooking temperatures
- Dishes that only work with specialty equipment
- Anything requiring more than one cooking vessel

What You Will Find:

- Complete meals from one pan
- Minimal prep and cleanup
- Proteins and vegetables cooked together
- Recipes that work on weeknights or meal prep Sundays
- Food that actually tastes like you tried (even though you barely did)

Let's cook the easiest dinners you'll ever make.

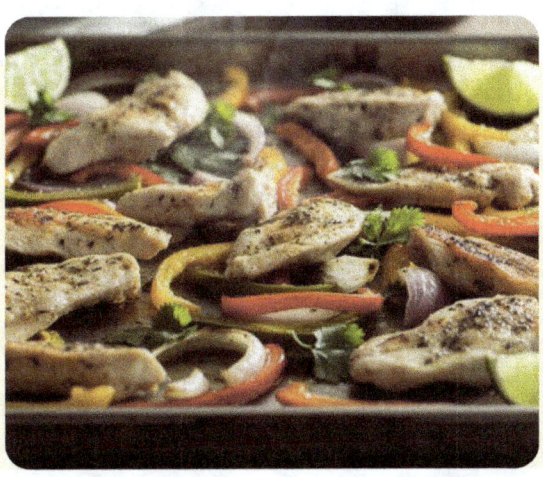

Sheet Pan Chicken Fajitas

Quick   One-Pan   Budget-Friendly

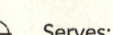 Serves: 4

 Prep Time: 10 min

 Cook Time: 20 min

 Total: 30 min

MACROS PER SERVING:

Calories: 340 | Protein: 38g |
Fat: 16g | Net Carbs: 7g

Ingredients:

- 2 pounds boneless, skinless chicken breasts, cut into strips
- 3 bell peppers (mix of colors), sliced into strips
- 1 large onion, sliced into strips
- 3 tablespoons olive oil
- 2 tablespoons lime juice
- 3 cloves garlic, minced
- 2 teaspoons chili powder
- 1½ teaspoons cumin
- 1 teaspoon paprika
- 1 teaspoon salt
- ½ teaspoon black pepper
- ½ teaspoon oregano

Instructions:

1. Preheat oven to 425°F. Line a large baking sheet with parchment paper or foil.
2. In a small bowl, whisk together olive oil, lime juice, garlic, chili powder, cumin, paprika, salt, pepper, and oregano.
3. Place chicken strips, bell peppers, and onion on the baking sheet. Pour the seasoned oil mixture over everything.
4. Toss with your hands or two spatulas until everything is evenly coated.
5. Spread everything in a single layer, trying not to overlap too much.
6. Roast for 20-22 minutes, stirring halfway through, until chicken is cooked through (165°F internal temperature) and vegetables are tender with some charred edges.
7. Remove from oven and let rest for 2-3 minutes.

Tips:

Make it a complete meal: Serve over cauliflower rice or shredded lettuce. Or use low-carb tortillas if you have room in your carb budget (add 4-6g net carbs per tortilla).

Meal prep: These fajitas reheat beautifully. Make a double batch and portion into containers. Add fresh toppings when serving.

Spice level: This is mild to medium. Add ½ teaspoon cayenne for more heat, or use jalapeño peppers instead of all bell peppers.

Chicken thighs option: Use 2 pounds boneless, skinless thighs cut into strips. Same cooking time, juicier results, often cheaper.

Leftovers: Use in breakfast scrambles, taco bowls, or salads throughout the week.

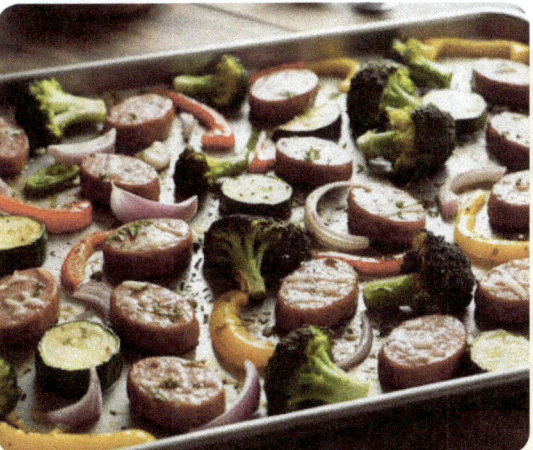

Sausage & Veggie Bake

  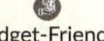

Quick   One-Pan   Budget-Friendly

 Serves: 4

 Prep Time: 10 min

 Cook Time: 25 min

Total: 35 min

MACROS PER SERVING:

Calories: 410 | Protein: 26g |
Fat: 30g | Net Carbs: 8g

Ingredients:

- 1½ pounds smoked sausage (kielbasa or similar), cut into 1-inch pieces
- 3 cups broccoli florets
- 2 medium zucchini, cut into half-moons
- 1 red bell pepper, cut into 1-inch pieces
- 1 yellow bell pepper, cut into 1-inch pieces
- 1 red onion, cut into wedges
- 3 tablespoons olive oil
- 1 tablespoon Italian seasoning
- 1 teaspoon garlic powder
- ¾ teaspoon salt
- ½ teaspoon black pepper
- ¼ teaspoon red pepper flakes (optional)

Instructions:

1. Preheat oven to 400°F. Line a large baking sheet with parchment paper.
2. Place sausage pieces, broccoli, zucchini, bell peppers, and onion on the baking sheet.
3. Drizzle with olive oil and sprinkle with Italian seasoning, garlic powder, salt, pepper, and red pepper flakes (if using).
4. Toss everything together until evenly coated. Spread in a single layer.
5. Roast for 25-30 minutes, stirring halfway through, until vegetables are tender and sausage is lightly browned.
6. Remove from oven and sprinkle with Parmesan cheese if desired. Let the residual heat melt it for 1-2 minutes.

Tips:

Sausage options: Any pre-cooked smoked sausage works. Kielbasa, andouille, Italian sausage, or chicken sausage. Check labels for added sugars.

Already cooked: Since the sausage is pre-cooked, you're really just roasting everything together. This makes it even easier.

Swap vegetables: Green beans, cauliflower, Brussels sprouts, or asparagus all work. Just keep pieces similar in size.

Storage: Refrigerate for up to 4 days. Reheat in a hot oven (425°F) for 5-7 minutes for best results.

Budget win: This feeds 4 people for under $12-15 total, depending on where you shop.

Greek Chicken Tray Bake

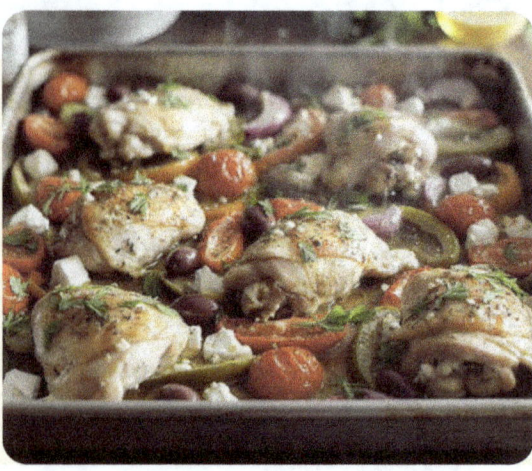

Quick   One-Pan

 Serves: 4

Prep Time: 10 min

Cook Time: 25 min

Total: 35 min

MACROS PER SERVING:

Calories: 395 | Protein: 40g | Fat: 22g | Net Carbs: 6g

Ingredients:

- 2 pounds boneless, skinless chicken thighs, cut into 2-inch pieces
- 2 cups cherry tomatoes
- 1 medium red onion, cut into wedges
- 1 red bell pepper, cut into 1-inch pieces
- 1 yellow bell pepper, cut into 1-inch pieces
- ½ cup pitted Kalamata olives
- 4 tablespoons olive oil
- Juice of 1 lemon
- 4 cloves garlic, minced
- 2 teaspoons dried oregano
- 1 teaspoon salt
- ½ teaspoon black pepper
- ½ cup crumbled feta cheese
- Fresh parsley for garnish

Instructions:

1. Preheat oven to 425°F. Line a large baking sheet with parchment paper.
2. In a small bowl, whisk together olive oil, lemon juice, garlic, oregano, salt, and pepper.
3. Place chicken pieces, cherry tomatoes, onion, bell peppers, and olives on the baking sheet.
4. Pour the olive oil mixture over everything and toss to coat evenly.
5. Spread in a single layer, ensuring chicken pieces aren't completely covered by vegetables.
6. Roast for 22-25 minutes, stirring halfway through, until chicken reaches 165°F internal temperature and vegetables are tender.
7. Remove from oven and immediately sprinkle with crumbled feta cheese. The heat will slightly soften it.

Tips:

Make it extra lemony: Add lemon zest to the olive oil mixture before tossing. Finish with a squeeze of fresh lemon juice.

Serve it with: This is delicious over cauliflower rice or with a simple cucumber and tomato salad on the side.

Cucumber yogurt sauce: Mix ½ cup Greek yogurt with ¼ cup diced cucumber, 1 minced garlic clove, and fresh dill. Drizzle over the finished dish. Adds 2g net carbs per serving.

Chicken breast option: Use 4 chicken breasts cut into large chunks. Reduce cooking time by 3-4 minutes.

Storage: Refrigerate for up to 4 days. Feta gets slightly softer when reheated but still tastes great.

Pork Chops & Asparagus Sheet Pan

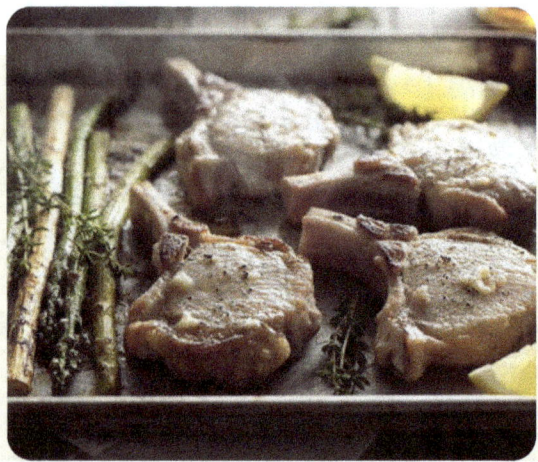

Quick   One-Pan

 Serves: 4

 Prep Time: 8 min

Cook Time: 20 min

 Total: 28 min

MACROS PER SERVING:

Calories: 385 | Protein: 38g | Fat: 23g | Net Carbs: 4g

Ingredients:

- 4 bone-in pork chops (8-10 oz each, about ¾ inch thick)
- 1½ pounds asparagus, trimmed
- 3 tablespoons olive oil, divided
- 3 tablespoons butter, melted
- 4 cloves garlic, minced
- 1 teaspoon dried thyme
- 1 teaspoon paprika
- ¾ teaspoon salt, divided
- ½ teaspoon black pepper, divided
- Lemon wedges for serving

Instructions:

1. Preheat oven to 425°F. Line a large baking sheet with foil.
2. Pat pork chops dry with paper towels. Rub with 1 tablespoon olive oil and season both sides with paprika, ½ teaspoon salt, and ¼ teaspoon pepper.
3. Place pork chops on one side of the baking sheet.
4. In a bowl, toss asparagus with remaining 2 tablespoons olive oil, melted butter, garlic, thyme, remaining ¼ teaspoon salt, and remaining ¼ teaspoon pepper.
5. Arrange asparagus on the other side of the baking sheet.
6. Roast for 18-20 minutes until pork chops reach 145°F internal temperature and asparagus is tender with some crispy tips.
7. Let pork chops rest for 3-5 minutes before serving.

Tips:

Even cooking: If your pork chops are thicker than ¾ inch, add 2-3 minutes to cooking time. Use a thermometer to be sure.

Asparagus thickness: Thick asparagus takes longer than thin. If yours are very thin, add them 5 minutes into cooking time.

Boneless option: Boneless pork chops work too. Reduce cooking time by 2-3 minutes.

Swap the vegetable: Green beans, broccoli, or Brussels sprouts (halved) all work with the same cooking time.

Garlic butter finish: After removing from oven, brush everything with extra melted garlic butter for maximum flavor.

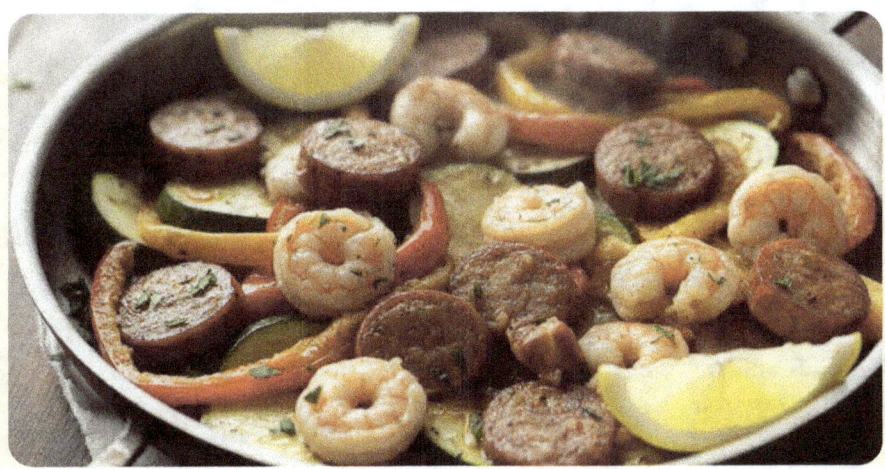

Cajun Shrimp & Sausage Skillet

Quick One-Pan

 Serves: 4

 Prep Time: 10 min

 Cook Time: 15 min

 Total: 25 min

MACROS PER SERVING:

Calories: 420 | Protein: 35g | Fat: 28g | Net Carbs: 7g

Ingredients:

- 1 pound large shrimp, peeled and deveined
- 12 oz andouille sausage, sliced into ½-inch rounds
- 1 red bell pepper, cut into strips
- 1 yellow bell pepper, cut into strips
- 1 medium zucchini, sliced into half-moons
- 1 small onion, sliced
- 3 tablespoons olive oil, divided
- 4 cloves garlic, minced
- 2 tablespoons Cajun seasoning (store-bought or homemade)
- ½ teaspoon salt
- ¼ teaspoon black pepper
- 2 tablespoons butter
- Juice of ½ lemon
- Fresh parsley for garnish

Homemade Cajun Seasoning (optional):

- 1 tablespoon paprika
- 1 teaspoon garlic powder
- 1 teaspoon onion powder
- 1 teaspoon dried oregano
- 1 teaspoon dried thyme
- ½ teaspoon cayenne pepper
- ½ teaspoon black pepper
- ½ teaspoon salt

Instructions:

1. Pat shrimp completely dry with paper towels. Season with 1 tablespoon Cajun seasoning.

2. Heat 1 tablespoon olive oil in a large skillet over high heat.

3. Add sausage slices and cook for 3-4 minutes until browned. Transfer to a plate.

4. Add another tablespoon olive oil to the skillet. Add shrimp in a single layer and cook for 2 minutes per side until pink and cooked through. Transfer to the plate with sausage.

5. Add remaining tablespoon olive oil to the skillet. Reduce heat to medium-high.

6. Add bell peppers, zucchini, and onion. Cook for 5-6 minutes, stirring occasionally, until vegetables are tender-crisp.

7. Add garlic and remaining tablespoon Cajun seasoning. Cook for 30 seconds.

8. Return shrimp and sausage to the skillet. Add butter and lemon juice. Toss everything together and cook for 1 minute until heated through.

Tips:

Spice level: Cajun seasoning varies by brand. Tony Chachere's is medium heat. Zatarain's is milder. Adjust to your preference or make your own.

Frozen shrimp: Works great. Thaw under cold running water for 5 minutes, then pat very dry.

Serve it over: Cauliflower rice to make it more filling, or just eat it as-is for a lighter meal.

Storage: Refrigerate for up to 3 days. Shrimp can get slightly rubbery when reheated, so reheat gently.

Make it creamier: Add ¼ cup heavy cream with the butter and lemon juice for a sauce.

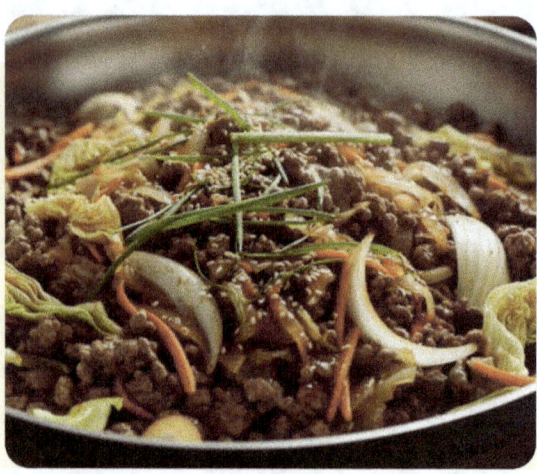

Beef & Cabbage Stir-Fry

 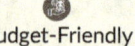
Quick   One-Pan   Budget-Friendly

 Serves: 4

 Prep Time: 10 min

 Cook Time: 15 min

 Total: 25 min

MACROS PER SERVING:

Calories: 380 | Protein: 32g |
Fat: 24g | Net Carbs: 8g

Ingredients:

- 1½ pounds ground beef (80/20)
- 6 cups shredded cabbage (about ½ medium head)
- 2 cups shredded carrots
- 1 medium onion, sliced
- 3 tablespoons sesame oil or avocado oil
- 4 cloves garlic, minced
- 1 tablespoon fresh ginger, grated
- ¼ cup soy sauce (or coconut aminos)
- 2 tablespoons rice vinegar
- 1 tablespoon sesame oil
- 1 teaspoon red pepper flakes (optional)
- 3 green onions, sliced
- 1 tablespoon sesame seeds

Instructions:

1. Heat oil in a large skillet or wok over high heat.
2. Add ground beef and cook, breaking it up with a spatula, for 6-8 minutes until browned and cooked through. Drain excess fat if there's more than 2 tablespoons.
3. Push beef to one side of the skillet. Add onion to the empty side and cook for 2 minutes.
4. Add cabbage and carrots. Stir everything together and cook for 5-6 minutes, stirring occasionally, until cabbage is wilted and tender.
5. Add garlic and ginger. Cook for 30 seconds until fragrant.
6. Pour in soy sauce, rice vinegar, and sesame oil. Add red pepper flakes if using. Toss everything together and cook for 1-2 minutes.
7. Remove from heat. Top with sliced green onions and sesame seeds.

Tips:

Coleslaw mix: Buy pre-shredded coleslaw mix (cabbage and carrots already mixed) to save time. You'll need about 8 cups total.

Ground turkey option: Use ground turkey instead of beef for a leaner version. Add 1 tablespoon of oil to keep it from drying out.

Make it saucier: Double the soy sauce and vinegar if you like more sauce.

Storage: This reheats beautifully for up to 4 days. Actually tastes better the next day as flavors meld.

Budget superstar: This entire meal costs about $10-12 to feed 4 people. Ground beef and cabbage are budget-friendly staples.

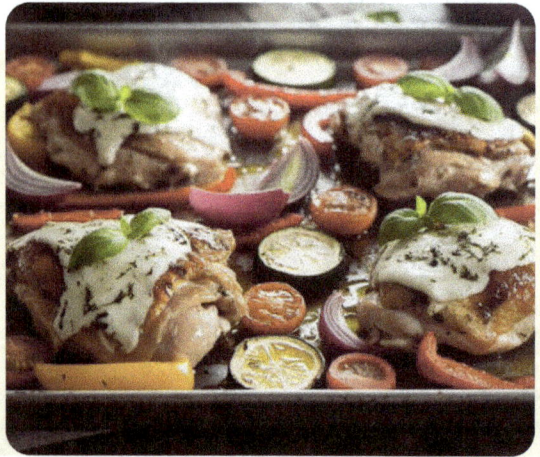

Italian Chicken & Vegetables

 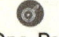
Quick   One-Pan

 Serves: 4

Prep Time: 10 min

 Cook Time: 25 min

 Total: 35 min

MACROS PER SERVING:

Calories: 380 | Protein: 39g |
Fat: 21g | Net Carbs: 7g

Ingredients:

- 2 pounds boneless, skinless chicken thighs
- 2 medium zucchini, sliced into rounds
- 1 pint cherry tomatoes
- 1 red bell pepper, cut into 1-inch pieces
- 1 yellow bell pepper, cut into 1-inch pieces
- 1 red onion, cut into wedges
- 4 tablespoons olive oil
- 4 cloves garlic, minced
- 2 tablespoons balsamic vinegar
- 2 teaspoons Italian seasoning
- 1 teaspoon salt
- ½ teaspoon black pepper
- ½ cup shredded mozzarella cheese
- Fresh basil for garnish

Instructions:

1. Preheat oven to 425°F. Line a large baking sheet with parchment paper.
2. In a small bowl, whisk together olive oil, garlic, balsamic vinegar, Italian seasoning, salt, and pepper.
3. Place chicken thighs, zucchini, tomatoes, bell peppers, and onion on the baking sheet.
4. Pour the olive oil mixture over everything and toss to coat.
5. Arrange chicken thighs in a single layer with vegetables around them.
6. Roast for 22-25 minutes until chicken reaches 165°F internal temperature and vegetables are tender.
7. Remove from oven and immediately sprinkle mozzarella cheese over the chicken. Let it melt for 1-2 minutes.

Tips:

Balsamic glaze: After cooking, drizzle with reduced balsamic vinegar for an elegant finish. Adds minimal carbs but big flavor.

Chicken breast option: Use 4 chicken breasts instead. Reduce cooking time by 3-4 minutes.

Make it creamy: Add a few dollops of ricotta cheese or goat cheese on top after cooking.

Storage: Refrigerate for up to 4 days. The tomatoes will release some liquid, but it just creates a delicious sauce.

Serve it with: Cauliflower rice or zucchini noodles to soak up all the flavorful juices.

Salmon & Brussels Sprouts

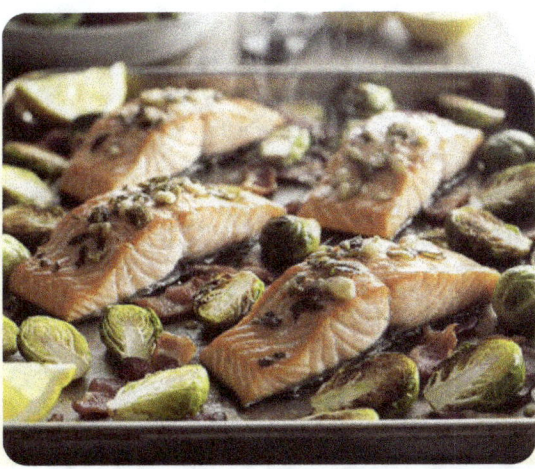

Quick   One-Pan

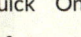 Serves: 4

 Prep Time: 10 min

 Cook Time: 18 min

 Total: 28 min

MACROS PER SERVING:

Calories: 445 | Protein: 36g | Fat: 30g | Net Carbs: 6g

Ingredients:

- 4 salmon fillets (6 oz each)
- 1½ pounds Brussels sprouts, trimmed and halved
- 4 strips bacon, chopped
- 3 tablespoons olive oil
- 3 cloves garlic, minced
- 1 teaspoon Dijon mustard
- ¾ teaspoon salt, divided
- ½ teaspoon black pepper, divided
- ¼ teaspoon red pepper flakes (optional)
- Lemon wedges for serving

Instructions:

1. Preheat oven to 425°F. Line a large baking sheet with parchment paper.
2. Spread Brussels sprouts and chopped bacon on the baking sheet. Drizzle with 2 tablespoons olive oil and season with ½ teaspoon salt and ¼ teaspoon pepper. Toss to coat.
3. Roast for 10 minutes.
4. While Brussels sprouts roast, pat salmon fillets dry. In a small bowl, mix remaining tablespoon olive oil with garlic and Dijon mustard. Brush over salmon fillets and season with remaining ¼ teaspoon salt and ¼ teaspoon pepper.
5. Remove baking sheet from oven. Stir Brussels sprouts and bacon. Make space for salmon fillets.
6. Place salmon fillets on the baking sheet among the Brussels sprouts.
7. Return to oven and roast for 8-10 minutes until salmon is opaque and flakes easily, and Brussels sprouts are crispy and caramelized.

Tips:

Crispy Brussels sprouts: Don't overcrowd them. If your baking sheet is too small, use two sheets.

Bacon renders fat: The bacon fat helps crisp up the Brussels sprouts beautifully. Don't drain it.

No bacon option: Skip the bacon and add an extra tablespoon of olive oil to the Brussels sprouts. Still delicious.

Frozen Brussels sprouts: Thaw completely and pat very dry before roasting. Add 3-4 minutes to initial roasting time.

Storage: Refrigerate for up to 3 days. Brussels sprouts lose some crispness but salmon reheats well.

Breakfast Hash

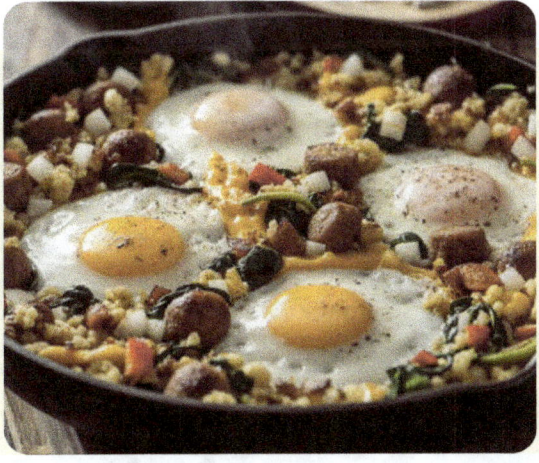

  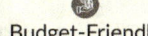
Quick   One-Pan   Budget-Friendly

 Serves: 4

 Prep Time: 10 min

 Cook Time: 20 min

Total: 30 min

MACROS PER SERVING:

Calories: 485 | Protein: 32g | Fat: 36g | Net Carbs: 6g

Ingredients:

- 1 pound breakfast sausage (bulk or removed from casings)
- 4 cups riced cauliflower (fresh or frozen)
- 1 red bell pepper, diced
- 1 small onion, diced
- 2 cups fresh spinach, chopped
- 3 tablespoons olive oil, divided
- 4 large eggs
- ¾ teaspoon salt, divided
- ½ teaspoon black pepper, divided
- ½ teaspoon garlic powder
- ½ teaspoon paprika
- 1 cup shredded cheddar cheese
- Optional: hot sauce, avocado slices

Instructions:

1. Heat 1 tablespoon olive oil in a large oven-safe skillet over medium-high heat.
2. Add sausage and cook, breaking it up, for 6-8 minutes until browned and cooked through.
3. Add bell pepper and onion. Cook for 3-4 minutes until softened.
4. Add cauliflower rice, remaining 2 tablespoons olive oil, ½ teaspoon salt, ¼ teaspoon pepper, garlic powder, and paprika. Cook for 4-5 minutes, stirring occasionally, until cauliflower is tender.
5. Stir in spinach and cook for 1 minute until wilted.
6. Make 4 wells in the hash. Crack an egg into each well. Season eggs with remaining ¼ teaspoon salt and ¼ teaspoon pepper.
7. Sprinkle shredded cheese over everything.
8. Transfer skillet to oven and broil for 3-5 minutes until eggs are set to your liking and cheese is melted and bubbly.
9. Let cool for 2 minutes before serving. Serve with hot sauce and avocado if desired.

Tips:

No oven-safe skillet: Cook everything on the stovetop, then cover the skillet with a lid to cook the eggs through (about 5-7 minutes).

Frozen cauliflower rice: Use it frozen. It cooks perfectly from frozen and prevents excess moisture.

Make it ahead: Cook the hash mixture (everything except eggs and cheese) on Sunday. Reheat in a skillet, add eggs and cheese, and finish under the broiler. Breakfast in 10 minutes.

Protein options: Ground beef, turkey, or chorizo all work instead of breakfast sausage.

Storage: Store hash and eggs separately. Refrigerate hash for up to 4 days, fry fresh eggs when serving.

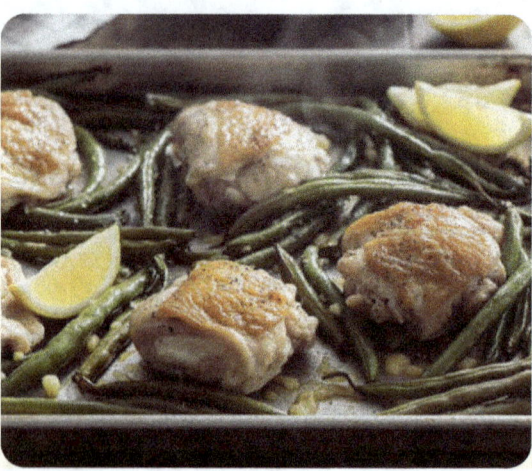

Chicken Thigh & Green Bean Bake

  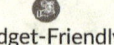
Quick   One-Pan   Budget-Friendly

 Serves: 4

 Prep Time: 10 min

 Cook Time: 25 min

 Total: 35 min

MACROS PER SERVING:

Calories: 420 | Protein: 38g | Fat: 27g | Net Carbs: 6g

Ingredients:

- 8 bone-in, skin-on chicken thighs (about 2½ pounds)
- 1½ pounds green beans, trimmed
- 3 tablespoons olive oil
- 4 tablespoons butter, melted
- 6 cloves garlic, minced
- 1 tablespoon lemon juice
- 1 teaspoon dried thyme
- 1 teaspoon paprika
- ¾ teaspoon salt
- ½ teaspoon black pepper
- Lemon wedges for serving

Instructions:

1. Preheat oven to 425°F. Line a large baking sheet with foil.
2. Pat chicken thighs dry with paper towels. Season skin side with paprika, ½ teaspoon salt, and ¼ teaspoon pepper.
3. Place chicken thighs skin-side up on one side of the baking sheet.
4. In a bowl, toss green beans with olive oil, melted butter, garlic, lemon juice, thyme, remaining ¼ teaspoon salt, and remaining ¼ teaspoon pepper.
5. Arrange green beans on the other side of the baking sheet.
6. Roast for 25-30 minutes until chicken skin is crispy and internal temperature reaches 165°F, and green beans are tender with some crispy edges.

Tips:

Crispy skin: Make sure chicken is completely dry before seasoning. Pat with paper towels thoroughly.

Boneless option: Use boneless, skinless thighs. Reduce cooking time to 20-22 minutes.

Green bean tip: Thicker green beans hold up better to high-heat roasting than thin ones.

Make it fancy: Add ¼ cup sliced almonds to the green beans for the last 5 minutes of cooking. Adds crunch and healthy fats.

Storage: Refrigerate for up to 4 days. Reheat in a hot oven (425°F) for 5-7 minutes to re-crisp the chicken skin.

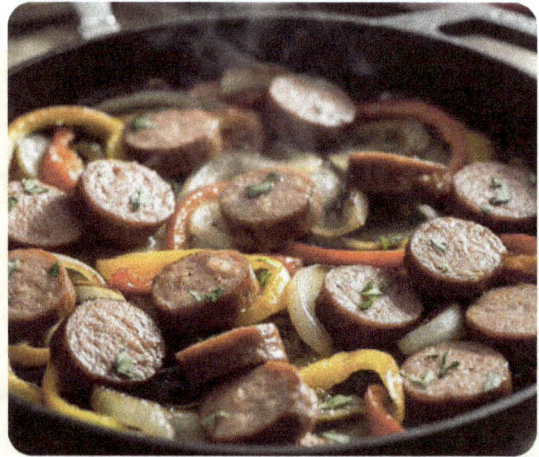

Kielbasa & Peppers Skillet

  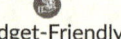
Quick   One-Pan   Budget-Friendly

 Serves: 4

 Prep Time: 8 min

 Cook Time: 18 min

 Total: 26 min

MACROS PER SERVING:

Calories: 395 | Protein: 24g | Fat: 29g | Net Carbs: 8g

Ingredients:

- 1½ pounds kielbasa sausage, sliced into ½-inch rounds
- 3 bell peppers (mix of colors), sliced into strips
- 2 medium onions, sliced
- 3 tablespoons olive oil
- 4 cloves garlic, minced
- 1 teaspoon paprika
- ½ teaspoon dried oregano
- ½ teaspoon salt
- ¼ teaspoon black pepper
- ¼ teaspoon red pepper flakes (optional)
- 2 tablespoons fresh parsley, chopped

Instructions:

1. Heat 1 tablespoon olive oil in a large skillet over medium-high heat.
2. Add kielbasa slices and cook for 4-5 minutes, stirring occasionally, until browned. Transfer to a plate.
3. Add remaining 2 tablespoons olive oil to the skillet.
4. Add bell peppers and onions. Cook for 8-10 minutes, stirring occasionally, until softened and starting to caramelize.
5. Add garlic, paprika, oregano, salt, pepper, and red pepper flakes (if using). Cook for 1 minute.
6. Return kielbasa to the skillet. Toss everything together and cook for 2-3 minutes until heated through.

Tips:

Already cooked: Kielbasa is pre-cooked, so you're just browning and heating everything together.

Make it mustard-y: Serve with spicy brown mustard or Dijon on the side for dipping.

Serve it over: Cauliflower rice, zucchini noodles, or just eat it as-is.

Cabbage addition: Add 2 cups shredded cabbage with the peppers and onions for more volume and fiber. Adds 2g net carbs per serving.

Storage: Refrigerate for up to 4 days. Reheats beautifully in a skillet or microwave.

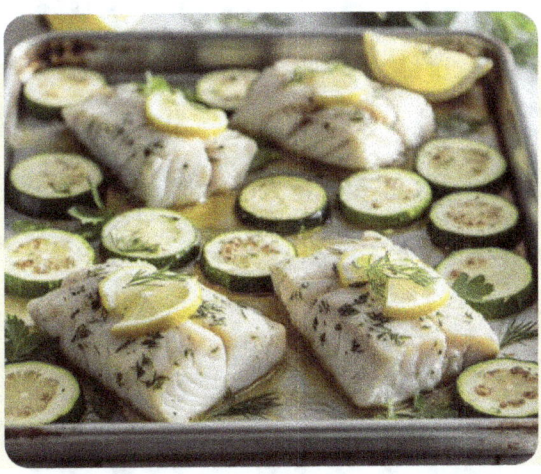

Lemon Herb Cod with Zucchini

 Quick One-Pan

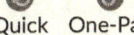 Serves: 4

 Prep Time: 10 min

 Cook Time: 15 min

 Total: 25 min

MACROS PER SERVING:

Calories: 265 | Protein: 32g | Fat: 13g | Net Carbs: 4g

Ingredients:

- 4 cod fillets (6 oz each)
- 3 medium zucchini, sliced into rounds
- 4 tablespoons olive oil, divided
- 4 tablespoons butter, melted
- 4 cloves garlic, minced
- Juice and zest of 1 lemon
- 2 tablespoons fresh parsley, chopped
- 1 tablespoon fresh dill, chopped (or 1 teaspoon dried)
- ¾ teaspoon salt, divided
- ½ teaspoon black pepper, divided
- Lemon wedges for serving

Instructions:

1. Preheat oven to 425°F. Line a large baking sheet with parchment paper.
2. Toss zucchini rounds with 2 tablespoons olive oil, ¼ teaspoon salt, and ¼ teaspoon pepper. Spread on one side of the baking sheet.
3. Pat cod fillets dry with paper towels and place on the other side of the baking sheet.
4. In a small bowl, mix remaining 2 tablespoons olive oil, melted butter, garlic, lemon juice, lemon zest, parsley, and dill.
5. Brush this mixture generously over the cod fillets. Season with remaining ½ teaspoon salt and ¼ teaspoon pepper.
6. Roast for 12-15 minutes until cod is opaque and flakes easily with a fork, and zucchini is tender.

Tips:

Don't overcook: Cod is done when it's opaque and flakes easily. Overcooked fish is dry and rubbery.

Other white fish: Halibut, tilapia, mahi-mahi, or any firm white fish works with the same cooking time.

Make it richer: Add ¼ cup heavy cream to the butter mixture before brushing on the fish. Creates a light sauce.

Frozen fish: Works fine. Thaw completely in the fridge overnight, then pat very dry before cooking.

Storage: Best eaten fresh, but leftovers can be refrigerated for 1-2 days. Fish doesn't reheat as well as other proteins.

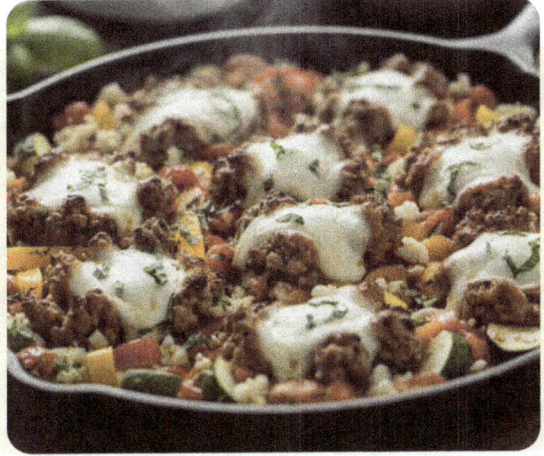

Ground Turkey Skillet

 Quick One-Pan Budget-Friendly

 Serves: 4

 Prep Time: 8 min

 Cook Time: 18 min

Total: 26 min

MACROS PER SERVING:

Calories: 350 | Protein: 34g | Fat: 20g | Net Carbs: 7g

Ingredients:

- 1½ pounds ground turkey
- 1 red bell pepper, diced
- 1 green bell pepper, diced
- 1 medium zucchini, diced
- 1 small onion, diced
- 2 cups cauliflower rice (fresh or frozen)
- 3 tablespoons olive oil, divided
- 4 cloves garlic, minced
- 2 teaspoons Italian seasoning
- 1 teaspoon paprika
- ¾ teaspoon salt
- ½ teaspoon black pepper
- 1 cup diced tomatoes (canned or fresh)
- 1 cup shredded mozzarella cheese
- Fresh basil for garnish

Instructions:

1. Heat 1 tablespoon olive oil in a large oven-safe skillet over medium-high heat.
2. Add ground turkey and cook, breaking it up, for 6-8 minutes until browned and cooked through. Transfer to a plate.
3. Add remaining 2 tablespoons olive oil to the skillet. Add bell peppers, zucchini, and onion. Cook for 5-6 minutes until softened.
4. Add cauliflower rice, garlic, Italian seasoning, paprika, salt, and pepper. Cook for 3-4 minutes, stirring occasionally.
5. Return turkey to the skillet. Add diced tomatoes. Stir everything together and cook for 2 minutes.
6. Sprinkle mozzarella cheese over the top.
7. Transfer skillet to oven and broil for 2-3 minutes until cheese is melted and bubbly.

Tips:

No oven-safe skillet: After adding cheese, just cover the skillet with a lid and let it sit off heat for 2-3 minutes. The steam will melt the cheese.

Ground turkey is lean: Add an extra tablespoon of olive oil when cooking it to prevent dryness.

Make it spicy: Use diced tomatoes with green chiles, or add ¼ teaspoon red pepper flakes.

Storage: Refrigerate for up to 4 days. This actually tastes better the next day as flavors meld.

Budget tip: Ground turkey often goes on sale. Stock up and freeze in 1½ pound portions.

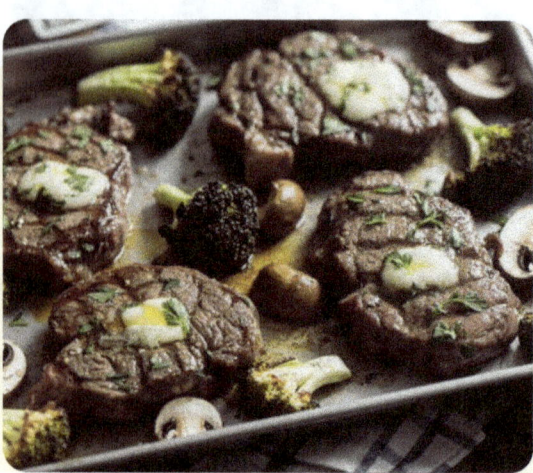

Steak & Mushroom Sheet Pan

 Quick   One-Pan

 Serves: 4

 Prep Time: 10 min

 Cook Time: 15 min

 Total: 25 min

MACROS PER SERVING:

Calories: 485 | Protein: 42g | Fat: 32g | Net Carbs: 5g

Ingredients:

- 1½ pounds sirloin steak (about 1 inch thick), cut into 4 portions
- 1 pound mushrooms (cremini or button), halved
- 2 cups broccoli florets
- 3 tablespoons olive oil, divided
- 4 tablespoons butter, divided
- 6 cloves garlic, minced
- 1 teaspoon dried thyme
- 1 teaspoon salt, divided
- ¾ teaspoon black pepper, divided
- 2 tablespoons fresh parsley, chopped

Instructions:

1. Preheat oven to 450°F. Line a large baking sheet with foil.
2. Pat steaks dry with paper towels. Rub with 1 tablespoon olive oil and season both sides with ½ teaspoon salt and ½ teaspoon pepper.
3. Place steaks on one side of the baking sheet.
4. In a bowl, toss mushrooms and broccoli with remaining 2 tablespoons olive oil, 2 tablespoons melted butter, garlic, thyme, remaining ½ teaspoon salt, and remaining ¼ teaspoon pepper.
5. Arrange mushrooms and broccoli on the other side of the baking sheet.
6. Roast for 12-15 minutes for medium-rare (130-135°F internal temperature), or adjust time for your preferred doneness. Vegetables should be tender and slightly charred.
7. Remove from oven. Let steaks rest for 5 minutes.
8. Top each steak with ½ tablespoon of the remaining butter and garnish with fresh parsley.

Tips:

Steak doneness: Medium-rare: 12-15 minutes. Medium: 15-18 minutes. Medium-well: 18-20 minutes. Always use a thermometer.

Let it rest: Don't skip the 5-minute rest. This keeps the steak juicy.

Cheaper cuts: Flank steak or flat iron also work. Slice thin against the grain after cooking.

Swap vegetables: Asparagus, green beans, or Brussels sprouts all work with the same method.

Garlic butter: Make extra garlic butter and keep it in the fridge. Perfect for topping any protein.

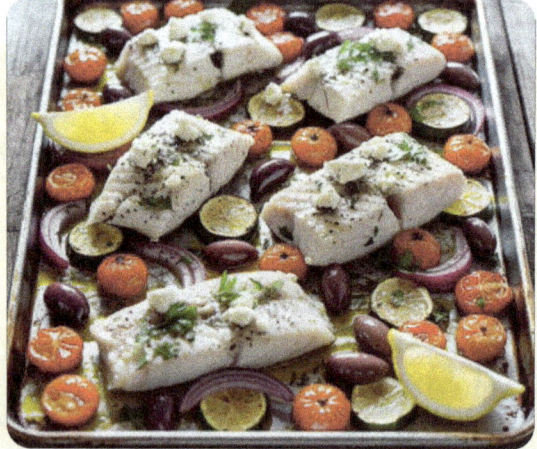

Mediterranean Baked Fish

 Quick   One-Pan

 Serves: 4

 Prep Time: 10 min

 Cook Time: 18 min

 Total: 28 min

MACROS PER SERVING:

Calories: 320 | Protein: 34g | Fat: 18g | Net Carbs: 6g

Ingredients:

- 4 white fish fillets (cod, halibut, or snapper, 6 oz each)
- 2 cups cherry tomatoes, halved
- 1 cup pitted Kalamata olives, halved
- 1 red onion, thinly sliced
- 1 medium zucchini, sliced into half-moons
- 4 tablespoons olive oil
- 4 cloves garlic, minced
- 2 teaspoons dried oregano
- ¾ teaspoon salt
- ½ teaspoon black pepper
- ½ cup crumbled feta cheese
- 2 tablespoons fresh parsley, chopped
- Lemon wedges for serving

Instructions:

1. Preheat oven to 400°F. Line a large baking sheet with parchment paper.
2. Arrange cherry tomatoes, olives, onion, and zucchini on the baking sheet.
3. In a small bowl, mix olive oil, garlic, oregano, salt, and pepper. Reserve 2 tablespoons of this mixture.
4. Drizzle the remaining mixture over the vegetables and toss to coat.
5. Make space for the fish fillets and place them on the baking sheet among the vegetables.
6. Brush the reserved olive oil mixture over the fish fillets.
7. Roast for 15-18 minutes until fish is opaque and flakes easily, and vegetables are tender.
8. Remove from oven and immediately sprinkle feta cheese over everything.

Tips:

Fish thickness: Thicker fillets need 18-20 minutes. Thin fillets need only 12-15 minutes.

Tomatoes create sauce: The cherry tomatoes break down slightly and create a delicious sauce. Don't drain it.

Make it more Greek: Add ¼ cup chopped fresh dill and serve with tzatziki sauce on the side (adds minimal carbs).

Storage: Best eaten fresh, but leftovers can be refrigerated for 1-2 days.

Budget option: Use frozen fish. Thaw completely and pat very dry before cooking.

Pork & Cauliflower Sheet Pan

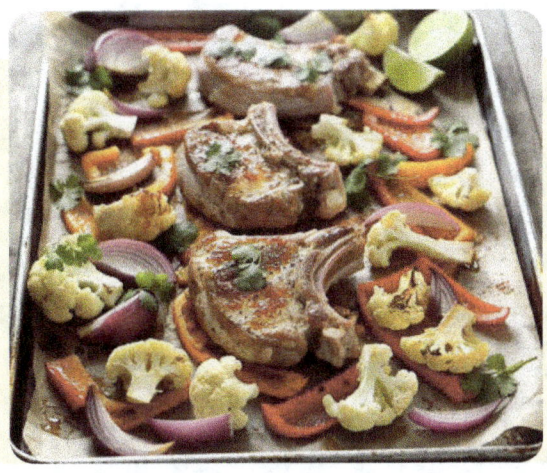

Quick   One-Pan   Budget-Friendly

 Serves: 4

 Prep Time: 10 min

 Cook Time: 25 min

 Total: 35 min

MACROS PER SERVING:

Calories: 395 | Protein: 36g | Fat: 24g | Net Carbs: 6g

Ingredients:

- 4 boneless pork chops (6-8 oz each, about ¾ inch thick)
- 1 large head cauliflower, cut into florets (about 6 cups)
- 1 red bell pepper, cut into 1-inch pieces
- 1 small red onion, cut into wedges
- 4 tablespoons olive oil, divided
- 4 cloves garlic, minced
- 2 teaspoons smoked paprika, divided
- 1 teaspoon cumin
- 1 teaspoon salt, divided
- ¾ teaspoon black pepper, divided
- ¼ teaspoon cayenne pepper (optional)
- Fresh cilantro for garnish
- Lime wedges for serving

Instructions:

1. Preheat oven to 425°F. Line a large baking sheet with parchment paper.
2. Pat pork chops dry. Rub with 1 tablespoon olive oil and season both sides with 1 teaspoon smoked paprika, ½ teaspoon salt, and ¼ teaspoon pepper.
3. In a large bowl, toss cauliflower florets, bell pepper, and onion with remaining 3 tablespoons olive oil, garlic, remaining teaspoon smoked paprika, cumin, remaining ½ teaspoon salt, remaining ½ teaspoon pepper, and cayenne (if using).
4. Spread vegetables on the baking sheet. Place pork chops on top of the vegetables.
5. Roast for 22-25 minutes until pork reaches 145°F internal temperature and cauliflower is tender and caramelized with crispy edges.
6. Let pork rest for 3-5 minutes.

Tips:

Even cooking: If pork chops are thicker than ¾ inch, add 2-3 minutes to cooking time.

Crispy cauliflower: Don't overcrowd the pan. Cauliflower needs space to caramelize rather than steam.

Bone-in option: Bone-in pork chops work great. Add 3-5 minutes to cooking time.

Make it spicy: Double the cayenne pepper or serve with hot sauce.

Storage: Refrigerate for up to 4 days. Reheat in a hot oven (425°F) for 5-7 minutes for best results.

Chicken Drumstick Dinner

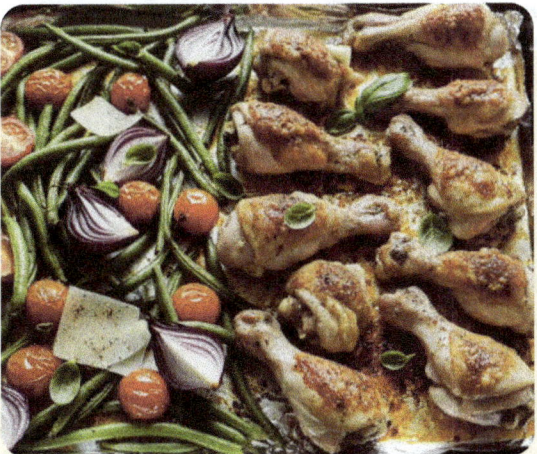

 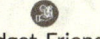
Quick   One-Pan   Budget-Friendly

 Serves: 4

 Prep Time: 10 min

 Cook Time: 35 min

 Total: 45 min

MACROS PER SERVING:

Calories: 420 | Protein: 38g | Fat: 26g | Net Carbs: 7g

Ingredients:

- 8 chicken drumsticks (about 2½ pounds)
- 1 pound green beans, trimmed
- 3 cups cherry tomatoes
- 1 red onion, cut into wedges
- 4 tablespoons olive oil, divided
- 4 cloves garlic, minced
- 2 teaspoons Italian seasoning
- 1 teaspoon paprika
- 1 teaspoon salt, divided
- ¾ teaspoon black pepper, divided
- ¼ cup grated Parmesan cheese
- Fresh basil for garnish

Instructions:

1. Preheat oven to 425°F. Line a large baking sheet with foil.
2. Pat drumsticks dry with paper towels. Rub with 2 tablespoons olive oil and season with Italian seasoning, paprika, ½ teaspoon salt, and ½ teaspoon pepper.
3. Place drumsticks on one side of the baking sheet.
4. In a bowl, toss green beans, cherry tomatoes, and onion with remaining 2 tablespoons olive oil, garlic, remaining ½ teaspoon salt, and remaining ¼ teaspoon pepper.
5. Arrange vegetables on the other side of the baking sheet.
6. Roast for 35-40 minutes, stirring vegetables halfway through, until drumsticks reach 165°F internal temperature and skin is crispy.
7. Remove from oven and sprinkle Parmesan cheese over the vegetables. Let the heat melt it for 1-2 minutes.

Tips:

Crispy skin: Make sure drumsticks are completely dry before seasoning. This helps skin crisp up.

Budget superstar: Chicken drumsticks are often the cheapest chicken cut (sometimes under $1/pound). Perfect for feeding a family on a budget.

Spice it up: Add ½ teaspoon cayenne to the drumstick seasoning, or use hot paprika instead of regular.

Make ahead: Cook drumsticks and vegetables on Sunday. Reheat portions throughout the week for quick lunches or dinners.

Storage: Refrigerate for up to 4 days. Reheat in a hot oven (425°F) for 8-10 minutes to re-crisp the skin.

Shrimp Scampi Skillet

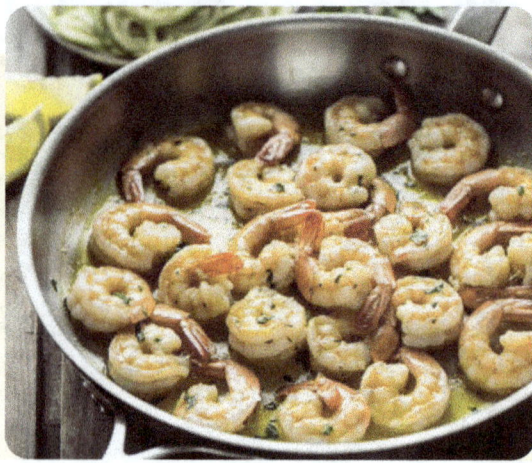

Quick   One-Pan

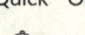 Serves: 4

 Prep Time: 8 min

Cook Time: 12 min

Total: 20 min

MACROS PER SERVING:

Calories: 285 | Protein: 28g | Fat: 18g | Net Carbs: 3g

Ingredients:

- 1½ pounds large shrimp, peeled and deveined
- 4 tablespoons butter
- 3 tablespoons olive oil
- 8 cloves garlic, minced
- ½ cup chicken broth
- Juice of 1 lemon
- ¼ cup white wine (optional, or use more broth)
- ¼ teaspoon red pepper flakes
- ½ teaspoon salt
- ¼ teaspoon black pepper
- 3 tablespoons fresh parsley, chopped
- Optional: zucchini noodles or cauliflower rice for serving

Instructions:

1. Pat shrimp completely dry with paper towels. Season with salt and pepper.
2. Heat olive oil in a large skillet over high heat.
3. Add shrimp in a single layer (work in batches if needed). Cook for 2 minutes per side until pink and cooked through. Transfer to a plate.
4. Reduce heat to medium. Add butter to the skillet.
5. Once butter melts, add garlic and red pepper flakes. Cook for 1 minute until fragrant.
6. Add chicken broth, lemon juice, and white wine (if using). Bring to a simmer and cook for 2-3 minutes until sauce reduces slightly.
7. Return shrimp to the skillet. Toss to coat in sauce and cook for 1 minute until heated through.
8. Remove from heat. Stir in fresh parsley.
9. Serve immediately, over zucchini noodles or cauliflower rice if desired.

Tips:

Wine substitute: Skip the wine and use extra chicken broth plus 1 teaspoon white wine vinegar for acidity.

Frozen shrimp: Works great. Thaw under cold running water for 5 minutes, then pat completely dry.

Make it saucier: Double the butter and broth. The sauce is delicious, so make extra for drizzling.

Serve it over: Zucchini noodles are traditional, but this is also great over cauliflower rice or spaghetti squash.

Storage: Best eaten fresh. Shrimp gets rubbery when reheated, but it's still edible for up to 2 days refrigerated.

Beef & Broccoli Sheet Pan

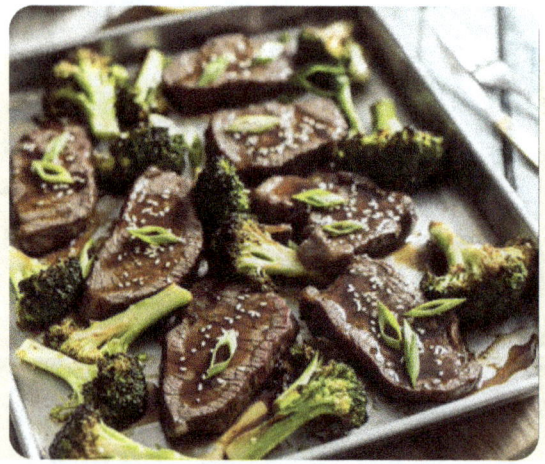

Quick   One-Pan

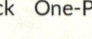 Serves: 4

 Prep Time: 10 min

 Cook Time: 15 min

 Total: 25 min

MACROS PER SERVING:

Calories: 420 | Protein: 36g | Fat: 26g | Net Carbs: 7g

Ingredients:

- 1½ pounds sirloin steak, sliced thin against the grain
- 6 cups broccoli florets
- 3 tablespoons sesame oil or avocado oil, divided
- 4 cloves garlic, minced
- 1 tablespoon fresh ginger, grated
- ¼ cup soy sauce (or coconut aminos)
- 2 tablespoons rice vinegar
- 1 tablespoon sesame oil
- 1 teaspoon erythritol or 5-6 drops liquid stevia (optional)
- ½ teaspoon salt
- ¼ teaspoon black pepper
- ¼ teaspoon red pepper flakes (optional)
- 2 green onions, sliced
- 1 tablespoon sesame seeds

Instructions:

1. Preheat oven to 450°F. Line a large baking sheet with parchment paper.
2. In a bowl, whisk together 2 tablespoons oil, garlic, ginger, soy sauce, rice vinegar, sesame oil, sweetener (if using), and red pepper flakes (if using).
3. Add sliced beef to the bowl and toss to coat. Let sit for 5 minutes while you prep broccoli.
4. Toss broccoli florets with remaining tablespoon oil, salt, and pepper. Spread on half of the baking sheet.
5. Arrange beef slices on the other half of the baking sheet, shaking off excess marinade.
6. Roast for 12-15 minutes until beef is cooked through and broccoli is tender with crispy edges.

Tips:

Slice it thin: Partially freeze the beef for 20 minutes before slicing. This makes it much easier to cut thin, even slices.

High heat is key: 450°F creates that slightly charred, restaurant-quality flavor.

Serve it over: Cauliflower rice to make it a more complete meal, or eat it as-is for a lighter option.

Storage: Refrigerate for up to 3 days. Reheats well in the microwave or on the stovetop.

Ground beef option: Can't slice steak thin? Use ground beef instead. Brown it in a skillet first, then spread on the sheet pan with broccoli and roast.

Sausage Breakfast Bake

Make-Ahead   One-Pan   Budget-Friendly

 Serves: 6

 Prep Time: 15 min

 Cook Time: 35 min

Total: 50 min

MACROS PER SERVING:

Calories: 395 | Protein: 28g | Fat: 29g | Net Carbs: 5g

Ingredients:

- 1 pound breakfast sausage (bulk or removed from casings)
- 12 large eggs
- ½ cup heavy cream
- 2 cups riced cauliflower (fresh or frozen)
- 1 red bell pepper, diced
- 1 small onion, diced
- 2 cups fresh spinach, chopped
- 2 cups shredded cheddar cheese, divided
- 1 teaspoon garlic powder
- ¾ teaspoon salt
- ½ teaspoon black pepper
- Cooking spray

Instructions:

1. Preheat oven to 375°F. Spray a 9x13-inch baking dish with cooking spray.

2. Heat a large skillet over medium-high heat. Add sausage and cook, breaking it up, for 6-8 minutes until browned and cooked through.

3. Add bell pepper and onion to the skillet with sausage. Cook for 3-4 minutes until softened.

4. Add cauliflower rice and cook for 2-3 minutes. If using frozen, cook until thawed and any excess moisture evaporates.

5. Stir in spinach and cook for 1 minute until wilted. Remove from heat.

6. In a large bowl, whisk together eggs, heavy cream, garlic powder, salt, and pepper.

7. Add the sausage and vegetable mixture to the egg mixture. Stir in 1½ cups of the shredded cheese.

8. Pour everything into the prepared baking dish. Spread evenly.

9. Top with remaining ½ cup cheese.

10. Bake for 30-35 minutes until eggs are set in the center and top is golden brown.

Tips:

Make ahead: Assemble everything the night before (through step 8). Cover and refrigerate. In the morning, bake as directed, adding 5-10 minutes to cooking time since it's cold.

Freeze it: Cut into portions, wrap individually in plastic wrap, then place in a freezer bag. Freeze for up to 2 months. Reheat from frozen for 2-3 minutes in the microwave.

Meal prep Sunday: Make this on Sunday. Cut into 6 portions. Grab and reheat for breakfast all week.

Variations: Use any vegetables you like. Mushrooms, zucchini, tomatoes, or jalapeños all work great.

Storage: Refrigerate for up to 5 days. Reheat individual portions in the microwave for 60-90 seconds.

CHAPTER 3 SUMMARY

You now have 20 one-pan recipes that eliminate the worst part of cooking: the cleanup. Here's how to make these recipes work for you:

The One-Pan Strategy:
Sheet pan meals work best when you:

- Cut everything into similar sizes
- Use high heat (400-425°F) for browning and caramelization
- Don't overcrowd the pan
- Flip or stir halfway through for even cooking

Skillet meals work best when you:
- Use a large skillet (12 inches or bigger)
- Layer ingredients by cooking time (protein first, quick vegetables last)
- Keep heat medium-high to high for proper browning
- Have an oven-safe skillet so you can finish dishes under the broiler

My Weekly One-Pan Rotation:
I don't make these every single night, but when I'm exhausted or just want minimal cleanup, these are my go-to recipes:

- **Monday:** Sheet Pan Chicken Fajitas (no brain power required)
- **Tuesday:** Sausage & Veggie Bake (dump and roast)
- **Wednesday:** Leftovers or something ultra-simple
- **Thursday:** Cajun Shrimp & Sausage Skillet (tastes fancy, super easy)
- **Friday:** Takeout or something I can broil in 10 minutes
- **Weekend:** Cook if I feel like it, or make the Sausage Breakfast Bake for the upcoming week

Meal Prep with One-Pan Meals:
Several of these recipes are perfect for Sunday meal prep:

- Sausage Breakfast Bake: Make Sunday, eat all week
- Greek Chicken Tray Bake: Makes great leftovers
- Beef & Cabbage Stir-Fry: Actually better the next day
- Sheet Pan Chicken Fajitas: Perfect for meal prep containers

Equipment Investment:
If you're going to cook one-pan meals regularly, invest in:

1. **Two large rimmed baking sheets** (also called half-sheet pans) - $15-20 each
2. **A large (12-inch) oven-safe skillet** - $30-50 for a good one

3. **Heavy-duty aluminum foil or parchment paper** - Makes cleanup even easier

That's it. You don't need anything else.

Common Mistakes to Avoid:
1. **Overcrowding the pan.** Everything steams instead of roasts. Use two pans if needed.
2. **Not preheating the oven.** If the oven isn't hot enough, food steams instead of browning.
3. **Cutting ingredients different sizes.** Small pieces overcook while large pieces undercook. Keep everything uniform.
4. **Using non-stick spray on high heat.** It can smoke and leave residue. Use parchment paper or foil instead.
5. **Not patting proteins dry.** Wet chicken/beef/fish will steam, not brown. Always pat dry.

Time-Saving Shortcuts:
*   Buy pre-cut vegetables when they're on sale
*   Use frozen cauliflower rice (cooks perfectly from frozen)
*   Buy pre-marinated meats occasionally when you're too tired to season
*   Double recipes and freeze half for later
*   Keep sheet pans lined with foil ready to go

The Real Benefits:
One-pan cooking isn't just about less cleanup (though that's huge). It's about:

*   Less decision fatigue (one pan = simpler choices)
*   Less time in the kitchen overall
*   Less stress about dinner
*   More energy for other things in your life

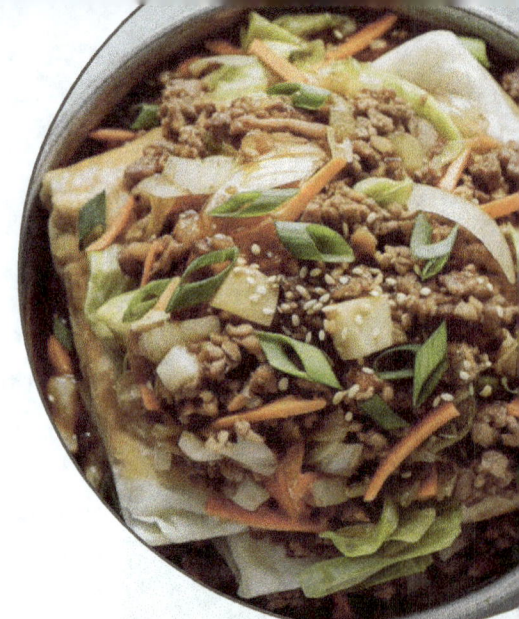

Let's talk about money.

Eating high-protein, low-carb doesn't have to be expensive, but I'm not going to lie to you: protein costs more than pasta. A pound of chicken costs more than a pound of rice. Steak costs more than potatoes.

But here's what I've learned after years of cooking this way: when you stop buying bread, cereal, pasta, rice, chips, crackers, cookies, and all the other carb-heavy fillers that used to pad out your grocery cart, you free up money for better protein. When you stop eating out because you're too tired to cook complicated meals, you save even more.

This chapter is about feeding yourself (or your family) well without breaking the bank. Every recipe costs less than $3 per serving using regular grocery store prices. Most cost under $2 per serving.

These aren't "stretch the meat with breadcrumbs" recipes. They're actual satisfying meals built around affordable proteins and vegetables. The recipes use cheaper cuts of meat, economical proteins like eggs and canned fish, and vegetables that won't drain your wallet.

The Budget Protein Hierarchy:

From cheapest to most expensive, here's what you need to know:

Under $0.25 per serving:
- Eggs (the absolute MVP)
- Canned sardines (don't dismiss them until you try them)

$0.50-$1.00 per serving:
- Chicken leg quarters (often under $1/pound)
- Pork shoulder (slow cook it into pulled pork)
- Ground beef when on sale (buy 80/20, never pay more than $3/pound)
- Canned tuna
- Chicken thighs

$1.00-$1.50 per serving:
- Ground turkey
- Pork chops
- Whole chickens (break them down yourself)
- Bone-in chicken breasts

$1.50-$2.50 per serving:
- Chuck roast
- Beef liver (extremely nutritious, very cheap)
- Boneless chicken thighs
- Bacon (when on sale)

Everything more expensive than this doesn't appear in this chapter.

The Budget Shopping Strategy:

1. **Plan around sales.** Check your store's weekly ad before meal planning. When chicken thighs hit $1.50/pound, buy 10 pounds and freeze them.

2. **Buy in bulk when prices are good.** Ground beef on sale? Buy 10 pounds. Portion into 1-1.5 pound packages and freeze.

3. **Use cheaper cuts.** Chicken thighs taste better than breasts and cost less. Pork shoulder is cheaper than tenderloin but becomes incredibly tender when cooked low and slow.

4. **Don't waste anything.** Save chicken bones for broth. Use bacon grease for cooking. Freeze vegetable scraps for stock.

5. **Buy whole, not pre-cut.** Whole chickens are cheaper per pound than parts. Whole heads of cabbage are cheaper than coleslaw mix. Pre-cut costs extra.

6. **Embrace eggs.** At $3 for a dozen, eggs provide 72 grams of protein for 50 cents. Nothing beats that ratio.

7. **Shop discount grocers.** Aldi, Lidl, and ethnic grocery stores often have better meat prices than major chains.

8. **Frozen vegetables are fine.** Often cheaper than fresh, already prepped, and just as nutritious.

The Reality Check:

I'm going to be honest: these recipes won't look like restaurant food. They're home cooking at its most practical. But they taste good, they fill you up, and they hit your protein targets without requiring you to choose between dinner and paying the electric bill.

Some of these recipes use organ meats. I know that's not for everyone, but liver is one of the most nutrient-dense and affordable proteins available. I include one recipe for those willing to try it, but you can skip it if you want.

What You'll Find in This Chapter:

- Complete meals under $3 per serving

- Recipes built around the cheapest proteins

- Bulk cooking options that freeze well

- Ways to use every part of what you buy

- No specialty ingredients or expensive substitutes

What You Won't Find:

- Grass-fed, organic, or specialty meats

- Expensive cheeses or imported ingredients

- Recipes requiring lots of fresh herbs

- Anything with a long list of single-use ingredients

Let's cook good food on a real budget.

Ground Beef & Egg Scramble

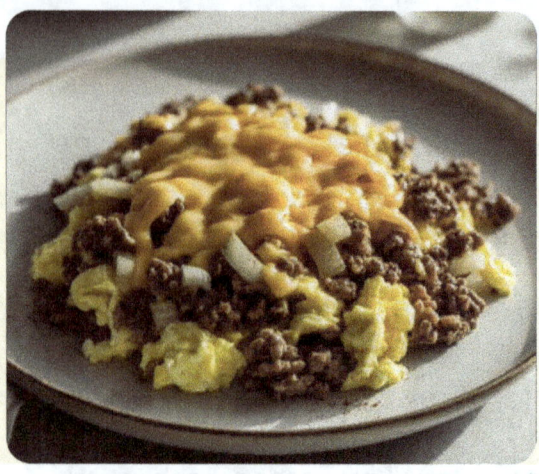

 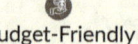
Quick   One-Pan   Budget-Friendly

 Serves: 4

 Prep Time: 5 min

 Cook Time: 12 min

Total: 17 min

Cost Per Serving: $1.75

MACROS PER SERVING:
Calories: 420 | Protein: 35g | Fat: 29g | Net Carbs: 3g

Ingredients:
- 1 pound ground beef (80/20)
- 8 large eggs
- 2 tablespoons butter
- 1 small onion, diced
- 2 cloves garlic, minced
- 1 teaspoon paprika
- ½ teaspoon cumin
- ¾ teaspoon salt
- ½ teaspoon black pepper
- 1 cup shredded cheddar cheese
- Optional: hot sauce for serving

Instructions:
1. Heat a large skillet over medium-high heat. Add ground beef and cook, breaking it up with a spatula, for 6-8 minutes until browned.
2. Add onion and cook for 2-3 minutes until softened.
3. Add garlic, paprika, cumin, ½ teaspoon salt, and ¼ teaspoon pepper. Cook for 1 minute.
4. Push beef mixture to one side of the skillet. Add butter to the empty side.
5. Crack eggs into a bowl, add remaining ¼ teaspoon salt and ¼ teaspoon pepper, and whisk.
6. Pour eggs into the buttered side of the skillet. Let sit for 30 seconds, then gently scramble for 2-3 minutes until just set.
7. Mix eggs into the beef. Remove from heat and sprinkle with cheese. Let the heat melt it for 1-2 minutes.
8. Serve with hot sauce if desired.

Tips:
Budget breakdown: Ground beef $4, eggs $2, cheese $1, onion/garlic/spices $0.50. Total: $7.50 for 4 servings.

Make it last: This reheats perfectly. Make it Sunday, portion into containers, and you have breakfast for 4 days.

Stretch it further: Add 2 cups of riced cauliflower with the beef. Increases volume, adds 1 more serving, barely changes macros.

Ground turkey: Often cheaper than ground beef. Works perfectly here.

Storage: Refrigerate for up to 4 days. Reheat in microwave for 60-90 seconds.

Chicken Thigh Curry

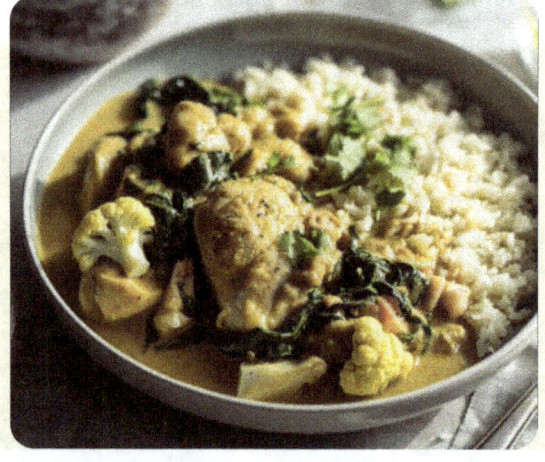

  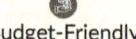
Quick   One-Pan   Budget-Friendly

 Serves: 6

 Prep Time: 10 min

 Cook Time: 25 min

 Total: 35 min

Cost Per Serving: $2.25

MACROS PER SERVING:
Calories: 445 | Protein: 32g | Fat: 32g | Net Carbs: 6g

Ingredients:
- 2 pounds boneless, skinless chicken thighs, cut into 2-inch pieces
- 1 can (14 oz) full-fat coconut milk
- 1 tablespoon coconut oil or olive oil
- 1 large onion, diced
- 4 cloves garlic, minced
- 1 tablespoon fresh ginger, grated (or 1 teaspoon ground)
- 2 tablespoons curry powder
- 1 teaspoon cumin
- 1 teaspoon paprika
- ½ teaspoon turmeric
- 1 teaspoon salt
- ½ teaspoon black pepper
- 2 cups cauliflower florets
- 1 cup diced tomatoes (canned or fresh)
- 2 cups fresh spinach
- Fresh cilantro for garnish (optional)

Instructions:
1. Heat oil in a large deep skillet or pot over medium-high heat.
2. Add chicken pieces and cook for 5-6 minutes until browned on all sides. Transfer to a plate.
3. Add onion to the skillet and cook for 3-4 minutes until softened.
4. Add garlic and ginger. Cook for 1 minute until fragrant.
5. Add curry powder, cumin, paprika, turmeric, salt, and pepper. Stir for 30 seconds until spices are fragrant.
6. Pour in coconut milk and add diced tomatoes. Stir to combine.
7. Return chicken to the skillet. Add cauliflower florets. Bring to a simmer.
8. Reduce heat to medium-low, cover, and simmer for 15 minutes until chicken is cooked through and cauliflower is tender.
9. Stir in spinach and cook for 1-2 minutes until wilted.

Tips:
Budget breakdown: Chicken thighs $6, coconut milk $2, vegetables $2, spices $1. Total: $11 for 6 servings.

Curry powder: Buy it in bulk from ethnic grocery stores. Much cheaper than grocery store spice aisles.

Coconut milk: Use full-fat for best flavor and texture. Light coconut milk makes the sauce thin and watery.

Serve it over: Cauliflower rice to make it more filling. Or just eat it as a stew with a spoon.

Meal prep: This actually gets better over time as flavors meld. Make Sunday, eat all week.

Storage: Refrigerate for up to 5 days or freeze for up to 3 months.

Cabbage Roll Bowl

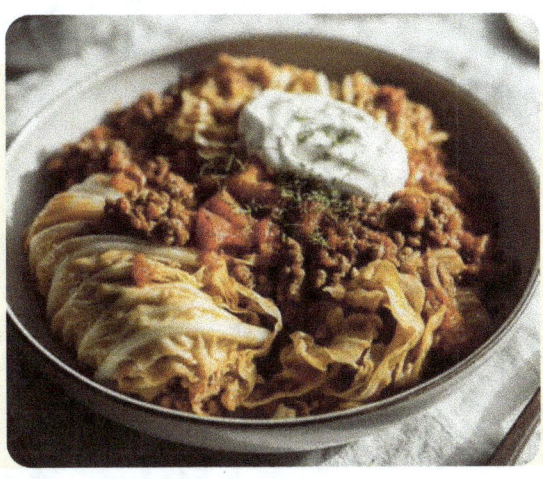

 Quick   One-Pan  Budget-Friendly

 Serves: 6

 Prep Time: 10 min

 Cook Time: 25 min

Total: 35 min

 Cost Per Serving: $1.85

MACROS PER SERVING:

Calories: 380 | Protein: 28g | Fat: 24g | Net Carbs: 8g

Ingredients:

- 1½ pounds ground beef (80/20)
- 6 cups shredded cabbage (about ½ large head)
- 1 can (14.5 oz) diced tomatoes, undrained
- 1 can (8 oz) tomato sauce
- 1 medium onion, diced
- 3 cloves garlic, minced
- 2 tablespoons olive oil
- 1 tablespoon paprika
- 1 teaspoon dried oregano
- 1 teaspoon salt
- ½ teaspoon black pepper
- ¼ teaspoon cayenne pepper (optional)
- 1 cup sour cream for serving

Instructions:

1. Heat olive oil in a large deep skillet over medium-high heat.
2. Add ground beef and cook, breaking it up, for 6-8 minutes until browned. Drain excess fat if there's more than 2 tablespoons.
3. Add onion and cook for 3-4 minutes until softened.
4. Add garlic, paprika, oregano, salt, pepper, and cayenne (if using). Cook for 1 minute.
5. Add cabbage and stir everything together. Cook for 3-4 minutes until cabbage starts to wilt.
6. Add diced tomatoes (with their juice) and tomato sauce. Stir to combine.
7. Bring to a simmer, then reduce heat to medium-low. Cover and cook for 12-15 minutes until cabbage is tender.
8. Taste and adjust seasoning if needed.
9. Serve in bowls with a dollop of sour cream on top.

Tips:

Budget breakdown: Ground beef $4.50, cabbage $1.50, tomatoes/sauce $2, sour cream $1.50, other ingredients $1.50. Total: $11 for 6 servings.

Why deconstructed: Traditional cabbage rolls take an hour to make. This tastes the same, takes 35 minutes, and dirties one pan.

Cabbage tip: Buy whole cabbages, not pre-shredded coleslaw mix. Whole cabbage costs half as much.

Ground turkey: Works great if it's cheaper than beef in your area.

Storage: Refrigerate for up to 5 days. This is one of those dishes that tastes even better the next day.

Freeze it: Freezes beautifully for up to 3 months. Thaw overnight in the fridge and reheat.

Tuna Salad Lettuce Boats

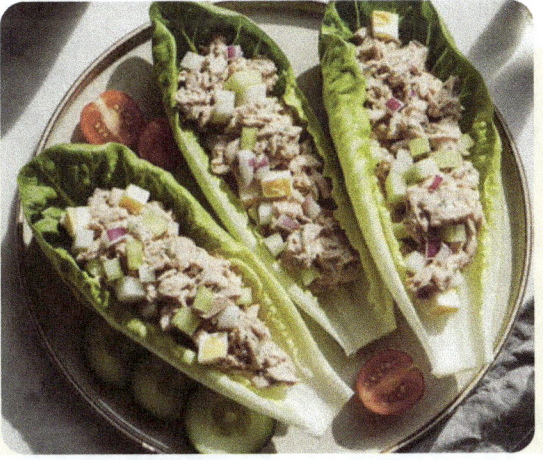

 Quick  Budget-Friendly

 Serves: 4

 Prep Time: 10 min

 Cook Time: 0 min

 Total: 10 min

 Cost Per Serving: $1.40

MACROS PER SERVING:

Calories: 285 | Protein: 26g | Fat: 18g | Net Carbs: 4g

Ingredients:

- 3 cans (5 oz each) tuna in water, drained
- ½ cup mayonnaise
- 2 tablespoons Dijon mustard
- ½ cup diced celery
- ¼ cup diced red onion
- 2 hard-boiled eggs, chopped
- 1 tablespoon lemon juice
- ½ teaspoon garlic powder
- ½ teaspoon salt
- ¼ teaspoon black pepper
- 12 large lettuce leaves (romaine or butter lettuce)
- Optional: cherry tomatoes, cucumber slices

Instructions:

1. In a large bowl, combine drained tuna, mayonnaise, and Dijon mustard. Mix well, breaking up any large chunks of tuna.
2. Add celery, red onion, chopped eggs, lemon juice, garlic powder, salt, and pepper. Mix until everything is evenly combined.
3. Taste and adjust seasoning if needed.
4. Wash and dry lettuce leaves.
5. Divide tuna salad among lettuce leaves (about ⅓ cup per leaf).
6. Serve with cherry tomatoes and cucumber slices if desired.

Tips:

Budget breakdown: Canned tuna $3, eggs $1, mayo $0.75, vegetables $1, lettuce $0.50. Total: $6.25 for 4 servings.

Canned tuna: Solid white albacore is more expensive. Chunk light tuna works fine and costs half as much.

Make the eggs ahead: Hard-boil a dozen eggs on Sunday. Use them throughout the week in recipes like this.

Mayo substitute: Greek yogurt works but changes the flavor. Half mayo, half Greek yogurt is a good compromise.

Storage: Tuna salad keeps for 3-4 days in the fridge. Store separately from lettuce. Assemble just before eating.

Not just boats: This tuna salad is great stuffed in tomatoes, bell peppers, or just eaten with a fork.

Egg Roll in a Bowl

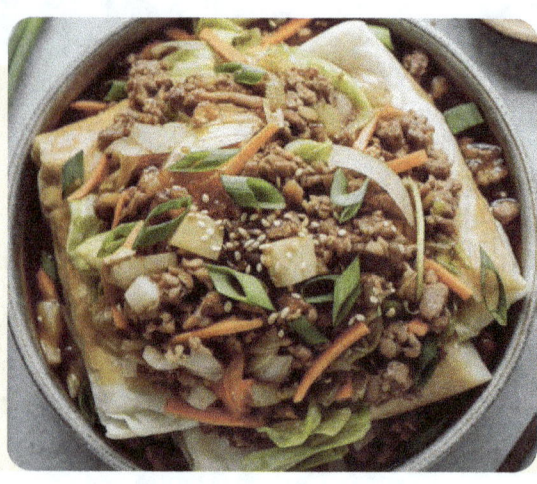

Quick | One-Pan | Budget-Friendly

🍲 Serves: 6

Prep Time: 10 min

Cook Time: 15 min

Total: 25 min

Cost Per Serving: $1.65

MACROS PER SERVING:

Calories: 365 | Protein: 26g |
Fat: 26g | Net Carbs: 7g

Ingredients:

- 1½ pounds ground pork (or ground turkey/beef)
- 6 cups shredded cabbage (about ½ large head)
- 2 cups shredded carrots
- 1 medium onion, diced
- 4 cloves garlic, minced
- 2 tablespoons sesame oil or vegetable oil
- 1 tablespoon fresh ginger, grated (or 1 teaspoon ground)
- ¼ cup soy sauce (or coconut aminos)
- 2 tablespoons rice vinegar
- 1 teaspoon red pepper flakes (optional)
- 4 green onions, sliced
- 2 tablespoons sesame seeds

Instructions:

1. Heat oil in a large skillet or wok over high heat.
2. Add ground pork and cook, breaking it up, for 6-8 minutes until browned and cooked through.
3. Add onion and cook for 2 minutes until starting to soften.
4. Add cabbage and carrots. Stir-fry for 5-6 minutes until cabbage is wilted and tender.
5. Add garlic and ginger. Cook for 1 minute until fragrant.
6. Pour in soy sauce and rice vinegar. Add red pepper flakes if using. Toss everything together and cook for 1-2 minutes.

Tips:

Budget breakdown: Ground pork $5, cabbage $1.50, carrots $1, other ingredients $2. Total: $9.50 for 6 servings.

Coleslaw mix: Buy pre-shredded coleslaw mix if you're short on time. Costs about $1 more but saves 10 minutes of chopping.

Ground pork: Often the cheapest ground meat. Buy it on sale and freeze in portions.

Soy sauce: Buy it at Asian grocery stores. Much cheaper than regular grocery stores.

Storage: Refrigerate for up to 5 days. This reheats beautifully and actually tastes better the next day.

Meal prep: Make a double batch on Sunday. Portion into containers for quick lunches all week.

Crack Slaw

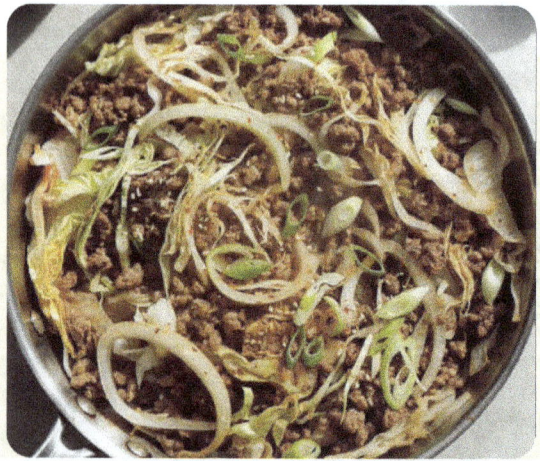

Quick | One-Pan | Budget-Friendly

🍲 Serves: 6

Prep Time: 8 min

Cook Time: 15 min

Total: 23 min

Cost Per Serving: $1.55

MACROS PER SERVING:

Calories: 340 | Protein: 24g |
Fat: 24g | Net Carbs: 6g

Ingredients:

- 1½ pounds ground pork
- 8 cups shredded cabbage (about ¾ large head)
- 1 medium onion, sliced thin
- 4 cloves garlic, minced
- 1 tablespoon fresh ginger, grated
- 3 tablespoons soy sauce
- 2 tablespoons rice vinegar
- 1 tablespoon sesame oil
- 1 teaspoon red pepper flakes
- 1 teaspoon salt
- ½ teaspoon black pepper
- 3 green onions, sliced
- 1 tablespoon sesame seeds

Instructions:

1. Heat a large skillet or wok over high heat. Add ground pork and cook, breaking it up, for 6-8 minutes until browned and cooked through.
2. Push pork to one side. Add onion to the empty side and cook for 2 minutes.
3. Add cabbage. It will seem like a lot, but it wilts down. Stir everything together and cook for 5-6 minutes until cabbage is tender.
4. Add garlic and ginger. Cook for 1 minute until fragrant.
5. In a small bowl, mix soy sauce, rice vinegar, sesame oil, red pepper flakes, salt, and pepper.
6. Pour sauce over the cabbage and pork. Toss everything together and cook for 1-2 minutes.

Tips:

Budget breakdown: Ground pork $5, cabbage $2, other ingredients $2. Total: $9 for 6 servings.

Why "crack" slaw: It's called this because people become addicted to it. It's that good.

High heat: This needs to cook at high heat to get slightly charred edges on the cabbage. Don't reduce the heat.

Make it spicier: Double the red pepper flakes or add sriracha when serving.

Storage: Refrigerate for up to 5 days. One of the best meal prep recipes in this entire book.

Ground beef: Works if ground pork isn't available. Same price, slightly different flavor.

Chicken Leg Quarters (Roasted)

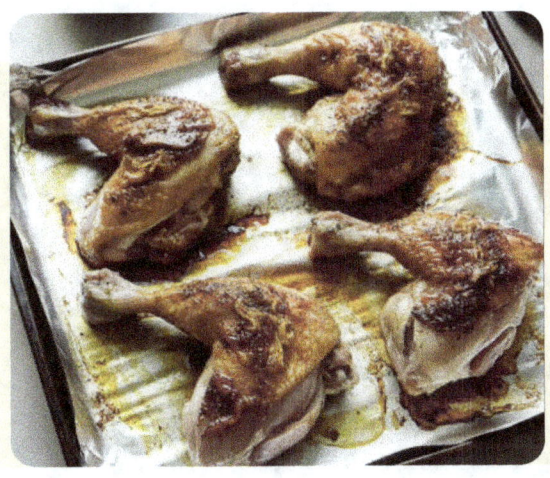

Quick Budget-Friendly

Serves: 4

Prep Time: 5 min

Cook Time: 45 min

Total: 50 min

Cost Per Serving: $1.25

MACROS PER SERVING:

Calories: 485 | Protein: 42g | Fat: 34g | Net Carbs: 0g

Ingredients:

- 4 chicken leg quarters (thigh and drumstick attached, about 3 pounds total)
- 2 tablespoons olive oil
- 2 teaspoons paprika
- 1 teaspoon garlic powder
- 1 teaspoon onion powder
- 1 teaspoon dried thyme
- 1 teaspoon salt
- ½ teaspoon black pepper
- ½ teaspoon cayenne pepper (optional)

Instructions:

1. Preheat oven to 425°F. Line a baking sheet with foil (makes cleanup easier).
2. Pat chicken leg quarters completely dry with paper towels. This is crucial for crispy skin.
3. Rub chicken all over with olive oil.
4. In a small bowl, mix paprika, garlic powder, onion powder, thyme, salt, pepper, and cayenne (if using).
5. Sprinkle seasoning mixture all over chicken, making sure to coat all sides. Pay special attention to the skin side.
6. Place chicken leg quarters skin-side up on the baking sheet, not touching each other.
7. Roast for 45-50 minutes until skin is crispy and golden, and internal temperature reaches 165°F.

Tips:

Budget breakdown: Chicken leg quarters are often $0.79-$1.29 per pound. 3 pounds costs about $3-4, plus $1 for seasonings and oil. Total: $5 for 4 servings.

Why leg quarters: They're the cheapest chicken cut available. Often under $1 per pound. And they're juicier than chicken breasts.

Crispy skin secret: Completely dry chicken + high heat = crispy skin. Don't skip the drying step.

Flavor variations: Try different spice blends. Cajun seasoning, Italian herbs, or just salt and pepper all work.

Storage: Refrigerate for up to 4 days. Eat cold, reheat gently, or shred the meat for other recipes.

Use the bones: Save the bones in the freezer. When you have enough, make chicken bone broth (Recipe 75).

Ground Beef Cauliflower Casserole

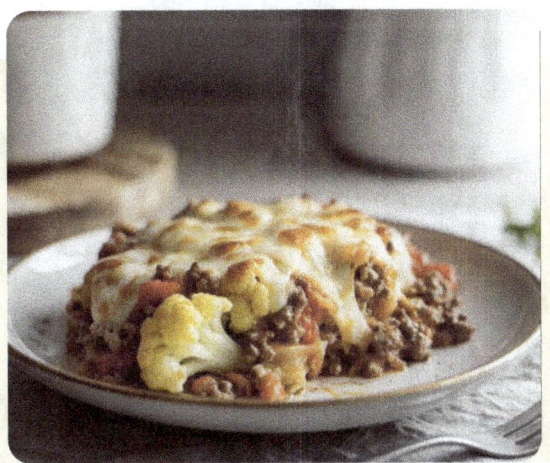

Make-Ahead Budget-Friendly

Serves: 6

Prep Time: 15 min

Cook Time: 30 min

Total: 45 min

Cost Per Serving: $2.15

MACROS PER SERVING:

Calories: 420 | Protein: 30g | Fat: 29g | Net Carbs: 7g

Ingredients:

- 1½ pounds ground beef (80/20)
- 1 large head cauliflower, cut into florets (about 6 cups)
- 1 can (14.5 oz) diced tomatoes, drained
- 1 medium onion, diced
- 3 cloves garlic, minced
- 2 tablespoons olive oil
- 1 tablespoon Italian seasoning
- 1 teaspoon paprika
- 1 teaspoon salt
- ½ teaspoon black pepper
- 2 cups shredded mozzarella cheese, divided
- ½ cup grated Parmesan cheese
- Cooking spray

Instructions:

1. Preheat oven to 375°F. Spray a 9x13-inch baking dish with cooking spray.
2. Bring a large pot of salted water to boil. Add cauliflower florets and cook for 5-6 minutes until tender but not mushy. Drain well and set aside.
3. While cauliflower cooks, heat olive oil in a large skillet over medium-high heat. Add ground beef and cook, breaking it up, for 6-8 minutes until browned.
4. Add onion and cook for 3 minutes until softened.
5. Add garlic, Italian seasoning, paprika, salt, and pepper. Cook for 1 minute.
6. Add drained tomatoes. Stir and cook for 2 minutes.
7. In the prepared baking dish, spread cauliflower florets in an even layer.
8. Pour beef mixture over the cauliflower, spreading evenly.
9. Sprinkle 1 cup mozzarella and all of the Parmesan cheese over the top.
10. Bake for 20 minutes until cheese is melted and bubbly.
11. Top with remaining 1 cup mozzarella. Bake for 5 more minutes until cheese is melted and starting to brown.

Tips:

Budget breakdown: Ground beef $4.50, cauliflower $3, cheese $3, tomatoes and other ingredients $2. Total: $12.50 for 6 servings.

Don't overcook cauliflower: It continues cooking in the oven. Stop when it's just tender.

Make ahead: Assemble everything (through step 9), cover, and refrigerate for up to 24 hours. Bake when ready, adding 5-10 minutes to cooking time since it's cold.

Freeze it: Freeze individual portions for up to 2 months. Thaw overnight in fridge and reheat.

Ground turkey: Works great if cheaper in your area. The cheese and seasonings give it plenty of flavor.

Storage: Refrigerate for up to 5 days. Reheat in microwave or oven.

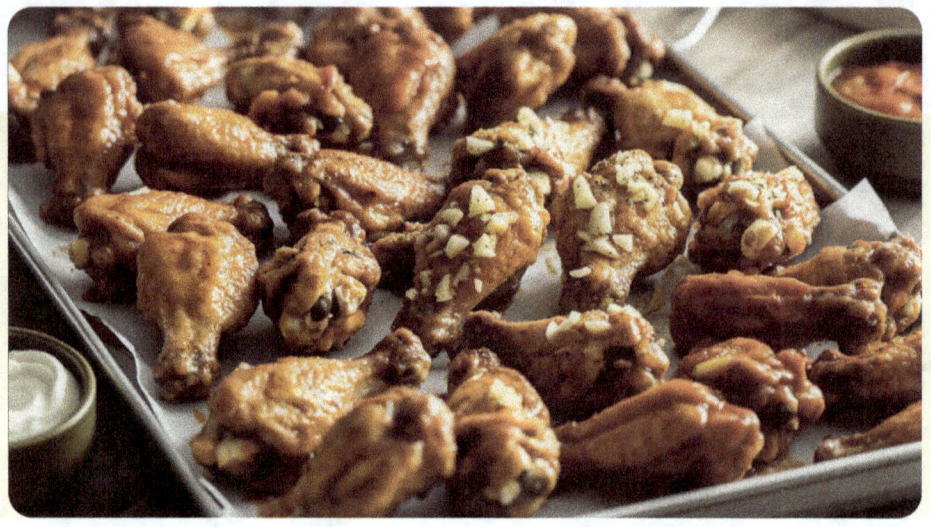

Baked Chicken Wings (Multiple Flavors)

Quick   Budget-Friendly

 Serves: 4

 Prep Time: 10 min

 Cook Time: 45 min

 Total: 55 min

 Cost Per Serving: $2.50

MACROS PER SERVING (plain):
Calories: 485 | Protein: 38g | Fat: 36g | Net Carbs: 1g

Instructions:

1. Preheat oven to 425°F. Line a baking sheet with foil and place a wire rack on top.
2. Pat wings completely dry with paper towels. This is crucial for crispy wings.
3. In a large bowl, toss wings with baking powder, salt, and pepper until evenly coated.
4. Arrange wings on the wire rack in a single layer, not touching.
5. Bake for 45-50 minutes, flipping halfway through, until skin is crispy and golden brown.
6. While wings bake, prepare your chosen sauce or dry rub.
7. For sauced wings (Buffalo or Garlic Parmesan): Transfer hot wings to a large bowl, add sauce, toss to coat.
8. For dry rub wings: Toss hot wings with dry rub mixture in a large bowl.

Tips:

Budget breakdown: Chicken wings $7.50 (often $2.50/pound on sale), sauce ingredients $1. Total: $8.50 for 4 servings, or $10 if you make all three flavors.

Baking powder secret: It raises the pH of the skin, making it extra crispy. Don't skip it, and make sure it's baking powder, not baking soda.

Wire rack: Elevates wings so air circulates all around. No wire rack? Flip wings more frequently during baking.

Buy on sale: Chicken wings often go on sale before major sporting events. Stock up and freeze.

Storage: Refrigerate plain or sauced wings for up to 4 days. Reheat in a 425°F oven for 5-7 minutes to re-crisp.

Blue cheese dip: Mix ½ cup sour cream with ¼ cup crumbled blue cheese for dipping. Adds 2g net carbs per serving.

Ingredients:

- 3 pounds chicken wings (about 24 wings)
- 2 tablespoons baking powder (not baking soda)
- 1 tablespoon salt
- 1 teaspoon black pepper

For Buffalo Wings:
- ½ cup Frank's RedHot sauce
- 4 tablespoons butter, melted

For Garlic Parmesan Wings:
- 4 tablespoons butter, melted
- 4 cloves garlic, minced
- ½ cup grated Parmesan cheese
- 2 tablespoons fresh parsley, chopped

For Dry Rub Wings:
- 2 tablespoons paprika
- 1 tablespoon garlic powder
- 1 tablespoon onion powder
- 1 teaspoon black pepper
- 1 teaspoon cayenne pepper

Pork Shoulder Slow Cooker Pulled Pork

 Make-Ahead   Budget-Friendly

Serves: 10

Prep Time: 10 min

Cook Time: 8 hours

Total: 8 hours 10 min

Cost Per Serving: $1.85

MACROS PER SERVING:

Calories: 380 | Protein: 32g | Fat: 26g | Net Carbs: 2g

Ingredients:

- 4 pounds pork shoulder (also called pork butt)
- 2 tablespoons olive oil
- 3 tablespoons chili powder
- 2 tablespoons paprika
- 2 tablespoons garlic powder
- 2 tablespoons onion powder
- 1 tablespoon cumin
- 1 tablespoon salt
- 1 tablespoon black pepper
- 1 teaspoon cayenne pepper (optional)
- 1 cup chicken broth
- ¼ cup apple cider vinegar

Instructions:

1. In a small bowl, mix chili powder, paprika, garlic powder, onion powder, cumin, salt, pepper, and cayenne (if using) to make a rub.
2. Pat pork shoulder dry with paper towels.
3. Rub the spice mixture all over the pork, coating all sides generously.
4. Heat olive oil in a large skillet over high heat. Sear pork on all sides until browned, about 3 minutes per side. This step is optional but adds flavor.
5. Place pork in slow cooker. Pour chicken broth and apple cider vinegar around it.
6. Cover and cook on low for 8-10 hours or on high for 5-6 hours, until pork is very tender and falls apart easily.
7. Remove pork from slow cooker. Shred with two forks, discarding large pieces of fat.
8. Return shredded pork to slow cooker and stir to coat with cooking liquid. Let sit for 5-10 minutes to absorb flavors.

Tips:

Budget breakdown: Pork shoulder is often $1.50-$2.50 per pound. 4 pounds costs $6-10, plus $2 for seasonings and broth. Total: $8-12 for 10 servings.

Set and forget: This cooks while you sleep or work. Perfect for meal prep.

Instant Pot: Pressure cook on high for 90 minutes with natural release. Same results in 2 hours total time.

Storage: Refrigerate for up to 5 days or freeze for up to 4 months. Portion into containers before freezing.

Use it for everything: Pulled pork works in breakfast scrambles, lettuce wraps, taco bowls, casseroles, or just eaten plain.

Save the fat: The fat that rises to the top of the liquid when refrigerated is pure gold. Save it for cooking eggs or vegetables.

Beef & Veggie Soup

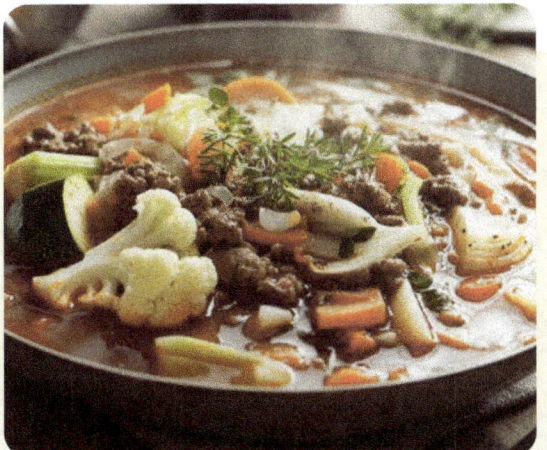

 One-Pan   Budget-Friendly

Serves: 8

Prep Time: 15 min

Cook Time: 45 min

Total: 60 min

Cost Per Serving: $1.95

MACROS PER SERVING:

Calories: 285 | Protein: 26g | Fat: 14g | Net Carbs: 8g

Ingredients:

- 1½ pounds ground beef (80/20)
- 8 cups beef broth
- 1 can (14.5 oz) diced tomatoes, undrained
- 3 cups cauliflower florets
- 2 cups diced zucchini
- 2 cups diced cabbage
- 1 large onion, diced
- 3 carrots, diced
- 4 cloves garlic, minced
- 2 tablespoons olive oil
- 2 teaspoons Italian seasoning
- 1 teaspoon paprika
- 1 teaspoon salt
- ½ teaspoon black pepper
- 2 bay leaves

Instructions:

1. Heat olive oil in a large pot or Dutch oven over medium-high heat.
2. Add ground beef and cook, breaking it up, for 6-8 minutes until browned. Don't drain.
3. Add onion and carrots. Cook for 5 minutes until starting to soften.
4. Add garlic, Italian seasoning, paprika, salt, and pepper. Cook for 1 minute.
5. Add beef broth, diced tomatoes (with juice), and bay leaves. Bring to a boil.
6. Reduce heat to medium-low and simmer for 20 minutes.
7. Add cauliflower, zucchini, and cabbage. Simmer for 15 more minutes until all vegetables are tender.

Tips:

Budget breakdown: Ground beef $4.50, broth $3 (or free if homemade), vegetables $4, tomatoes and seasonings $2. Total: $13.50 for 8 servings.

Make your own broth: Save bones from chicken or beef in the freezer. When you have enough, simmer with water, vegetables, and herbs for free broth.

Bulk it up: Add more cabbage and cauliflower to stretch this further. They're cheap and filling.

Storage: Refrigerate for up to 5 days or freeze for up to 3 months. Actually tastes better after a day as flavors meld.

Meal prep: Make a huge batch on Sunday. Portion into containers for easy lunches.

Instant Pot: Sauté beef and onions using sauté function, add everything else, pressure cook on high for 15 minutes with quick release.

Sardine Salad

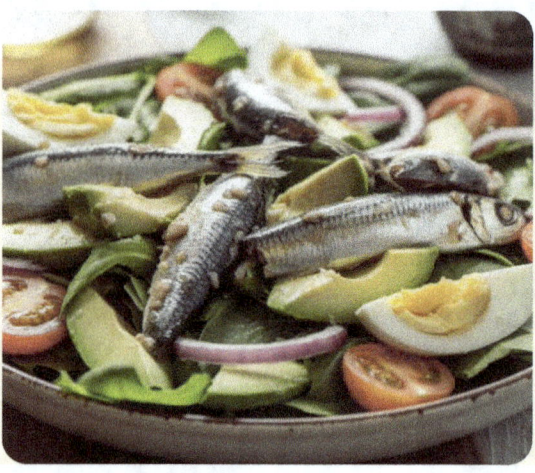

 Quick   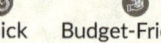 Budget-Friendly

 Serves: 2

Prep Time: 10 min

Cook Time: 0 min

Total: 10 min

Cost Per Serving: $2.25

MACROS PER SERVING:

Calories: 385 | Protein: 32g | Fat: 26g | Net Carbs: 4g

Ingredients:

- 2 cans (4.4 oz each) sardines in water or olive oil, drained
- 4 cups mixed salad greens
- 1 medium avocado, diced
- ½ cup cherry tomatoes, halved
- ¼ small red onion, sliced thin
- 2 hard-boiled eggs, sliced
- 2 tablespoons olive oil
- 1 tablespoon lemon juice
- 1 tablespoon Dijon mustard
- ½ teaspoon salt
- ¼ teaspoon black pepper

Instructions:

1. Divide salad greens between two large bowls.
2. Top each bowl with 1 can of drained sardines, half the avocado, half the cherry tomatoes, half the red onion, and 1 sliced egg.
3. In a small bowl, whisk together olive oil, lemon juice, Dijon mustard, salt, and pepper.
4. Drizzle dressing over each salad.

Tips:

Budget breakdown: Sardines $2 (often $1 per can), eggs $1, avocado $1.50, greens and vegetables $1. Total: $5.50 for 2 servings.

Give sardines a chance: They're nutritional powerhouses. High in omega-3s, protein, and calcium. And incredibly cheap.

Which sardines: Look for wild-caught sardines in water or olive oil. Avoid ones in tomato sauce (added sugar).

Don't like sardines: Use canned salmon or mackerel instead. Similar price and nutrition.

Make it heartier: Add a hard-boiled egg or two to each salad for extra protein.

Storage: Store components separately. Assemble fresh salads when ready to eat.

Liver & Onions

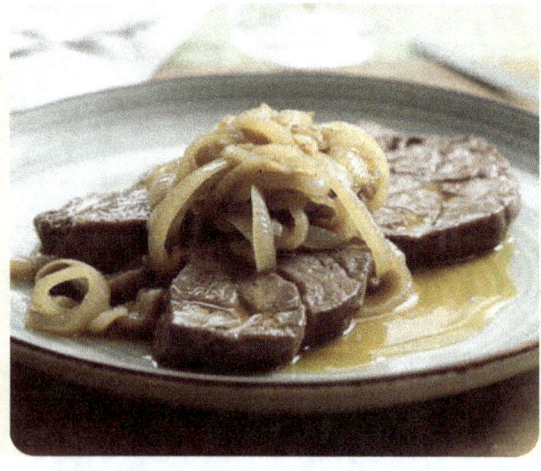

 Quick   Budget-Friendly

 Serves: 4

Prep Time: 10 min

Cook Time: 12 min

Total: 22 min

Cost Per Serving: $1.65

MACROS PER SERVING:

Calories: 285 | Protein: 28g | Fat: 16g | Net Carbs: 6g

Ingredients:

- 1 pound beef liver, sliced ½ inch thick
- 2 large onions, sliced thin
- ½ cup almond flour
- 4 tablespoons butter, divided
- 2 tablespoons olive oil
- ½ cup beef broth
- ¾ teaspoon salt
- ½ teaspoon black pepper
- ½ teaspoon paprika
- ¼ teaspoon garlic powder

Instructions:

1. Pat liver slices dry with paper towels. Season both sides with salt, pepper, paprika, and garlic powder.
2. Place almond flour in a shallow dish. Dredge each liver slice in almond flour, shaking off excess.
3. Heat 2 tablespoons butter and 1 tablespoon olive oil in a large skillet over medium-high heat.
4. Add liver slices (work in batches if needed) and cook for 3-4 minutes per side until browned on the outside but still slightly pink in the center. Transfer to a plate.
5. Add remaining tablespoon olive oil to the skillet. Add sliced onions and reduce heat to medium.
6. Cook onions, stirring occasionally, for 8-10 minutes until soft and caramelized.
7. Add beef broth and remaining 2 tablespoons butter to the skillet. Scrape up any browned bits from the bottom.
8. Return liver to the skillet and spoon onions and sauce over it. Cook for 1-2 minutes until heated through.

Tips:

Budget breakdown: Beef liver is typically $1.50-$2.50 per pound. 1 pound costs about $2, onions $1, almond flour and other ingredients $3. Total: $6 for 4 servings.

Why liver: It's one of the most nutrient-dense foods on earth. Loaded with vitamin A, iron, B vitamins, and protein. And dirt cheap.

Don't overcook: Liver gets tough and grainy when overcooked. Keep it slightly pink in the center.

Milk soak (optional): If you're sensitive to liver's strong flavor, soak slices in milk for 30 minutes before cooking. Rinse and pat dry.

Not for everyone: Liver has a distinctive flavor. If you hate it, you hate it. But it's worth trying once given the nutrition and price.

Storage: Refrigerate for up to 3 days. Best eaten fresh.

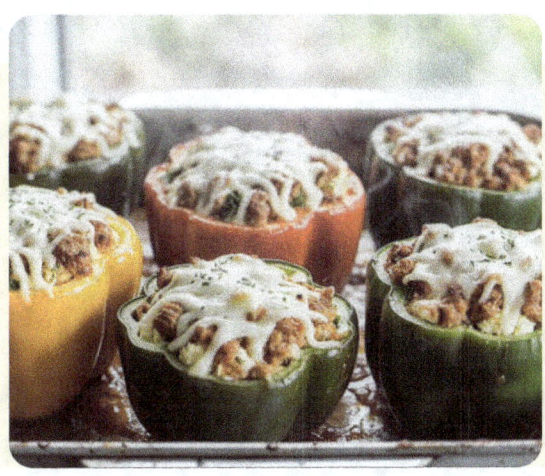

Ground Turkey Stuffed Peppers

 Make-Ahead   Budget-Friendly

 Serves: 6

Prep Time: 15 min

Cook Time: 35 min

Total: 50 min

Cost Per Serving: $2.15

MACROS PER SERVING:

Calories: 320 | Protein: 28g | Fat: 16g | Net Carbs: 9g

Ingredients:

- 1½ pounds ground turkey
- 6 large bell peppers (any color), tops cut off, seeds removed
- 1 can (14.5 oz) diced tomatoes, drained
- 2 cups riced cauliflower
- 1 small onion, diced
- 3 cloves garlic, minced
- 2 tablespoons olive oil
- 2 teaspoons Italian seasoning
- 1 teaspoon paprika
- 1 teaspoon salt
- ½ teaspoon black pepper
- 1½ cups shredded mozzarella cheese

Instructions:

1. Preheat oven to 375°F.
2. Heat olive oil in a large skillet over medium-high heat. Add ground turkey and cook, breaking it up, for 6-8 minutes until browned.
3. Add onion and cook for 3 minutes until softened.
4. Add cauliflower rice, garlic, Italian seasoning, paprika, salt, and pepper. Cook for 3-4 minutes.
5. Add diced tomatoes and stir to combine. Cook for 2 minutes. Remove from heat.
6. Stand bell peppers upright in a 9x13-inch baking dish. If they don't stand well, cut a thin slice off the bottom to create a flat base.
7. Divide turkey mixture evenly among the 6 peppers, packing it in.
8. Pour ½ cup water into the bottom of the baking dish (this helps steam the peppers).
9. Cover dish with foil and bake for 25 minutes.
10. Remove foil, top each pepper with shredded cheese, and bake uncovered for 10 more minutes until cheese is melted and peppers are tender.

Tips:

Budget breakdown: Ground turkey $5, bell peppers $3, cheese $2, cauliflower rice and other ingredients $2. Total: $12 for 6 servings.

Ground turkey tip: It's lean and can be dry. The tomatoes and cheese add moisture and flavor.

Make ahead: Stuff peppers, cover, and refrigerate for up to 24 hours before baking. Add 5-10 minutes to cooking time since they're cold.

Freeze it: Freeze stuffed peppers (before baking) for up to 3 months. Bake from frozen, adding 15-20 minutes to cooking time.

Ground beef: Works great if it's cheaper than turkey in your area.

Storage: Refrigerate for up to 5 days. Reheat in microwave or oven.

Chicken Bone Broth (From Scraps)

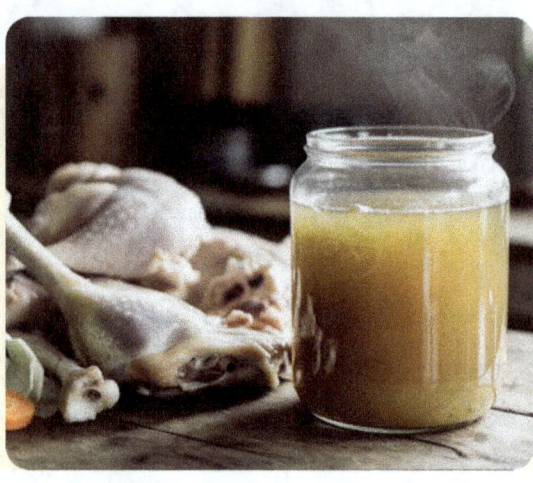

Make-Ahead   Budget-Friendly

🍽 Serves: 8 cups

✂ Prep Time: 10 min

🍲 Cook Time: 4-24 hours

🕐 Total: 4-24 hours

💲 Cost Per Serving (1 cup): $.15

MACROS PER SERVING (1 cup):

Calories: 40 | Protein: 10g | Fat: 0g | Net Carbs: 0g

Ingredients:

- Bones and carcass from 1-2 roasted chickens (or 2-3 pounds chicken bones)
- 2 tablespoons apple cider vinegar
- 1 large onion, quartered (no need to peel)
- 2 carrots, cut into large chunks
- 2 celery stalks, cut into large chunks
- 4 cloves garlic, smashed
- 2 bay leaves
- 1 tablespoon black peppercorns
- 1 tablespoon salt (or to taste)
- 12 cups cold water

Instructions:

Slow Cooker Method (recommended):

1. Place chicken bones and carcass in slow cooker.

2. Add vegetables, garlic, bay leaves, peppercorns, and apple cider vinegar.

3. Pour in cold water until bones are covered (about 12 cups).

4. Cover and cook on low for 12-24 hours. The longer it cooks, the richer and more gelatinous the broth.

5. In the last hour of cooking, add salt to taste.

6. Strain broth through a fine-mesh strainer or cheesecloth. Discard solids.

7. Let broth cool, then refrigerate. Fat will rise to the top and solidify. You can remove it or stir it back in.

Stovetop Method:

1. Place bones and all ingredients in a large pot.

2. Bring to a boil, then immediately reduce to a bare simmer.

3. Simmer for 4-6 hours, checking occasionally to ensure bones stay covered with water.

4. Strain and cool as above.

Instant Pot Method:

1. Place bones and all ingredients in Instant Pot.

2. Pressure cook on high for 120 minutes with natural release.

3. Strain and cool as above.

Tips:

Budget breakdown: If you save bones from chickens you already bought and cooked, this is essentially FREE. You're using what you'd otherwise throw away.

Save your bones: Every time you eat chicken, save the bones in a freezer bag. When the bag is full, make broth.

Vinegar is important: It helps extract minerals from the bones into the broth.

Gelatinous = good: When your broth cools, it should gel like Jello. This means it's rich in collagen and gelatin. That's what you want.

Storage: Refrigerate for up to 5 days or freeze for up to 6 months. Freeze in ice cube trays for small portions.

Uses: Drink it plain, use as a base for soups, cook cauliflower rice in it, add to sauces, or use anywhere you need liquid in cooking.

CHAPTER 4 SUMMARY

You now have 15 budget-friendly recipes that prove eating high-protein, low-carb doesn't require unlimited funds. Here's how to make these recipes work for your budget:

The Core Budget Strategy:

1. **Plan meals around sales.** Check weekly ads before shopping. When chicken thighs are $1.50/pound, plan 3 chicken recipes that week.
2. **Buy in bulk when prices drop.** Ground beef under $3/pound? Buy 10 pounds. Portion and freeze.
3. **Use the whole animal.** Save bones for broth. Use bacon grease for cooking. Nothing goes to waste.
4. **Embrace cheaper cuts.** Chicken leg quarters, pork shoulder, and ground meat are your friends. They taste just as good (often better) than expensive cuts.
5. **Make eggs central.** At $0.25-$0.50 per egg, they're the most economical protein on earth.

My Budget Weekly Meal Plan:

Here's what an actual budget week looks like at my house:

Total weekly cost for 2 people: $40-50

- **Monday:** Ground Beef & Egg Scramble ($1.75 per serving × 2 = $3.50)
- **Tuesday:** Egg Roll in a Bowl ($1.65 per serving × 2 = $3.30)
- **Wednesday:** Leftovers from Monday and Tuesday
- **Thursday:** Cabbage Roll Bowl ($1.85 per serving × 2 = $3.70)
- **Friday:** Tuna Salad Lettuce Boats ($2.25 per serving × 2 = $4.50)
- **Saturday:** Chicken Leg Quarters with roasted vegetables ($1.25 + $1 vegetables = $4.50)
- **Sunday:** Meal prep day - Make Pork Shoulder Pulled Pork for the following week

The Freezer is Your Friend:

These recipes freeze exceptionally well:

- Pork Shoulder Pulled Pork (up to 4 months)
- Ground Beef Cauliflower Casserole (up to 3 months)
- Beef & Veggie Soup (up to 3 months)
- Ground Turkey Stuffed Peppers (up to 3 months)
- Chicken Bone Broth (up to 6 months)

Cook once, eat for weeks.

Price Comparison: Budget Proteins

Here's what to expect to pay (per 4 oz cooked serving):

- **Eggs:** $0.50 for 2-3 eggs (18-21g protein)
- **Chicken leg quarters:** $0.50-$0.75 (35-40g protein)
- **Ground beef (on sale):** $0.75-$1.00 (20-25g protein)

- **Ground pork:** $0.60-$0.90 (20-25g protein)
- **Canned tuna:** $0.75-$1.00 (20-25g protein)
- **Pork shoulder:** $0.60-$0.80 (25-30g protein)
- **Chicken thighs:** $0.75-$1.25 (25-30g protein)

For comparison, that $8 fast food meal provides about 20-25g protein and costs more than these home-cooked options that give you 25-40g protein.

Where to Save More Money:

1. **Shop discount grocers:** Aldi, Lidl, ethnic markets often beat mainstream grocery stores by 20-40%.
2. **Buy manager's specials:** Meat marked down for quick sale is perfect for immediate cooking or freezing.
3. **Skip pre-cut everything:** Whole chickens, whole cabbages, block cheese. Do the cutting yourself and save 30-50%.
4. **Use frozen vegetables:** Often cheaper than fresh, already prepped, and just as nutritious.
5. **Make your own broth:** From bones you'd throw away anyway. Saves $3-5 per week.
6. **Buy generic brands:** Store brands are often identical to name brands at half the price.

Common Budget Mistakes:

1. **Buying boneless, skinless chicken breasts.** They're the most expensive chicken cut and the easiest to overcook. Thighs are cheaper and juicier.
2. **Shopping without a list.** Impulse purchases kill budgets. Plan first, buy only what's on the list.
3. **Throwing away bones and scraps.** That's free broth you're discarding.
4. **Not using your freezer.** Buy in bulk when prices are good, portion, and freeze.
5. **Buying "keto" products.** Expensive specialty foods aren't necessary. Real food is cheaper.

The Reality:

Yes, you can eat high-protein, low-carb on a tight budget. It requires:

- Planning around sales
- Doing some prep work yourself
- Using cheaper cuts and proteins
- Being willing to eat the same thing multiple times a week
- Making smart substitutions

But it's absolutely doable. These 15 recipes prove it.

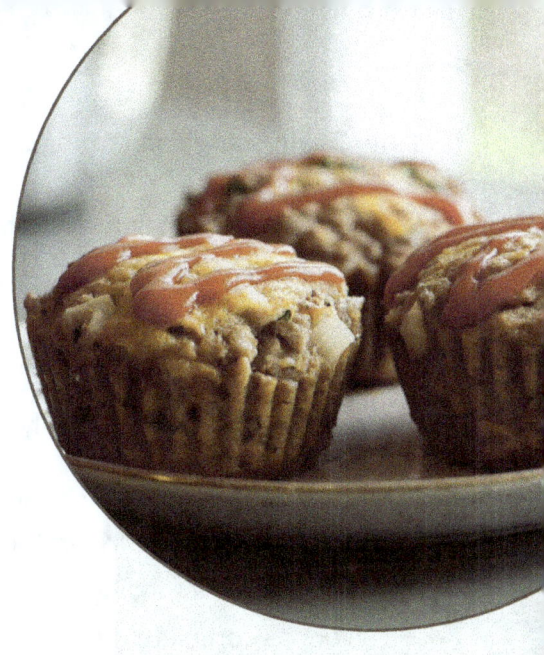

This is the chapter that will change your life.

I know that sounds dramatic, but I mean it. When I started batch cooking on Sundays, everything got easier. Weeknight dinners stopped being a source of stress. I stopped ordering takeout because I was too tired to cook. I saved money. I lost weight. I actually stuck to my eating plan because the food was just... there, ready to go.

Make-ahead meals and meal prep aren't about being some organized superhuman who has their entire life color-coded and scheduled. It's about being a regular person who's tired on Tuesday and doesn't want to think about what's for dinner.

The concept is simple: spend 2-3 hours one day cooking multiple meals or components. Store them properly. Reheat and eat throughout the week. That's it.

THE TWO APPROACHES TO MEAL PREP:

Approach 1: Full Meals Cook complete meals, portion them into containers, refrigerate or freeze. Grab a container, reheat, eat. This is perfect for lunches or if you eat alone.

Approach 2: Meal Components Cook proteins and vegetables separately. Mix and match throughout the week to create different meals. This prevents boredom and works better for families where people want variety.

Both work. Most people (including me) use a combination of both.

My Sunday Meal Prep Routine:
Here's what 2-3 hours on Sunday afternoon actually looks like:

Hour 1 (Oven does the work):
- Put a pork shoulder or beef roast in the slow cooker (10 minutes of hands-on time)
- Season and roast 3-4 pounds of chicken thighs (5 minutes prep, 40 minutes hands-off)
- While chicken roasts, hard-boil a dozen eggs (5 minutes prep, 12 minutes hands-off)
- Prep vegetables: wash lettuce, chop peppers and cucumbers, portion into containers

Hour 2 (Stovetop work):
- Brown 2 pounds of ground beef with taco seasoning (15 minutes)
- Make a batch of meatballs or meatloaf muffins (20 minutes prep, 20 minutes baking)
- Cook bacon in the oven (5 minutes prep, 15 minutes hands-off)
- Make cauliflower rice if running low (10 minutes)

Hour 3 (Finishing and storing):
- Shred the pork or beef
- Portion everything into containers
- Label with dates
- Clean up

The Recipes in This Chapter:
Every recipe here is specifically designed to:

- Make large batches (4-8+ servings)
- Store well in the refrigerator (4-5 days) or freezer (2-3 months)
- Reheat without losing quality
- Work as complete meals or components for other dishes
- Actually taste good on day 4

These aren't just "recipes that make leftovers." These are recipes engineered for meal prep success.

Storage and Food Safety:
Let me be clear about this because it matters:

Refrigerator (40°F or below):
- Cooked proteins: 3-4 days
- Hard-boiled eggs: 1 week
- Cooked vegetables: 3-4 days
- Soups and stews: 4-5 days

Freezer (0°F or below):
- Cooked meat: 2-3 months
- Soups and stews: 3-4 months
- Meatballs and meatloaf: 2-3 months
- Cooked egg dishes: 2-3 months

Critical Rules:
1. Cool food to room temperature before refrigerating (but don't leave out more than 2 hours)
2. Store in airtight containers
3. Label everything with dates
4. Reheat to 165°F internal temperature
5. If it smells off, throw it out

Containers That Actually Work:
After years of trial and error, here's what I use:

For refrigerator storage:
- Glass containers with locking lids (Pyrex, Glasslock)
- Meal prep containers with divided sections (for full meals)

- Mason jars (for soups, salads, overnight prep)

For freezer storage:
- Heavy-duty freezer bags (portion food, press out air, freeze flat)
- Aluminum pans with lids (for casseroles)
- Vacuum-sealed bags if you have a sealer (extends freezer life)

Don't use:
- Cheap plastic containers that warp in the microwave
- Containers without tight-sealing lids (causes freezer burn)
- Anything not labeled freezer-safe

Reheating Without Ruining Everything:
Microwave (fastest):

- Remove lid or vent container
- Heat on 70% power for longer time rather than 100% power quickly
- Stir halfway through if possible
- Add a tablespoon of water to prevent drying out

Oven (best for maintaining texture):
- Preheat to 350°F
- Cover with foil to prevent drying
- Heat until internal temperature reaches 165°F
- Remove foil for last 5 minutes if you want crispiness

Stovetop (best for soups and stews):
- Use low-medium heat
- Stir frequently
- Add liquid if needed

What Makes These Recipes Special:
Every recipe in this chapter has been tested for:

- **Reheating quality:** Tastes good on day 1 and day 4
- **Texture stability:** Doesn't get mushy or dry when stored
- **Versatility:** Can be used in multiple ways
- **Actual taste:** These aren't sad desk lunches. They're meals you'll look forward to eating.

Now let's cook some food that actually survives the week.

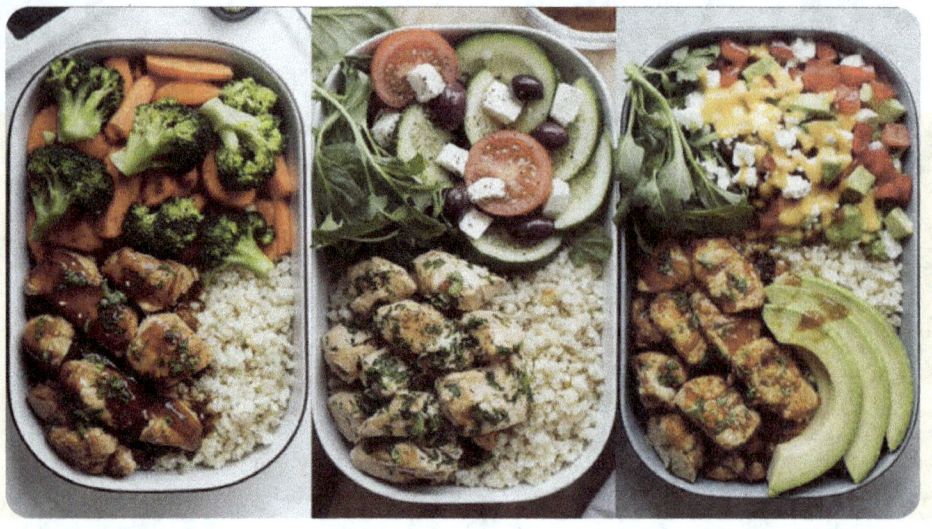

Meal Prep Chicken Bowls (3 Variations)

Make-Ahead   Budget-Friendly

Serves: 6 (2 of each variation)

Prep Time: 25 min

Cook Time: 40 min

Total: 65 min

Cost Per Serving: $2.75

MACROS PER SERVING (average):
Calories: 395 | Protein: 38g |
Fat: 22g | Net Carbs: 7g

Instructions:

Prep the chicken:
1. Preheat oven to 400°F. Line a baking sheet with parchment paper.
2. Pat chicken dry and season all sides with olive oil, salt, pepper, and garlic powder.
3. Arrange on baking sheet and bake for 25-30 minutes (breasts) or 30-35 minutes (thighs) until internal temperature reaches 165°F.
4. Let cool for 10 minutes, then slice, dice, or shred depending on which variations you're making.

Prep the vegetables:
1. Steam or roast broccoli for 5-7 minutes until tender-crisp.
2. Make or heat cauliflower rice according to package directions.
3. Dice cucumbers and tomatoes, shred carrots, wash greens.

Assemble the bowls:
1. Divide chicken into 6 portions (about 6 oz each).
2. Get 6 meal prep containers with lids.
3. Assemble 2 of each variation according to the ingredients listed above.
4. Keep any wet ingredients (dressings, salsa, sour cream) in small separate containers if you prefer, or add directly to the bowl.

Storage and reheating:
1. Seal containers and refrigerate for up to 4 days.
2. To reheat: Remove any ingredients you want cold (greens, avocado, sour cream). Microwave on 70% power for 2-3 minutes, stirring halfway. Add cold ingredients back.

Tips:

Budget breakdown: Chicken $9, vegetables $4, cheese/feta $2, other ingredients $2. Total: $17 for 6 meals, or $2.75 per meal.

Make it easier: Buy a rotisserie chicken. Skip the cooking, just shred and portion. Saves 30 minutes.

Customize: Don't like these variations? Create your own. Formula is: protein + vegetable + healthy fat + sauce/seasoning.

Keep dressings separate: If you meal prep more than 2 days ahead, pack dressings in small containers to prevent sogginess.

Freeze it: These don't freeze well due to the fresh vegetables. Make only what you'll eat in 4 days.

Switch proteins: Ground beef, pork, shrimp, or tofu all work using the same bowl structure.

Base Ingredients (for all bowls):
- 3 pounds boneless, skinless chicken breasts or thighs
- 2 tablespoons olive oil
- 2 teaspoons salt
- 1 teaspoon black pepper
- 1 teaspoon garlic powder

Variation 1: Teriyaki Bowl
Per bowl:
- 6 oz cooked chicken, sliced
- 1 cup cauliflower rice
- ½ cup broccoli florets, steamed
- ¼ cup shredded carrots
- 2 tablespoons teriyaki sauce (sugar-free or homemade)
- 1 teaspoon sesame seeds

Variation 2: Mediterranean Bowl
Per bowl:
- 6 oz cooked chicken, diced
- 1 cup mixed greens
- ¼ cup cucumber, diced
- ¼ cup cherry tomatoes, halved
- 2 tablespoons crumbled feta cheese
- 2 tablespoons Greek vinaigrette
- 5 Kalamata olives

Variation 3: Tex-Mex Bowl
Per bowl:
- 6 oz cooked chicken, shredded
- 1 cup cauliflower rice
- ¼ cup black beans (optional, adds 5g net carbs)
- ¼ cup shredded cheese
- 2 tablespoons salsa
- 2 tablespoons sour cream
- ¼ avocado, sliced

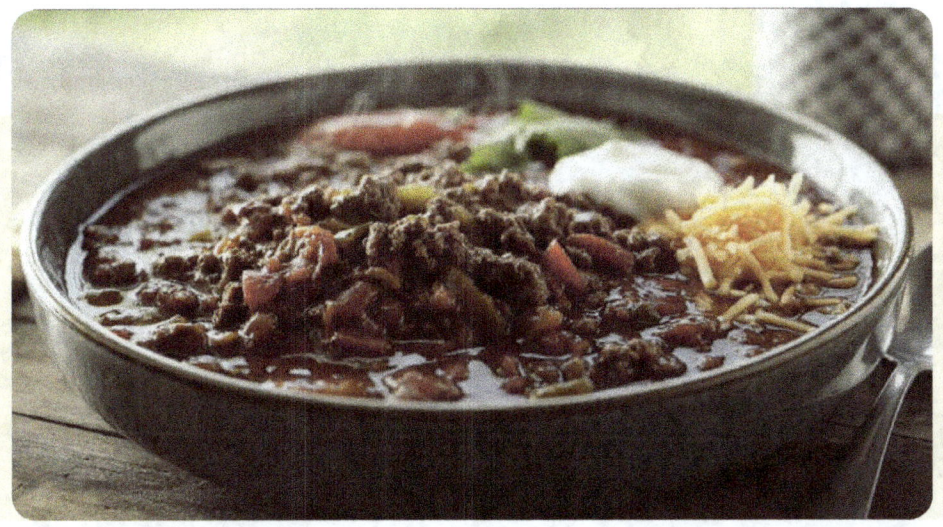

Beef Chili (No Beans)

Make-Ahead   One-Pan   Budget-Friendly

Serves: 8
Prep Time: 15 min
Cook Time: 45 min
Total: 60 min
Cost Per Serving: $2.25

MACROS PER SERVING:
Calories: 380 | Protein: 32g | Fat: 24g | Net Carbs: 8g

Instructions:

1. Heat olive oil in a large pot or Dutch oven over medium-high heat.

2. Add ground beef and cook, breaking it up with a spoon, for 8-10 minutes until browned. Don't drain the fat.

3. Add onion and bell peppers. Cook for 5 minutes until softened.

4. Add garlic, chili powder, cumin, paprika, oregano, salt, pepper, and cayenne (if using). Stir for 1 minute until spices are fragrant.

5. Add crushed tomatoes, diced tomatoes (with juice), tomato paste, and beef broth. Stir to combine everything.

6. Bring to a boil, then reduce heat to low. Partially cover and simmer for 30-40 minutes, stirring occasionally. The longer it simmers, the better it tastes.

7. Taste and adjust seasoning if needed. If it's too thick, add more broth. If too thin, simmer uncovered to reduce.

Tips:

Budget breakdown: Ground beef $7.50, tomatoes $4, peppers and onion $2, spices $1.50, broth $1. Total: $16 for 8 servings.

Why no beans: Keeps carbs low. If you want beans, add 1-2 cans of drained black or kidney beans (adds 5-8g net carbs per serving).

Slow cooker method: Brown beef first, then transfer everything to slow cooker. Cook on low for 6-8 hours or high for 3-4 hours.

Instant Pot method: Use sauté function to brown beef and cook vegetables. Add everything else, pressure cook on high for 15 minutes with quick release.

Storage: Refrigerate for up to 5 days or freeze for up to 4 months. Gets better with time as flavors meld.

Serving suggestions: Top with cheese, sour cream, and avocado. Serve over cauliflower rice or eat as a stew.

Meal prep: Portion into containers. Grab one, heat, top with your favorites. Perfect easy lunch or dinner.

Ingredients:

- 2½ pounds ground beef (80/20)
- 1 can (28 oz) crushed tomatoes
- 1 can (14.5 oz) diced tomatoes, undrained
- 1 can (6 oz) tomato paste
- 2 cups beef broth
- 2 large bell peppers (any color), diced
- 1 large onion, diced
- 4 cloves garlic, minced
- 3 tablespoons chili powder
- 2 tablespoons cumin
- 1 tablespoon paprika
- 1 teaspoon oregano
- 1 teaspoon salt
- ½ teaspoon black pepper
- ½ teaspoon cayenne pepper (optional)
- 2 tablespoons olive oil

For serving (optional):
- Shredded cheddar cheese
- Sour cream
- Diced avocado
- Sliced jalapeños
- Fresh cilantro

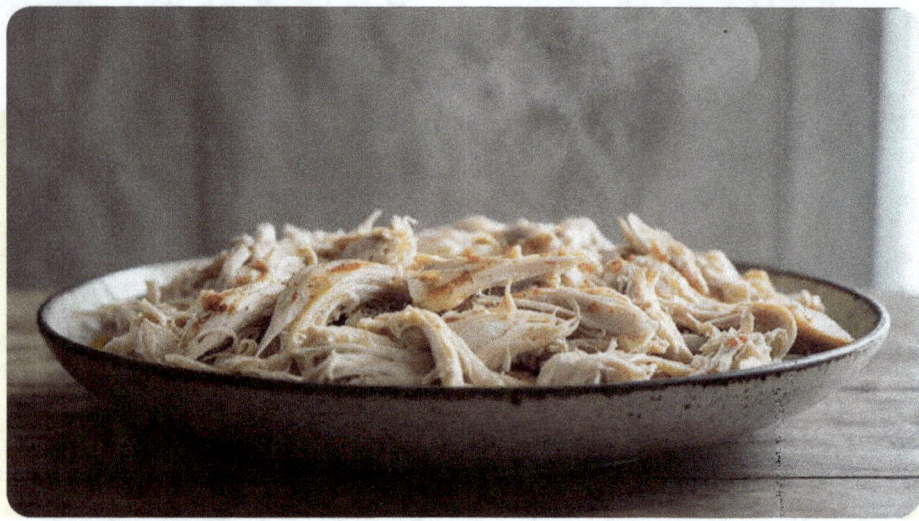

Pulled Chicken (Multiple Uses)

Make-Ahead   Budget-Friendly

🍽 Serves: 8

✂ Prep Time: 10 min

🍲 Cook Time: 4-6 hours (slow cooker)

⏱ Total: 4-6 hours

$ Cost Per Serving: $1.75

MACROS PER SERVING:
Calories: 245 | Protein: 36g | Fat: 10g | Net Carbs: 2g

Ingredients:

- 4 pounds boneless, skinless chicken breasts or thighs
- 1 cup chicken broth
- 2 tablespoons olive oil
- 1 tablespoon paprika
- 1 tablespoon garlic powder
- 1 tablespoon onion powder
- 2 teaspoons cumin
- 2 teaspoons salt
- 1 teaspoon black pepper
- ½ teaspoon cayenne pepper (optional)

Instructions:

Slow Cooker Method:
1. Place chicken in slow cooker.
2. In a small bowl, mix paprika, garlic powder, onion powder, cumin, salt, pepper, and cayenne (if using).
3. Rub spice mixture all over chicken.
4. Drizzle with olive oil and pour chicken broth around the chicken.
5. Cover and cook on low for 6-8 hours or on high for 3-4 hours, until chicken is very tender and shreds easily.
6. Remove chicken from slow cooker and shred with two forks.
7. Return shredded chicken to slow cooker and stir to coat with cooking liquid. Let sit for 5-10 minutes.
8. Use a slotted spoon to portion chicken, leaving most of the liquid behind (or keep it for moisture if storing).

Instant Pot Method:
1. Season chicken with spice mixture.
2. Place chicken in Instant Pot with olive oil and broth.
3. Pressure cook on high for 15 minutes with natural release.
4. Shred and proceed as above.

Oven Method:
1. Preheat oven to 350°F.
2. Place seasoned chicken in a baking dish. Add broth and drizzle with olive oil.
3. Cover tightly with foil.
4. Bake for 45-60 minutes until chicken shreds easily.
5. Shred and proceed as above.

Tips:

Budget breakdown: Chicken $12 (often on sale for $2-3/pound), broth $1, spices $1. Total: $14 for 8 servings.

Thighs vs. breasts: Thighs stay moister and have more flavor. Breasts are leaner. Both work perfectly.

Storage: Refrigerate for up to 5 days or freeze for up to 4 months. Portion into 1-2 cup containers for easy use.

Ways to use pulled chicken:
- Taco bowls or lettuce wraps
- Chicken salad (mix with mayo, celery, onion)
- Breakfast scrambles
- On top of salads
- Stuffed in peppers or tomatoes
- Mixed into cauliflower rice
- Buffalo chicken dip
- Chicken soup (add to broth with vegetables)
- Pizza topping
- Straight out of the container with hot sauce

Flavor variations:
- **Mexican:** Add 2 tablespoons chili powder and juice of 1 lime
- **BBQ:** Toss shredded chicken with sugar-free BBQ sauce
- **Buffalo:** Mix with buffalo sauce and butter
- **Italian:** Use Italian seasoning instead of cumin

Meal prep star: Make this every 2 weeks. Use it for 8+ different meals. Never gets boring because you can flavor it differently each time.

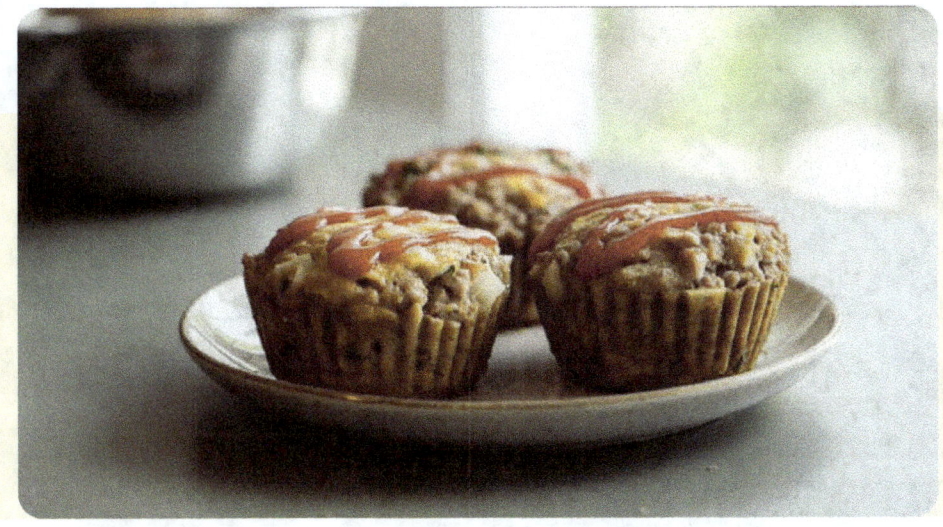

Meatloaf Muffins

Make-Ahead Budget-Friendly

Serves: 12 (1 muffin per serving)

Prep Time: 15 min

Cook Time: 25 min

Total: 40 min

Cost Per Serving: $0.85

MACROS PER SERVING:
Calories: 215 | Protein: 18g | Fat: 14g | Net Carbs: 3g

Ingredients:

- 2 pounds ground beef (80/20)
- 2 large eggs
- ½ cup almond flour
- ½ cup grated Parmesan cheese
- ½ cup diced onion
- 2 cloves garlic, minced
- ¼ cup sugar-free ketchup
- 2 tablespoons Worcestershire sauce
- 1 tablespoon Dijon mustard
- 1 teaspoon salt
- ½ teaspoon black pepper
- 1 teaspoon Italian seasoning
- Cooking spray

For topping (optional):
- ¼ cup sugar-free ketchup
- 1 tablespoon Dijon mustard

Instructions:

1. Preheat oven to 375°F. Spray a 12-cup muffin tin generously with cooking spray.
2. In a large bowl, combine ground beef, eggs, almond flour, Parmesan cheese, onion, garlic, ketchup, Worcestershire sauce, Dijon mustard, salt, pepper, and Italian seasoning.
3. Mix with your hands until just combined. Don't overmix or the meatloaf will be tough.
4. Divide mixture evenly among the 12 muffin cups, pressing down gently and rounding the tops.
5. If using topping, mix ketchup and mustard in a small bowl. Brush over the top of each muffin.
6. Bake for 22-25 minutes until internal temperature reaches 160°F.
7. Let cool in the pan for 5 minutes, then run a butter knife around the edges and pop them out.
8. Cool completely before storing.

Tips:

Budget breakdown: Ground beef $6, eggs $1, almond flour $2, cheese $1, other ingredients $1. Total: $11 for 12 muffins.

Why muffins instead of loaf: They cook faster, portion control is built-in, they freeze individually, and they're portable.

Storage: Refrigerate for up to 4 days or freeze for up to 3 months. Freeze on a baking sheet first, then transfer to a freezer bag.

Reheating: From fridge, microwave 1 muffin for 45-60 seconds. From frozen, microwave for 90 seconds to 2 minutes.

Meal prep use: Pair with roasted vegetables for a complete meal, or eat cold as a snack.

Ground turkey: Works great for a leaner version. Add 1 tablespoon olive oil to the mixture to keep them moist.

Add vegetables: Mix in ½ cup diced bell peppers, mushrooms, or zucchini for extra nutrition.

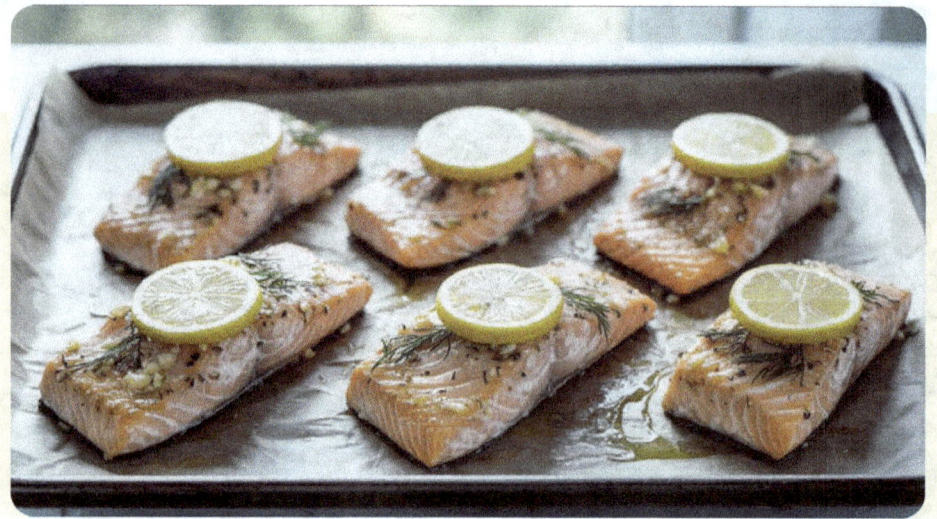

Baked Salmon Portions

Make-Ahead

 Serves: 6

Prep Time: 5 min

Cook Time: 12 min

Total: 17 min

Cost Per Serving: $3.50
(when salmon is on sale)

MACROS PER SERVING:
Calories: 320 | Protein: 34g |
Fat: 19g | Net Carbs: 1g

Ingredients:
- 2 pounds salmon fillet, cut into 6 portions
- 3 tablespoons olive oil
- 2 tablespoons lemon juice
- 4 cloves garlic, minced
- 2 teaspoons dried dill
  (or 1 tablespoon fresh)
- 1 teaspoon paprika
- ¾ teaspoon salt
- ½ teaspoon black pepper
- Lemon slices for garnish

Instructions:

1. Preheat oven to 425°F. Line a large baking sheet with parchment paper.

2. Pat salmon portions dry with paper towels. Place on baking sheet, skin-side down if skin-on.

3. In a small bowl, whisk together olive oil, lemon juice, garlic, dill, paprika, salt, and pepper.

4. Brush mixture generously over each salmon portion.

5. Place a thin lemon slice on top of each portion if desired.

6. Bake for 10-12 minutes until salmon is opaque and flakes easily with a fork. Don't overcook.

Tips:

Budget breakdown: Salmon is expensive ($8-12/pound) but often goes on sale. Stock up when it's under $8/pound and freeze.

Storage: Refrigerate cooked salmon for up to 3 days. It doesn't freeze as well as other proteins, but you can freeze for up to 2 months if needed.

Eat cold or hot: Cooked salmon is delicious cold on salads or reheated gently.

Reheating: Don't overcook it again. Microwave on 50% power for 30-60 seconds just until warm, or eat cold.

Meal prep uses:
- On top of salads
- With roasted vegetables
- In scrambled eggs for breakfast
- Flaked into cauliflower rice
- Mixed with mayo and celery for salmon salad
- With steamed asparagus and butter

Flavor variations:
- **Asian:** Use soy sauce, ginger, and sesame oil instead of lemon and dill
- **Mediterranean:** Use oregano, basil, and sun-dried tomatoes
- **Cajun:** Use Cajun seasoning instead of dill and paprika

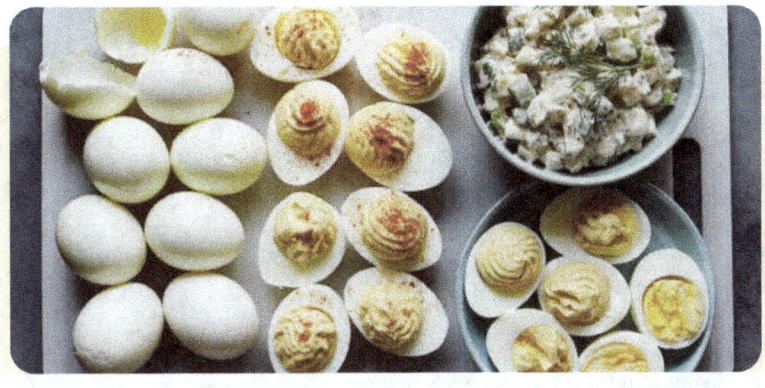

Hard-Boiled Egg Variations

Quick · Make-Ahead · Budget-Friendly

🍽 Serves: 12 eggs

🍳 Cook Time: 12 min

💲 COST PER SERVING (per egg): $0.30

✂ Prep Time: 5 min

⏱ Total: 17 min

MACROS PER EGG (plain):
Calories: 70 | Protein: 6g | Fat: 5g | Net Carbs: 1g

Base Instructions for Perfect Hard-Boiled Eggs:

Stovetop Method (recommended):
1. Place eggs in a single layer in a pot. Cover with cold water by 1 inch.
2. Bring to a rolling boil over high heat.
3. As soon as water boils, remove from heat, cover, and let sit for 12 minutes.
4. Transfer eggs to an ice bath (bowl of ice water) and let cool for 5 minutes.
5. Peel when ready to use, or store unpeeled in the refrigerator for up to 1 week.

Instant Pot Method:
1. Place eggs on the trivet in Instant Pot. Add 1 cup water.
2. Pressure cook on high for 5 minutes with quick release.
3. Transfer to ice bath immediately.

Peeling Tip:

Gently crack egg all over, then roll between your hands. Start peeling from the wider end where the air pocket is.

VARIATION 1: Classic Deviled Eggs

🍽 Makes: 24 deviled egg halves

Additional Macros per half: +15 calories, +1g fat

Instructions:
1. Cut eggs in half lengthwise. Remove yolks to a bowl.
2. Mash yolks with a fork until crumbly.
3. Add mayonnaise, mustard, vinegar, salt, and pepper. Mix until smooth and creamy.
4. Spoon or pipe mixture back into egg white halves.
5. Sprinkle with paprika.
6. Refrigerate for up to 3 days in an airtight container.

Additional Ingredients:
- 12 hard-boiled eggs, peeled
- ½ cup mayonnaise
- 2 teaspoons Dijon mustard
- 1 teaspoon white vinegar or lemon juice
- ¼ teaspoon salt
- ⅛ teaspoon black pepper
- Paprika for garnish

VARIATION 2: Egg Salad

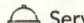 Serves: 4

Macros per serving: Calories: 285 | Protein: 18g | Fat: 22g | Net Carbs: 2g

Instructions:
1. In a large bowl, chop hard-boiled eggs into chunks (not too fine).
2. Add mayonnaise, mustard, celery, red onion, dill, salt, and pepper.
3. Mix gently until combined.
4. Taste and adjust seasoning.
5. Refrigerate for at least 30 minutes before serving.
6. Store in an airtight container for up to 4 days.

Serving suggestions:

In lettuce wraps, stuffed in tomatoes or avocados, on cucumber slices, or with a fork straight from the container.

Additional Ingredients:
- 8 hard-boiled eggs, peeled and chopped
- ½ cup mayonnaise
- 1 tablespoon Dijon mustard
- ¼ cup diced celery
- 2 tablespoons diced red onion
- 1 tablespoon fresh dill, chopped (or 1 teaspoon dried)
- ½ teaspoon salt
- ¼ teaspoon black pepper

VARIATION 3: Jammy Eggs (for salad toppings)

For runny yolks, adjust cooking time:

- Stovetop: 8-9 minutes instead of 12
- Instant Pot: 3 minutes instead of 5

Use for:

- Topping salads
- Serving with roasted vegetables
- Adding to ramen or soup
- Protein snack with everything bagel seasoning

Tips:

Fresh vs. old eggs: Older eggs (1-2 weeks old) peel easier than very fresh eggs.

Meal prep strategy: Hard-boil a dozen eggs every Sunday. They last all week and provide instant protein.

Quick breakfast: Eat 2-3 plain hard-boiled eggs with salt and pepper. Takes 30 seconds.

Portable protein: Pack hard-boiled eggs in your lunch. Easy, affordable protein that doesn't need refrigeration for a few hours.

Color the yolks: Add beet juice or turmeric to the boiling water for colorful deviled eggs (great for parties).

Storage: Store hard-boiled eggs in the refrigerator for up to 1 week. Keep them in the shell until ready to use for best freshness.

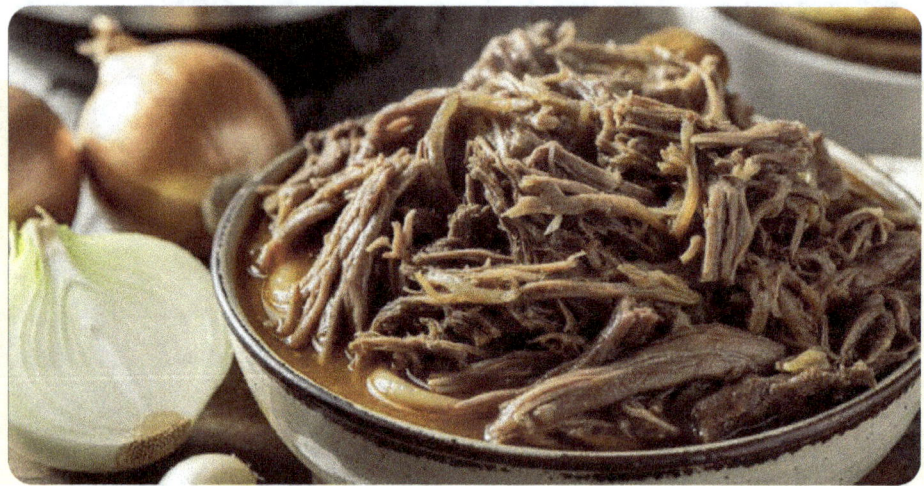

Shredded Beef (Slow Cooker)

Make-Ahead   Budget-Friendly

Serves: 10

Prep Time: 10 min

Cook Time: 8 hours

Total: 8 hours 10 min

Cost Per Serving: $2.15

MACROS PER SERVING:
Calories: 340 | Protein: 35g | Fat: 20g | Net Carbs: 3g

Instructions:

1. Trim excess fat from chuck roast (leave some for flavor). Pat dry with paper towels.
2. In a small bowl, mix paprika, cumin, chili powder, salt, pepper, and oregano. Rub all over the roast.
3. Optional but recommended: Sear the roast in a hot skillet with 1 tablespoon oil for 3-4 minutes per side until browned. This adds flavor but can be skipped if you're short on time.
4. Place onion and garlic in the bottom of slow cooker.
5. Place roast on top of onions and garlic.
6. In a bowl, whisk together beef broth, Worcestershire sauce, apple cider vinegar, and tomato paste. Pour around the roast.
7. Add bay leaves.
8. Cover and cook on low for 8-10 hours or on high for 5-6 hours, until beef is very tender and shreds easily.
9. Remove beef from slow cooker. Shred with two forks, discarding any large pieces of fat.
10. Remove bay leaves from liquid. Skim excess fat from the surface if desired.
11. Return shredded beef to slow cooker and stir to coat with liquid. Let sit for 5-10 minutes.

Ingredients:

- 4 pounds beef chuck roast
- 2 cups beef broth
- 1 large onion, sliced
- 6 cloves garlic, smashed
- 3 tablespoons Worcestershire sauce
- 2 tablespoons apple cider vinegar
- 2 tablespoons tomato paste
- 1 tablespoon paprika
- 1 tablespoon cumin
- 1 tablespoon chili powder
- 2 teaspoons salt
- 1 teaspoon black pepper
- 1 teaspoon oregano
- 3 bay leaves

Tips:

Budget breakdown: Chuck roast $20-25 (often on sale for $4-6/pound), broth $1.50, other ingredients $2. Total: $23.50 for 10 servings.

Chuck roast: This is an economical cut that becomes incredibly tender when slow-cooked. Buy on sale and freeze until needed.

Instant Pot method: Sear meat using sauté function, add all ingredients, pressure cook on high for 60 minutes with natural release.

Storage: Refrigerate for up to 5 days or freeze for up to 4 months. The liquid helps keep it moist.

Ways to use shredded beef:

- Taco bowls or lettuce wraps
- On top of cauliflower rice
- Stuffed in peppers
- Mixed into scrambled eggs
- Beef and cabbage bowls
- Philly cheesesteak bowls (add sautéed peppers and onions, top with cheese)
- Soup (add to broth with vegetables)
- Italian beef (add Italian seasoning and pepperoncini)

Flavor the liquid: Save the cooking liquid. It's flavorful and can be used as a base for soup or reduced into a gravy.

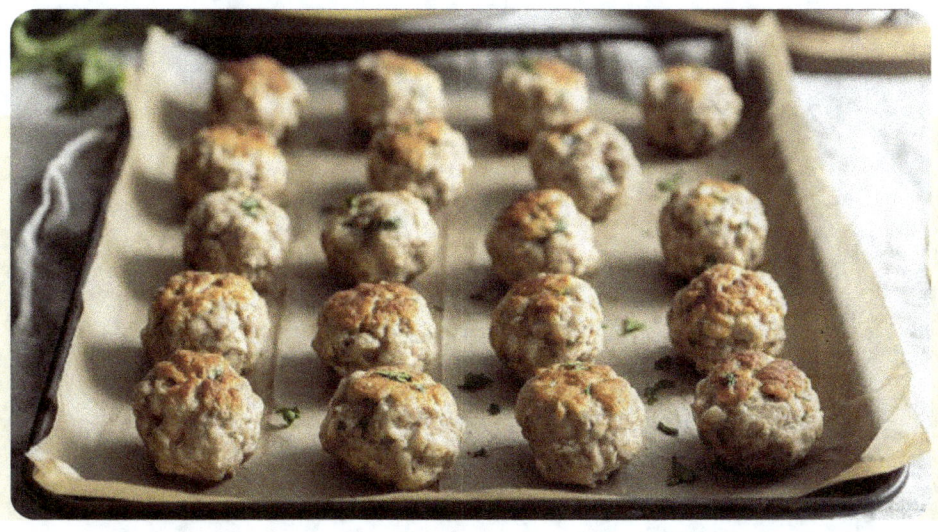

Turkey Meatballs

Make-Ahead   Budget-Friendly

Serves: 8 (4 meatballs per serving)

Prep Time: 15 min

Cook Time: 20 min

Total: 35 min

Cost Per Serving: $1.85

MACROS PER SERVING (4 meatballs):
Calories: 255 | Protein: 28g |
Fat: 14g | Net Carbs: 3g

Instructions:

1. Preheat oven to 400°F. Line two baking sheets with parchment paper.

2. In a large bowl, combine ground turkey, eggs, almond flour, Parmesan cheese, parsley, garlic, Italian seasoning, salt, pepper, red pepper flakes (if using), and olive oil.

3. Mix gently with your hands until just combined. Don't overmix.

4. Using a cookie scoop or your hands, form into 32 meatballs (about 2 tablespoons each).

5. Place meatballs on prepared baking sheets, spacing them about 1 inch apart.

6. Bake for 18-20 minutes until golden brown and cooked through (internal temperature 165°F).

Ingredients:

- 2 pounds ground turkey
- 2 large eggs
- ½ cup almond flour
- ½ cup grated Parmesan cheese
- ¼ cup fresh parsley, chopped (or 2 tablespoons dried)
- 4 cloves garlic, minced
- 1 tablespoon Italian seasoning
- 1 teaspoon salt
- ½ teaspoon black pepper
- ¼ teaspoon red pepper flakes (optional)
- 2 tablespoons olive oil (for added moisture)

Tips:

Budget breakdown: Ground turkey $6, eggs $1, almond flour $2, cheese $1.50, other ingredients $1.50. Total: $12 for 8 servings.

Keep them moist: Ground turkey is lean. The olive oil, eggs, and Parmesan add moisture so they don't dry out.

Uniform size: Use a cookie scoop to make evenly-sized meatballs. This ensures they all cook at the same rate.

Storage: Refrigerate for up to 4 days or freeze for up to 3 months. Freeze on a baking sheet first, then transfer to freezer bags.

Reheating: From fridge, microwave 4 meatballs for 60-90 seconds. From frozen, microwave for 2-3 minutes.

Ways to use turkey meatballs:
- With marinara sauce and zucchini noodles
- In egg scrambles (chop them up)
- On top of cauliflower rice
- In soup
- As a snack with mustard
- In lettuce wraps with sauce
- With Swedish "cream" sauce (heavy cream, beef broth, Dijon)

Flavor variations:
- Asian: Replace Italian seasoning with ginger, garlic, and green onions. Use soy sauce instead of cheese.
- Mexican: Use cumin, chili powder, and cilantro instead of Italian herbs.
- Greek: Add oregano, lemon zest, and feta cheese.

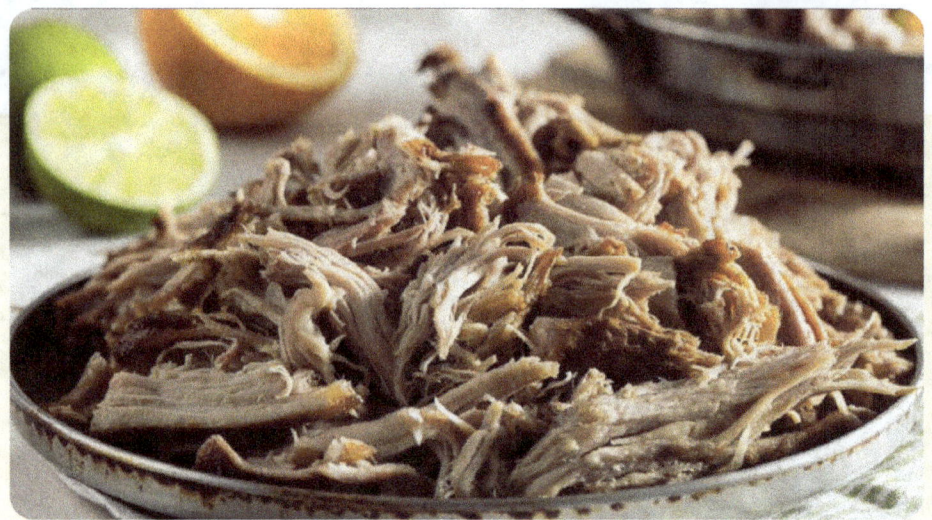

Pork Carnitas

Make-Ahead   Budget-Friendly

- Serves: 10
- Prep Time: 10 min
- Cook Time: 3 hours
- Total: 3 hours 10 min
- Cost Per Serving: $1.95

MACROS PER SERVING:
Calories: 365 | Protein: 32g |
Fat: 24g | Net Carbs: 2g

Ingredients:

- 4 pounds pork shoulder (pork butt), cut into 3-inch chunks
- 2 tablespoons lard or olive oil
- Juice of 2 oranges
- Juice of 2 limes
- 6 cloves garlic, smashed
- 1 tablespoon cumin
- 1 tablespoon oregano
- 1 tablespoon salt
- 1 teaspoon black pepper
- 1 teaspoon chili powder
- 1 bay leaf

For finishing (optional but recommended):
- 2 tablespoons reserved pork fat

Instructions:

Oven Method:
1. Preheat oven to 300°F.
2. In a large bowl, combine orange juice, lime juice, garlic, cumin, oregano, salt, pepper, and chili powder.
3. Add pork chunks and toss to coat. Let marinate for 10 minutes (or up to overnight in the fridge).
4. Heat lard or oil in a large Dutch oven over high heat. Working in batches, sear pork on all sides until golden brown, about 2-3 minutes per side. Transfer to a plate.
5. Return all pork to the Dutch oven. Add marinade and bay leaf. Cover tightly.
6. Bake for 2½ to 3 hours until pork is very tender and falls apart easily.
7. Remove pork and shred with two forks. Discard bay leaf.
8. Optional but delicious: Heat a large skillet over high heat. Add shredded pork in batches and cook undisturbed for 2-3 minutes until crispy on the bottom. Flip and crisp the other side.

Slow Cooker Method:
1. Sear pork as directed above.
2. Place all ingredients in slow cooker.
3. Cook on low for 8-10 hours or high for 4-5 hours until very tender.
4. Proceed with shredding and crisping as above.

Tips:

Budget breakdown: Pork shoulder $16-20 (often $1.50-2/pound on sale), oranges and limes $2, other ingredients $2. Total: $20-24 for 10 servings.

Why carnitas: The traditional Mexican preparation creates tender, flavorful pulled pork with crispy edges.

The crispy step: Don't skip crisping the edges in a hot skillet. This is what makes carnitas special.

Storage: Refrigerate for up to 5 days or freeze for up to 4 months.

Ways to use pork carnitas:
- Taco bowls or lettuce wraps
- On top of cauliflower rice
- In breakfast scrambles
- Carnitas salad
- Stuffed in peppers
- Mixed with eggs and cheese for a breakfast burrito bowl
- Straight with sour cream, guacamole, and hot sauce

Save the fat: The rendered pork fat is amazing for cooking. Store it in a jar and use it to cook eggs or vegetables.

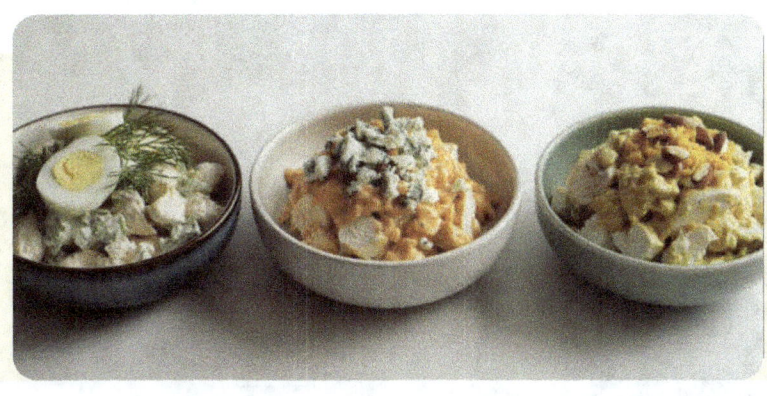

Chicken Salad (3 Ways)

 Quick   Make-Ahead

🍽️ Serves: 6   ✂️ Prep Time: 15 min

Cook Time: 0 min (using precooked chicken)   Total: 15 min

💲 COST PER SERVING: $2.25

Base Chicken Salad
Macros per serving:
Calories: 285 | Protein: 28g | Fat: 18g | Net Carbs: 3g

Base Instructions:

1. In a large bowl, combine mayonnaise, Dijon mustard, lemon juice, salt, and pepper. Mix well.
2. Add diced chicken, celery, and red onion. Stir until everything is evenly coated.
3. Taste and adjust seasoning if needed.
4. Refrigerate for at least 30 minutes before serving (flavors meld together).
5. Store in an airtight container for up to 4 days.

Base Ingredients:

- 3 cups cooked chicken, diced (from rotisserie chicken or meal prep)
- ½ cup mayonnaise
- 2 tablespoons Dijon mustard
- ½ cup diced celery
- ¼ cup diced red onion
- 1 tablespoon lemon juice
- ½ teaspoon salt
- ¼ teaspoon black pepper

VARIATION 1:
Classic Chicken Salad

Add to base recipe:

- 2 hard-boiled eggs, chopped
- 2 tablespoons fresh dill, chopped
- 1 tablespoon capers (optional)

VARIATION 2:
Buffalo Chicken Salad

Modify base recipe:

- Reduce mayonnaise to ¼ cup
- Add ¼ cup Frank's RedHot sauce
- Add ¼ cup crumbled blue cheese
- Omit lemon juice
- Add 2 tablespoons ranch dressing

VARIATION 3: Curry Chicken Salad

Add to base recipe:

- 2 tablespoons curry powder
- ¼ cup chopped almonds or pecans
- 2 tablespoons raisins (optional, adds 3g net carbs per serving)
- 1 teaspoon fresh ginger, grated

Tips:

Budget breakdown: Rotisserie chicken $6-8, mayo $1, celery and onion $2, other ingredients $2. Total: $11-13 for 6 servings.

Shortcut: Use rotisserie chicken or leftover cooked chicken to make this in 15 minutes.

From scratch: If making chicken specifically for this, poach 1½ pounds chicken breasts in simmering water for 15-20 minutes until cooked through. Let cool, then dice.

Make it ahead: Chicken salad actually improves after sitting in the fridge for a day. Make it Sunday, eat all week.

Ways to serve:
- In lettuce wraps (butter lettuce or romaine)
- Stuffed in tomatoes or avocados
- On cucumber slices
- Wrapped in deli meat
- On a bed of greens
- With celery sticks for dipping
- Straight from the container with a fork

Meal prep: Portion into 6 containers. Pair with vegetables or eat alone for a quick protein-packed lunch.

Storage: The onions and celery will soften over time. If you plan to eat this over 4-5 days, add fresh celery and onion to each portion when serving.

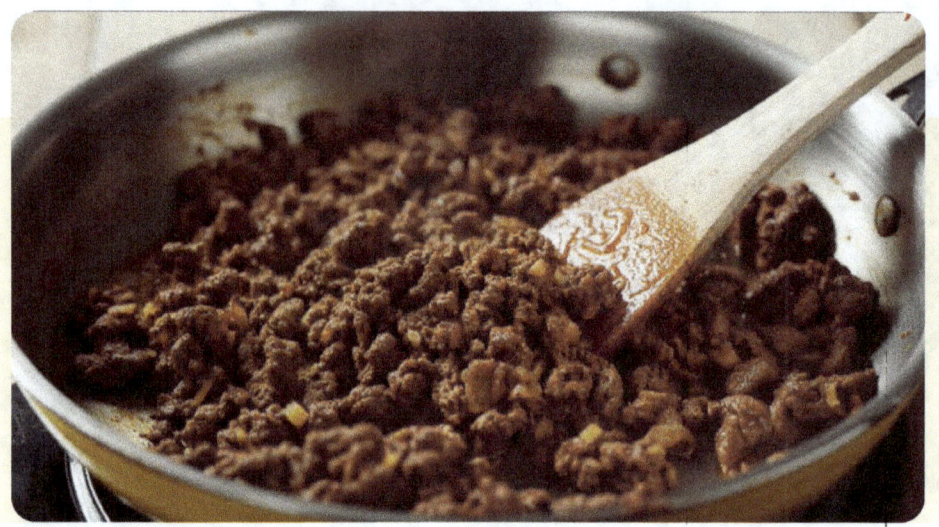

Taco Meat (Seasoning from Scratch)

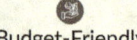

Quick   Make-Ahead   Budget-Friendly

- Serves: 6
- Prep Time: 5 min
- Cook Time: 12 min
- Total: 17 min
- Cost Per Serving: $1.65

MACROS PER SERVING:
Calories: 285 | Protein: 26g |
Fat: 19g | Net Carbs: 2g

Ingredients:

For the taco seasoning (makes about ½ cup):
- 4 tablespoons chili powder
- 2 tablespoons cumin
- 2 tablespoons paprika
- 1 tablespoon garlic powder
- 1 tablespoon onion powder
- 1 tablespoon oregano
- 2 teaspoons salt
- 1 teaspoon black pepper
- 1 teaspoon cayenne pepper (optional)

For the taco meat:
- 2 pounds ground beef (80/20)
- 3 tablespoons taco seasoning (from above)
- ½ cup water
- 1 tablespoon olive oil (if beef is very lean)

Instructions:

Make the seasoning:
1. Combine all seasoning ingredients in a small jar or container.
2. Shake or stir to mix well.
3. Store in an airtight container for up to 6 months.

Cook the taco meat:
1. Heat a large skillet over medium-high heat. Add ground beef and cook, breaking it up with a spatula, for 8-10 minutes until browned and cooked through.
2. Drain excess fat if there's more than 2 tablespoons in the pan.
3. Add 3 tablespoons taco seasoning and ½ cup water. Stir well to coat all the meat.
4. Reduce heat to medium and simmer for 2-3 minutes until water evaporates and meat is well-coated with seasoning.
5. Taste and add more seasoning if desired.

Tips:

Budget breakdown: Ground beef $6, spices $2. Total: $8 for 6 servings. Much cheaper than taco seasoning packets.

Why make your own seasoning: Store-bought packets often contain sugar, fillers, and anti-caking agents. Homemade is cheaper, tastes better, and has no hidden carbs.

Storage: Cooked taco meat keeps for up to 5 days in the fridge or 3 months in the freezer.

Portion it: Divide into 6 containers (about ⅔ cup each). Grab one for a quick meal.

Ways to use taco meat:
- Taco bowls with lettuce, cheese, sour cream, avocado
- Breakfast scrambles
- Stuffed in peppers or tomatoes
- On top of cauliflower rice
- In egg muffins or frittatas
- Taco salad
- Mixed with cauliflower rice and cheese for a quick casserole
- Lettuce wraps
- Topped with fried eggs for breakfast

Ground turkey or chicken: Works great if you want a leaner option. Add 1 tablespoon olive oil to keep it from drying out.

Spice level: This recipe is medium heat. Reduce or omit cayenne for mild. Double it for spicy.

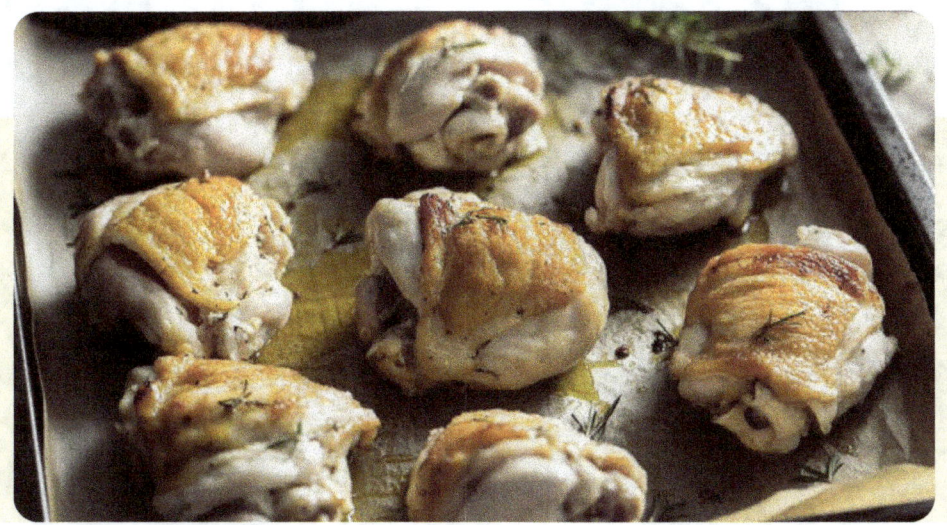

Make-Ahead   Budget-Friendly

Serves: 6

Prep Time: 10 min (plus marinating)

Cook Time: 30 min

Total: 40 min + marinating

Cost Per Serving: $2.15

MACROS PER SERVING:
Calories: 385 | Protein: 38g |
Fat: 24g | Net Carbs: 2g

Ingredients:

- 3 pounds boneless, skinless chicken thighs
- ½ cup olive oil
- ¼ cup lemon juice
- ¼ cup soy sauce (or coconut aminos)
- 6 cloves garlic, minced
- 2 tablespoons Dijon mustard
- 1 tablespoon dried oregano
- 1 tablespoon paprika
- 1 teaspoon black pepper
- 1 teaspoon salt
- ½ teaspoon red pepper flakes (optional)

Instructions:

Marinate the chicken:
1. In a large bowl or gallon-size freezer bag, whisk together olive oil, lemon juice, soy sauce, garlic, Dijon mustard, oregano, paprika, pepper, salt, and red pepper flakes (if using).
2. Add chicken thighs and turn to coat completely.
3. Marinate in the refrigerator for at least 2 hours, or up to 24 hours. The longer, the better.

Cook the chicken:

Oven method:
1. Preheat oven to 425°F. Line a baking sheet with parchment paper.
2. Remove chicken from marinade, shake off excess, and arrange on baking sheet in a single layer.
3. Roast for 25-30 minutes until internal temperature reaches 165°F and chicken is golden brown.
4. Let rest for 5 minutes before storing.

Grill method:
1. Preheat grill to medium-high heat (about 400°F).
2. Remove chicken from marinade and shake off excess.
3. Grill for 6-7 minutes per side until internal temperature reaches 165°F.

Stovetop method:
1. Heat 1 tablespoon oil in a large skillet over medium-high heat.
2. Remove chicken from marinade and shake off excess.
3. Cook chicken in batches, 6-7 minutes per side, until internal temperature reaches 165°F.

Tips:

Budget breakdown: Chicken thighs $9 (often on sale for $1.50-2/pound), marinade ingredients $2. Total: $11 for 6 servings.

Marinating time: 2 hours minimum, 24 hours maximum. Beyond 24 hours, the acid in the marinade can make the chicken mushy.

Freeze in marinade: Put raw chicken and marinade in a freezer bag, freeze flat. Thaw overnight in fridge. The chicken marinates as it thaws.

Storage: Refrigerate cooked chicken for up to 4 days. Reheat gently or eat cold on salads.

Ways to use marinated chicken:
- Slice for salads
- Chop for bowls with cauliflower rice and vegetables
- Shred for tacos or wraps
- Eat whole with roasted vegetables
- Dice for chicken salad
- Add to soups

Meal prep strategy: Marinate 3 pounds on Saturday, cook on Sunday, use throughout the week.

Burger Patties (Freezer-Friendly)

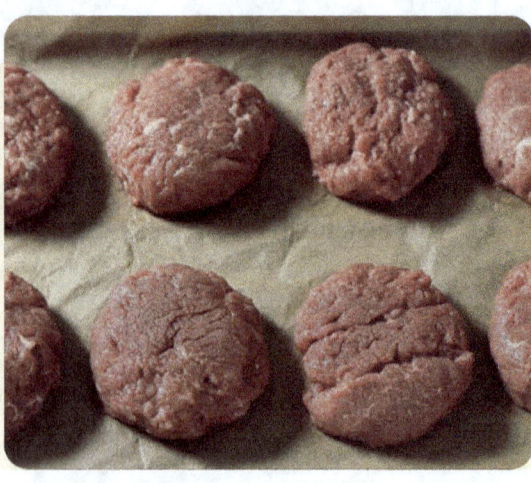

Make-Ahead   Budget-Friendly

🍽 Serves: 8 (1 patty per serving)

✂ Prep Time: 15 min

🍳 Cook Time: 10 min

⏲ Total: 25 min

💲 Cost Per Serving: $1.15

MACROS PER SERVING (1 patty):
Calories: 310 | Protein: 26g | Fat: 22g | Net Carbs: 1g

Ingredients:

- 2½ pounds ground beef (80/20)
- 1 tablespoon Worcestershire sauce
- 1 tablespoon Dijon mustard
- 2 teaspoons garlic powder
- 2 teaspoons onion powder
- 1½ teaspoons salt
- 1 teaspoon black pepper
- ½ teaspoon paprika

Instructions:

Form the patties:
1. In a large bowl, combine ground beef, Worcestershire sauce, Dijon mustard, garlic powder, onion powder, salt, pepper, and paprika.
2. Mix gently with your hands until just combined. Don't overmix or burgers will be dense.
3. Divide mixture into 8 equal portions (about 5 oz each).
4. Form each portion into a patty about ¾ inch thick and 4 inches in diameter.
5. Press a small indent in the center of each patty with your thumb (prevents puffing up during cooking).

To freeze (recommended):
1. Place parchment paper squares between patties so they don't stick together.
2. Stack patties and wrap tightly in plastic wrap, then place in a freezer bag.
3. Freeze for up to 4 months.
4. To cook from frozen, add 2-3 minutes to cooking time.

To cook immediately:

Grill method:
1. Preheat grill to medium-high heat (about 400°F). Oil grates.
2. Cook patties for 4-5 minutes per side for medium (160°F internal temperature).

Stovetop method:
1. Heat a large skillet over medium-high heat. Add 1 tablespoon oil.
2. Cook patties for 4-5 minutes per side for medium (160°F internal temperature).

Oven method:
1. Preheat oven to 400°F. Line a baking sheet with parchment.
2. Place patties on sheet and bake for 15-18 minutes until internal temperature reaches 160°F.

Tips:

Budget breakdown: Ground beef $7.50-9 (depending on sales). Total: About $9 for 8 burgers.

Why make your own: Pre-made frozen burgers often contain fillers and are more expensive. Make your own, freeze them, and you have burger night ready anytime.

Seasoning: This is a basic seasoning. Feel free to add other spices like cumin, chili powder, or cayenne.

Don't press them: When cooking, resist the urge to press down on burgers with a spatula. This squeezes out all the juices.

Cheese: Add cheese in the last minute of cooking, cover the pan/grill, and let it melt.

Storage: Cooked burgers refrigerate for up to 4 days. Reheat gently or eat cold.

Bunless serving ideas:
- On a bed of lettuce with all the fixings
- Crumbled over a salad
- Burger bowl with cauliflower rice, cheese, pickles, onions
- Wrapped in lettuce leaves
- With a fried egg on top for breakfast

Make it a meal prep: Cook all 8 on Sunday. Store in containers. Reheat for quick dinners or lunches.

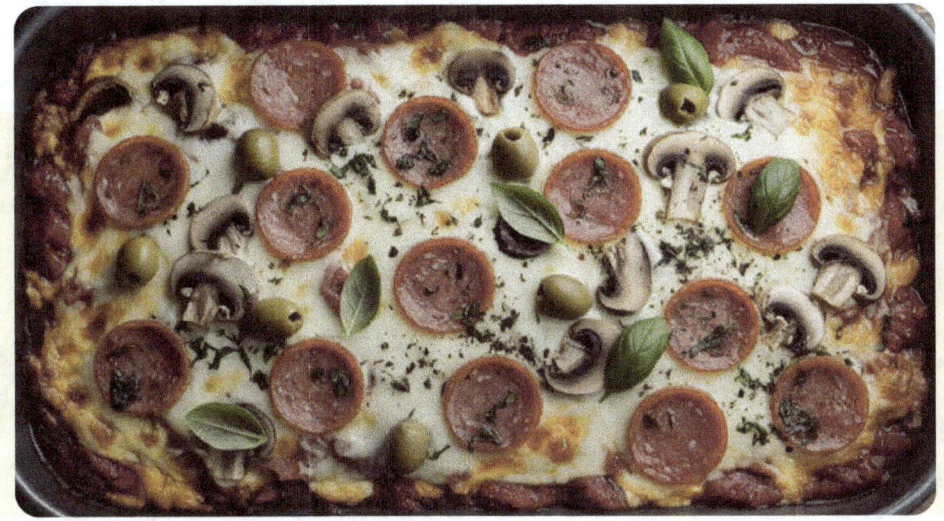

Pizza Casserole (Crustless)

 Make-Ahead   Budget-Friendly

- Serves: 8
- Prep Time: 15 min
- Cook Time: 30 min
- Total: 45 min
- Cost Per Serving: $2.35

MACROS PER SERVING:
Calories: 380 | Protein: 30g |
Fat: 25g | Net Carbs: 6g

Instructions:

1. Preheat oven to 375°F. Spray a 9x13-inch baking dish with cooking spray.
2. Heat a large skillet over medium-high heat. Add ground beef and cook, breaking it up, for 8-10 minutes until browned. Drain excess fat.
3. Add garlic, Italian seasoning, salt, pepper, and red pepper flakes (if using) to the beef. Cook for 1 minute.
4. Add diced tomatoes and marinara sauce. Stir and simmer for 5 minutes. Remove from heat.
5. In a separate bowl, mix softened cream cheese, heavy cream, and ½ cup mozzarella until smooth.
6. Spread half of the meat sauce in the bottom of the prepared baking dish.
7. Drop spoonfuls of the cream cheese mixture over the meat sauce and spread gently (it doesn't have to be perfect).
8. Top with remaining meat sauce.
9. Sprinkle with remaining 1½ cups mozzarella and Parmesan cheese.
10. Add any optional toppings.
11. Bake for 25-30 minutes until cheese is melted and bubbly and edges are golden brown.

Tips:

Budget breakdown: Ground beef $6, cheeses $6, marinara $2, other ingredients $3. Total: $17 for 8 servings.

Italian sausage: Use bulk Italian sausage instead of ground beef for more authentic pizza flavor.

Make ahead: Assemble everything (through step 10), cover tightly, and refrigerate for up to 24 hours. Bake when ready, adding 5-10 minutes to cooking time since it's cold.

Freeze it: Freeze unbaked casserole for up to 3 months. Thaw overnight in fridge, then bake. Or bake from frozen, adding 20-25 minutes to cooking time (cover with foil for first 20 minutes).

Storage: Refrigerate for up to 5 days. Reheat individual portions in microwave for 2-3 minutes.

Serve with: A simple side salad is all you need.

Meal prep: Cut into 8 portions and store in containers. Grab one for a quick dinner or lunch.

Ingredients:

- 2 pounds ground beef (80/20) or Italian sausage
- 1 can (14.5 oz) diced tomatoes, drained
- 1 cup sugar-free marinara sauce
- 8 oz cream cheese, softened
- ½ cup heavy cream
- 2 cups shredded mozzarella cheese, divided
- ½ cup grated Parmesan cheese
- 3 cloves garlic, minced
- 2 teaspoons Italian seasoning
- 1 teaspoon salt
- ½ teaspoon black pepper
- ½ teaspoon red pepper flakes (optional)
- Cooking spray

Toppings (all optional):
- Sliced pepperoni
- Sliced mushrooms
- Diced bell peppers
- Sliced olives
- Fresh basil

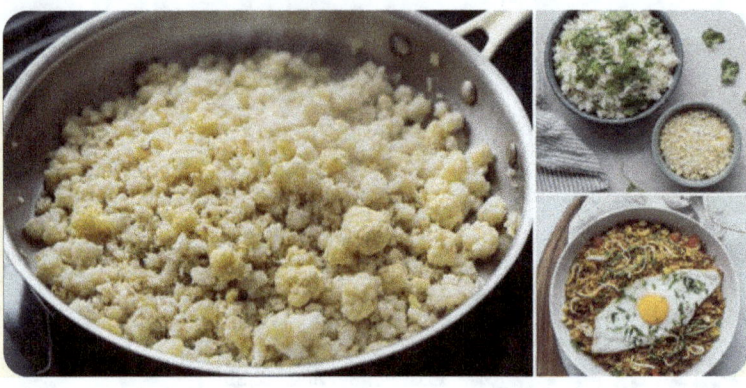

Cauliflower Rice Base (Flavored 3 Ways)

Quick   Make-Ahead   Budget-Friendly

Serves: 6 (1 cup per serving)

Cook Time: 8 min

COST PER SERVING: $1.15

Prep Time: 5 min

Total: 13 min

Base Cauliflower Rice
Macros per serving (plain):
Calories: 60 | Protein: 3g | Fat: 5g | Net Carbs: 3g

Base Instructions:

1. If using frozen cauliflower rice, no need to thaw.
2. Heat butter or oil in a large skillet over medium-high heat.
3. Add cauliflower rice, salt, and pepper. Stir well.
4. Cook for 6-8 minutes, stirring occasionally, until cauliflower is tender and any excess moisture has evaporated.

Base Ingredients:

- 6 cups cauliflower rice (fresh or frozen)
- 2 tablespoons butter or olive oil
- ½ teaspoon salt
- ¼ teaspoon black pepper

VARIATION 1:
Cilantro Lime Cauliflower Rice

Add to cooked base:

- Juice of 1 lime
- Zest of 1 lime
- ¼ cup fresh cilantro, chopped
- 1 clove garlic, minced (cook with the rice)

Additional macros: +5 calories, +1g net carbs

VARIATION 2:
Garlic Herb Cauliflower Rice

Add to base while cooking:

- 4 cloves garlic, minced
- 1 tablespoon fresh parsley, chopped (or 1 teaspoon dried)
- 1 teaspoon dried thyme
- ¼ cup grated Parmesan cheese (stir in at the end)

Additional macros: +25 calories, +2g fat, +2g protein, +1g net carbs

VARIATION 3: "Fried Rice" Style Cauliflower Rice

Add to base:

- 2 eggs, beaten
- 2 tablespoons soy sauce (or coconut aminos)
- 1 teaspoon sesame oil
- 2 cloves garlic, minced

- 1 teaspoon fresh ginger, grated
- ½ cup frozen peas and carrots (optional, adds 3g net carbs)
- 2 green onions, sliced

Instructions:

1. Cook cauliflower rice as directed in base recipe.
2. Push to one side. Add beaten eggs to empty side and scramble.
3. Mix eggs into rice. Add soy sauce, sesame oil, garlic, ginger.
4. Cook for 1-2 minutes more.

Additional macros: +50 calories, +4g fat, +4g protein, +2g net carbs

Tips:

Budget breakdown: Cauliflower rice (fresh or frozen) $4-6, butter and seasonings $1. Total: $5-7 for 6 cups.

Fresh vs. frozen: Both work great. Frozen is already riced and often cheaper. Fresh requires a food processor or box grater.

Make fresh cauliflower rice: Cut cauliflower into florets. Pulse in food processor until rice-sized (don't over-process or it becomes mushy). Store raw for up to 5 days or blanch and freeze.

Get it dry: The key to good cauliflower rice is cooking out the moisture. Don't cover the pan while cooking.

Storage: Refrigerate cooked cauliflower rice for up to 5 days. Reheat in microwave or skillet.

Uses for cauliflower rice:
- Base for any bowl (burrito bowls, teriyaki bowls, curry)
- Side dish instead of regular rice
- Mixed into soups or casseroles
- Base for fried "rice"
- In place of grains in any recipe

Meal prep strategy: Make a big batch of plain cauliflower rice. Portion into containers. Reheat and flavor differently each day.

CHAPTER 5 SUMMARY

You now have 15 make-ahead recipes that will transform how you eat throughout the week. Here's how to actually implement meal prep in your life:

Start Small:
Don't try to prep everything at once. Start with:

- Week 1: Make one batch protein (pulled chicken or shredded beef)
- Week 2: Add hard-boiled eggs
- Week 3: Add one full meal (chili or curry)
- Week 4: Add burger patties or meatballs to your freezer

Build the habit gradually.

My Realistic Sunday Meal Prep:
Here's what I actually do most Sundays (takes 2-3 hours):

Proteins (pick 2):
- Pulled chicken in slow cooker (10 min prep, cooks while I do other things)
- Hard-boil a dozen eggs (5 min prep, 12 min cook, hands-off)
- Ground beef or turkey for taco meat (15 min total)

Vegetables:
- Wash and chop lettuce, peppers, cucumbers (15 min)
- Make 2 batches of cauliflower rice (20 min)

Optional:
- Batch of meatballs or burger patties for the freezer (30 min)

What This Gets Me:
- Proteins for 15+ meals
- Eggs for snacks all week
- Prepped vegetables for quick cooking
- Future meals in the freezer

Total active time: About 60-90 minutes. The rest is hands-off cooking.

The Meal Prep Containers You Actually Need:
Don't buy expensive "meal prep systems." Here's what works:

For refrigerator:
- 6-8 rectangular glass containers with lids (for full meals)
- 4-6 round glass containers (for components like taco meat, pulled chicken)
- Mason jars (for eggs, salad dressings, cauliflower rice)

For freezer:
- Gallon freezer bags (for burger patties, meatballs, shredded meat)
- Quart freezer bags (for individual portions)
- Aluminum pans with lids (for casseroles)

Total investment: $30-50 one time.

The Meal Prep Formula:
Every Sunday, aim to prep:

- 2 proteins (cooked or marinated)
- 1 complete meal (soup, chili, casserole)
- Hard-boiled eggs
- 2-3 vegetables (washed, chopped, or cooked)
- Optional: 1 batch for the freezer

Mix and match throughout the week.

Weekly Meal Plan Using These Recipes:

Sunday: Meal prep day (3 hours)
- Make: Beef chili, pulled chicken, hard-boiled eggs, cauliflower rice

Monday:
- Lunch: Meal prep chicken bowl (Teriyaki variation)
- Dinner: Beef chili with cheese and sour cream

Tuesday:
- Lunch: Beef chili leftovers
- Dinner: Pulled chicken tacos (lettuce wraps) with cauliflower rice

Wednesday:
- Lunch: Chicken salad (using pulled chicken) in lettuce wraps
- Dinner: Burger patties from freezer with roasted vegetables

Thursday:
- Lunch: Meal prep chicken bowl (Tex-Mex variation)
- Dinner: Turkey meatballs with marinara and zucchini noodles

Friday:
- Lunch: Hard-boiled eggs, deli meat, cheese, vegetables
- Dinner: Pizza casserole (made on Sunday, reheated)

Saturday:
- Cook something fresh or eat out
- Take a break from meal prep

The Financial Benefit:
Let's do the math:

Buying lunch 5 days/week: $10-15 per meal = $50-75/week = $200-300/month

Meal prepping lunches: $2-3 per meal = $10-15/week = $40-60/month

Savings: $160-240 per month = $1,920-2,880 per year

That's a nice vacation. Or a new wardrobe. Or just peace of mind.

Common Meal Prep Mistakes:
1. **Trying to prep every single meal.** Start with lunches only or just a few dinners. Don't overwhelm yourself.
2. **Making foods you don't actually like.** Just because something meal preps well doesn't mean you have to eat it. Prep foods you enjoy.
3. **Not labeling containers.** Two weeks later, you won't remember if that's chili or taco meat. Label everything with contents and date.
4. **Letting food go bad.** If you're not going to eat it within 4 days, freeze it. Don't let it sit in the fridge until it's science experiment.
5. **Making it complicated.** Meal prep doesn't need to be Instagram-perfect. It needs to be food you'll actually eat.

The Mindset:
Meal prep isn't about being perfect or organized. It's about:

- Trading 2-3 hours on Sunday for 10+ easy meals during the week
- Removing decision fatigue (no more "what's for dinner?")
- Saving money by not ordering takeout
- Actually sticking to your eating goals because the food is just... there

Some weeks you'll prep everything. Some weeks you'll prep one thing. Some weeks you'll skip it entirely. That's fine. It's a tool, not a mandate.

Next Chapter Preview:
Chapter 6 covers soups and stews. Because sometimes you just want a bowl of warm, comforting food that you made once and can eat for days.

But before we move on: Pick 3-4 recipes from this chapter. Try them over the next two Sundays. See which ones become staples in your rotation.

You don't need to master all 15 recipes. You need 4-5 make-ahead meals that fit your life and taste preferences.

Now let's talk about soup.

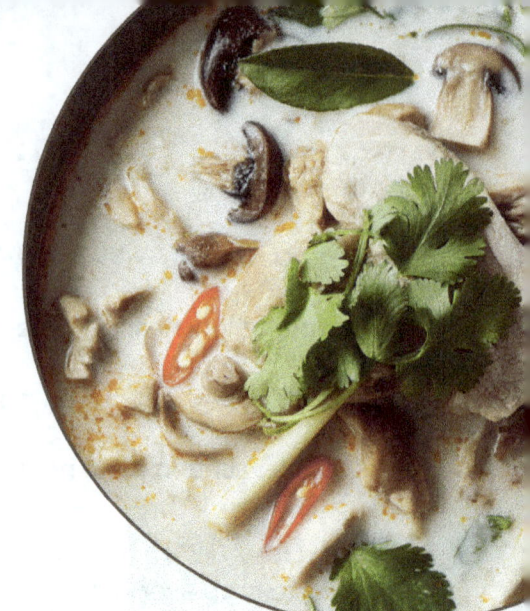

There's something deeply satisfying about a bowl of homemade soup.

Maybe it's the warmth. Maybe it's the fact that soup feels like someone cares about you (even when that someone is yourself, cooking for yourself). Maybe it's just that soup is one of the few foods that actually gets better when you make a huge batch and eat it for three days straight.

Whatever the reason, soup is the ultimate comfort food. And when you're eating high-protein, low-carb, it's also one of the easiest ways to get a complete, satisfying meal in a bowl.

This chapter is about soups and stews that don't rely on noodles, potatoes, or rice to fill you up. These recipes use protein, vegetables, and rich broths to create meals that are just as satisfying as their carb-heavy counterparts—sometimes more so.

Why Soup is Perfect for This Way of Eating:
1. **It's forgiving.** Soup doesn't require precise measurements or techniques. If you add too much of something, adjust the seasoning. If it's too thick, add broth. Too thin? Simmer longer. Hard to mess up.

2. **It scales easily.** All these recipes make 6-8 servings. Want more? Double it. The cooking time barely changes.

3. **It freezes beautifully.** Make a huge batch, freeze half, and you have soup ready for those nights when even opening the refrigerator feels like too much work.

4. **It's economical.** Soup stretches proteins and uses up vegetables that are past their prime. Cheaper cuts of meat become tender through slow cooking.

5. **It keeps you full.** The combination of protein, fat, and liquid volume means you stay satisfied for hours. No 10 AM hunger despite eating breakfast.

The Two Types of Soup in This Chapter:
Brothy Soups: Clear or semi-clear broth base with chunks of protein and vegetables floating in it. Examples: chicken soup, egg drop soup, Italian wedding soup. These are lighter and work well as first courses or when you want something warming but not heavy.

Creamy/Hearty Stews: Thick, rich soups that are almost stew-like. Examples: broccoli cheese soup, seafood chowder, beef stew. These are complete meals in a bowl. Pair with a simple salad and you're done.

Soup-Making Basics:
Build flavor in layers:

1. Sauté aromatics first (onion, garlic, celery)
2. Brown proteins if using meat
3. Add liquid and bring to a simmer

4. Add vegetables based on cooking time (hard vegetables like cauliflower first, soft vegetables like spinach last)

5. Season throughout, not just at the end

Use good broth: Homemade is best (see Recipe 75 for chicken bone broth), but store-bought works. Just buy good quality broth, not bouillon cubes with more salt than flavor.

Don't rush it: Most soups improve with time. Make soup in the morning or the night before and let it sit in the fridge. Flavors meld and deepen. Reheat when ready to eat.

Season properly: Soup needs more salt than you think. The large volume of liquid requires adequate seasoning. Taste and adjust before serving.

Equipment You Need:
- **Large pot or Dutch oven (6-8 quarts):** For making soup. Heavy-bottomed is best for even heat distribution.
- **Immersion blender (optional but useful):** For pureeing soups right in the pot. Makes creamy soups easier.
- **Ladle:** For serving and portioning.
- **Storage containers:** Quart-sized containers for refrigerator. Freezer bags or containers for freezer.

That's it. Soup doesn't require specialty equipment.

Storage and Reheating:
Refrigerator: Most soups keep 4-5 days refrigerated. Longer than other leftovers because the salt and acidity act as preservatives.

Freezer: Most soups freeze beautifully for 3-4 months. Exceptions: soups with cream (can separate), soups with lots of delicate vegetables (get mushy).

Freezer tips:
- Cool completely before freezing
- Freeze in portion sizes you'll actually use
- Leave 1-2 inches headspace in containers (liquid expands when frozen)
- Freeze flat in freezer bags for easier storage
- Label everything with contents and date

Reheating:
- Stovetop is best: low-medium heat, stir occasionally
- Microwave works: use 50-70% power for even heating
- Add liquid if needed: soup thickens as it sits
- Adjust seasonings after reheating: flavors can dull in the fridge

The Recipes:
Every soup in this chapter is:

- High in protein (at least 20g per serving)
- Low in net carbs (under 10g per serving, most under 8g)
- Makes 6-8 servings (enough for multiple meals)

- Stores well (refrigerator and freezer)
- Actually tastes good (not just "healthy")

Some take 30 minutes. Some take 2 hours. I'll tell you which is which so you can plan accordingly.

A Note on "No Noodles" and "No Potatoes":

You'll see several recipes that are versions of soups traditionally made with pasta or potatoes. I'm not trying to trick you into thinking cauliflower tastes like potatoes or that you won't notice the noodles are gone.

What I am saying is this: these soups are delicious in their own right. The flavors are there. The satisfaction is there. You might even find you prefer them this way because you're not feeling bloated and tired an hour later.

Give them a fair shot.

Now let's make some soup.

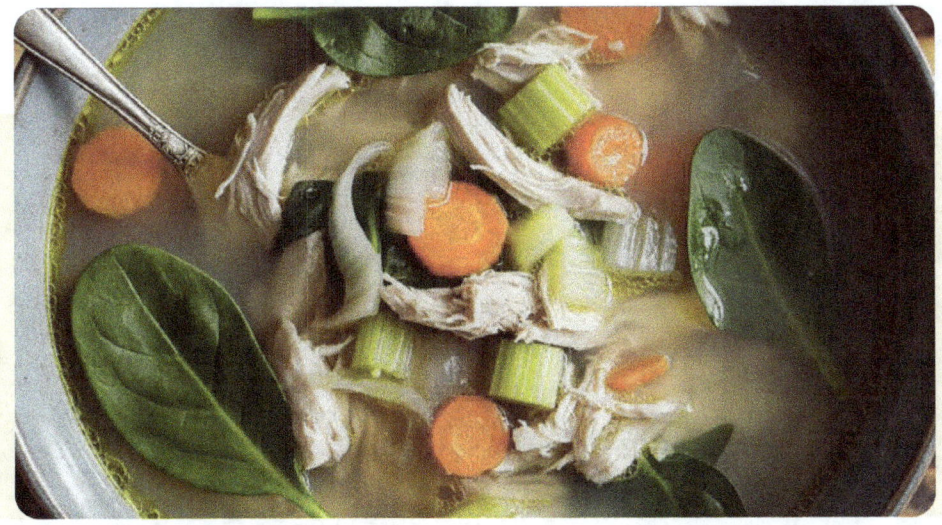

Chicken Soup (No Noodles)

Make-Ahead   Budget-Friendly

🍽 Serves: 8

✂ Prep Time: 15 min

⏲ Cook Time: 45 min

⏱ Total: 60 min

💲 Cost Per Serving: $2.15

MACROS PER SERVING:
Calories: 245 | Protein: 28g |
Fat: 11g | Net Carbs: 6g

Instructions:

1. Heat olive oil or butter in a large pot or Dutch oven over medium-high heat.
2. Add chicken pieces and season with salt and pepper. Cook for 3-4 minutes per side until lightly browned (doesn't need to be cooked through). Transfer to a plate.
3. In the same pot, add onion, carrots, and celery. Cook for 5-6 minutes until vegetables begin to soften.
4. Add garlic, thyme, and parsley. Cook for 1 minute until fragrant.
5. Pour in chicken broth and add bay leaves. Bring to a boil.
6. Return chicken to the pot. Reduce heat to medium-low and simmer for 25-30 minutes until chicken is cooked through and tender.
7. Remove chicken from pot and shred with two forks. Return shredded chicken to the pot.
8. If using spinach, stir it in and cook for 2 minutes until wilted.
9. Remove bay leaves. Stir in lemon juice.

Ingredients:

- 2 pounds boneless, skinless chicken thighs or breasts
- 8 cups chicken broth (homemade or store-bought)
- 3 medium carrots, sliced
- 3 celery stalks, sliced
- 1 medium onion, diced
- 4 cloves garlic, minced
- 2 bay leaves
- 2 teaspoons dried thyme
- 1 teaspoon dried parsley (or 2 tablespoons fresh)
- 1 teaspoon salt
- ½ teaspoon black pepper
- 2 tablespoons olive oil or butter
- 2 cups fresh spinach (optional)
- Juice of ½ lemon

Tips:

Budget breakdown: Chicken $6, broth $3 (or free if homemade), vegetables $3, seasonings $1. Total: $13 for 8 servings.

Use a rotisserie chicken: Skip steps 1-2 and 6. Add shredded rotisserie chicken in step 7. Ready in 30 minutes.

Noodle substitute: Add 2 cups cooked zucchini noodles or shirataki noodles in the last 5 minutes if you really want "noodles." Adds minimal carbs.

Storage: Refrigerate for up to 5 days or freeze for up to 4 months.

Make it creamier: Stir in ½ cup heavy cream or coconut milk at the end. Adds 2g fat, 1g carbs per serving.

Slow cooker method: Place all ingredients (raw chicken, vegetables, broth, seasonings) in slow cooker. Cook on low for 6-8 hours or high for 3-4 hours. Shred chicken in the pot.

Instant Pot method: Sauté vegetables using sauté function, add chicken and broth, pressure cook on high for 15 minutes with quick release. Shred chicken in the pot.

When you're sick: This is the soup to make. The warm broth, protein, and vegetables help you heal. Make a batch and freeze portions for when you need it.

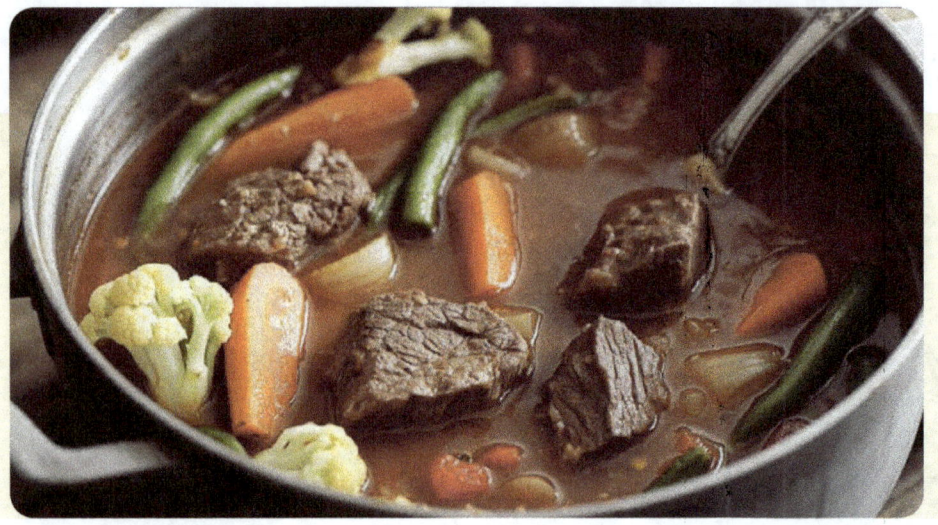

Beef Stew (No Potatoes)

Make-Ahead   Budget-Friendly

Serves: 8

Prep Time: 20 min

Cook Time: 2 hours

Total: 2 hours 20 min

Cost Per Serving: $3.25

MACROS PER SERVING:
Calories: 385 | Protein: 32g |
Fat: 22g | Net Carbs: 8g

Instructions:

1. Pat beef cubes dry with paper towels. Season all sides with salt, pepper, and paprika.
2. Heat olive oil in a large pot or Dutch oven over high heat.
3. Working in batches, sear beef cubes on all sides until browned, about 2-3 minutes per side. Don't overcrowd the pot. Transfer browned beef to a plate.
4. Reduce heat to medium. Add onions to the pot and cook for 3-4 minutes until slightly softened, scraping up any browned bits from the bottom.
5. Add garlic and cook for 1 minute until fragrant.
6. Stir in tomato paste and cook for 1 minute.
7. Add beef broth, diced tomatoes (with juice), Worcestershire sauce, bay leaves, and thyme. Stir to combine.
8. Return beef to the pot along with any accumulated juices. Bring to a boil.
9. Reduce heat to low, cover, and simmer for 1 hour, stirring occasionally.
10. Add carrots and cauliflower. Simmer covered for 30 more minutes.
11. Add green beans. Simmer uncovered for 15 more minutes until all vegetables are tender and stew has thickened slightly.
12. Remove bay leaves. Taste and adjust seasoning.

Tips:

Budget breakdown: Chuck roast $15-18, broth $3, vegetables $4, tomatoes and seasonings $2. Total: $24-27 for 8 servings.

Why chuck roast: It's an economical cut that becomes incredibly tender when slow-cooked. Don't use expensive steak cuts for stew.

The searing step matters: Browning the meat adds deep, savory flavor. Don't skip it.

Potato substitute: Cauliflower adds bulk and absorbs the flavors beautifully. Radishes also work (lose their sharp taste when cooked long).

Storage: Refrigerate for up to 5 days or freeze for up to 4 months. Actually tastes better the next day.

Slow cooker method: Sear beef first, then transfer everything to slow cooker. Cook on low for 8-10 hours or high for 4-5 hours.

Instant Pot method: Sear beef using sauté function. Add all ingredients except green beans. Pressure cook on high for 35 minutes with natural release. Stir in green beans and simmer on sauté for 5 minutes.

Thicken it more: If you want thicker stew, mash some of the cauliflower against the side of the pot or blend ½ cup of the soup and stir it back in.

Ingredients:

- 2½ pounds beef chuck roast, cut into 1½-inch cubes
- 6 cups beef broth
- 1 can (14.5 oz) diced tomatoes, undrained
- 3 cups cauliflower florets, cut into large chunks
- 3 medium carrots, cut into 1-inch pieces
- 2 cups green beans, cut into 1-inch pieces
- 2 medium onions, cut into wedges
- 4 cloves garlic, minced
- 3 tablespoons tomato paste
- 2 tablespoons Worcestershire sauce
- 2 tablespoons olive oil
- 2 bay leaves
- 2 teaspoons dried thyme
- 1 teaspoon paprika
- 1 teaspoon salt
- ½ teaspoon black pepper
- 2 tablespoons fresh parsley, chopped

Egg Drop Soup

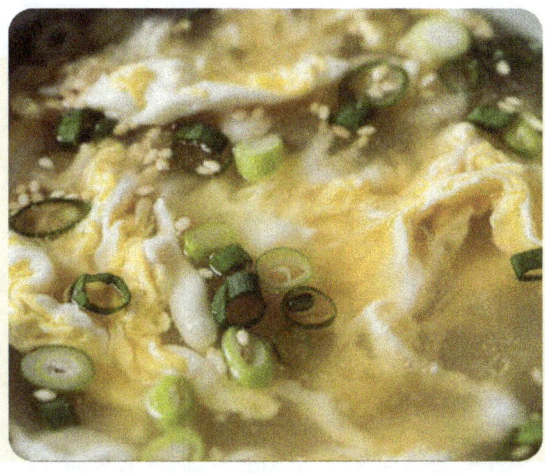

 Quick 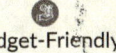 Budget-Friendly

 Serves: 6

 Prep Time: 5 min

 Cook Time: 10 min

Total: 15 min

 Cost Per Serving: $1.25

MACROS PER SERVING:

Calories: 95 | Protein: 8g | Fat: 5g | Net Carbs: 3g

Ingredients:

- 8 cups chicken broth
- 4 large eggs, beaten
- 2 tablespoons soy sauce (or coconut aminos)
- 1 tablespoon sesame oil
- 1 teaspoon fresh ginger, grated
- 2 cloves garlic, minced
- 3 green onions, sliced (white and green parts separated)
- ¼ teaspoon white pepper (or black pepper)
- ½ teaspoon salt (adjust based on broth saltiness)
- Optional: ½ teaspoon xanthan gum (for thicker soup)

Instructions:

1. In a large pot, bring chicken broth to a boil over high heat.
2. Add white parts of green onions, garlic, and ginger. Reduce heat to medium and simmer for 3 minutes.
3. Add soy sauce, sesame oil, white pepper, and salt. Stir to combine.
4. If using xanthan gum, sprinkle it over the soup while whisking continuously. This will thicken the soup slightly.
5. Bring soup back to a gentle boil.
6. While stirring the soup in a circular motion with a spoon, slowly drizzle in the beaten eggs. The eggs will cook immediately and form ribbons.
7. Remove from heat immediately once all eggs are added.
8. Taste and adjust seasoning if needed.

Tips:

Budget breakdown: Eggs $1, broth $3, green onions and seasonings $1. Total: $5 for 6 servings.

The stirring technique: The key to silky egg ribbons is continuously stirring while slowly drizzling the eggs. If you dump them all at once, you'll get chunks instead of ribbons.

Add protein: This soup is light on protein. Serve it as a starter, or add 2 cups of shredded cooked chicken for a more substantial meal (adds 15g protein per serving).

Add vegetables: Stir in 2 cups of baby spinach or bok choy with the eggs for extra nutrition and minimal carbs.

Storage: Refrigerate for up to 3 days. The eggs may get slightly chewier, but it still tastes good. Don't freeze this one.

Make it spicy: Add ½ teaspoon red pepper flakes or a drizzle of chili oil when serving.

Restaurant-style: Use homemade chicken broth instead of store-bought. The depth of flavor is incomparable.

Creamy Broccoli Cheese Soup

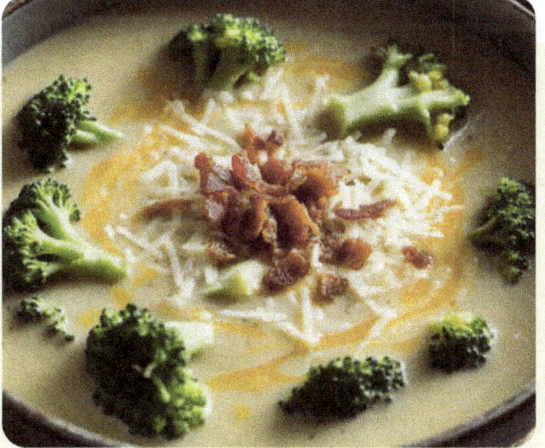

 Make-Ahead

 Serves: 8

 Prep Time: 15 min

 Cook Time: 30 min

Total: 45 min

 Cost Per Serving: $2.45

MACROS PER SERVING:

Calories: 320 | Protein: 14g | Fat: 26g | Net Carbs: 6g

Ingredients:

- 6 cups broccoli florets, chopped small
- 4 cups chicken broth
- 2 cups heavy cream
- 3 cups shredded sharp cheddar cheese
- ½ cup grated Parmesan cheese
- 1 medium onion, diced
- 3 cloves garlic, minced
- 4 tablespoons butter
- 1 teaspoon Dijon mustard
- ½ teaspoon paprika
- 1 teaspoon salt
- ½ teaspoon black pepper
- ¼ teaspoon nutmeg (optional but recommended)
- Optional: cooked bacon bits for topping

Instructions:

1. Melt butter in a large pot over medium heat.
2. Add onion and cook for 5-6 minutes until softened and translucent.
3. Add garlic and cook for 1 minute until fragrant.
4. Add broccoli florets and stir to coat with butter. Cook for 3-4 minutes.
5. Pour in chicken broth. Bring to a boil, then reduce heat and simmer for 12-15 minutes until broccoli is very tender.
6. Use an immersion blender to partially blend the soup, leaving some chunks for texture. Or transfer half the soup to a blender, puree, and return to pot. (Be careful blending hot liquids—leave the blender lid slightly open to vent steam.)
7. Stir in heavy cream, Dijon mustard, paprika, salt, pepper, and nutmeg (if using).
8. Reduce heat to low. Gradually add cheddar cheese and Parmesan, stirring constantly until melted and smooth.
9. Simmer (do not boil) for 5 more minutes, stirring occasionally, until soup reaches desired thickness.
10. Taste and adjust seasoning.

Tips:

Budget breakdown: Broccoli $4, cheese $6, cream $3, broth $2, other ingredients $2. Total: $17 for 8 servings.

Don't boil after adding cheese: High heat causes cheese to separate and get grainy. Keep it at a gentle simmer.

Consistency: This soup thickens as it sits. If reheating and it's too thick, add broth or cream to thin it out.

Cauliflower variation: Use half broccoli, half cauliflower for a milder flavor. Same carb count.

Storage: Refrigerate for up to 5 days. Can be frozen for up to 2 months, though cream soups sometimes separate when thawed (whisk vigorously when reheating to bring it back together).

Make it vegetarian: Use vegetable broth instead of chicken broth.

Add protein: Stir in 2 cups of diced cooked chicken for a more complete meal.

Slow cooker method: Add broccoli, onion, garlic, broth, and seasonings to slow cooker. Cook on low for 4-5 hours. Blend partially, then stir in cream and cheese. Cook on low for 15 more minutes.

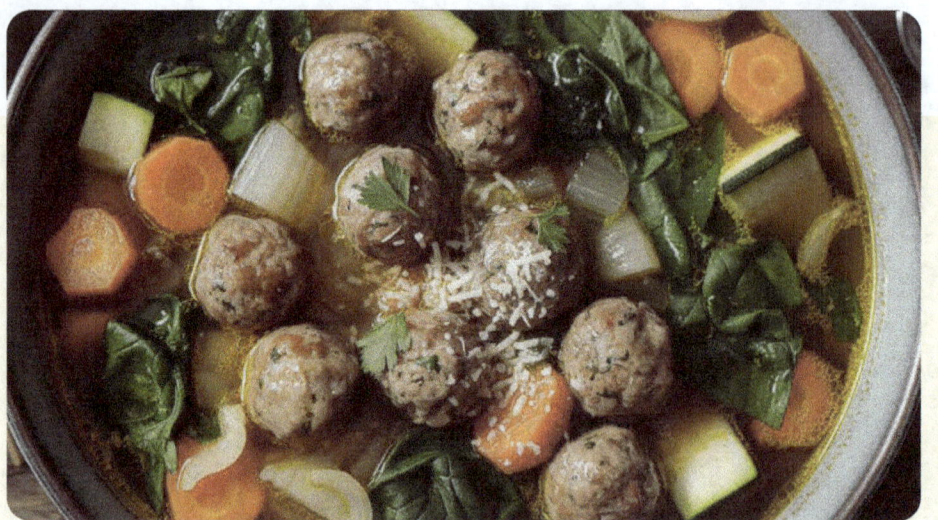

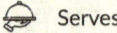
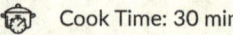

Make-Ahead   Budget-Friendly

Serves: 8

Prep Time: 20 min

Cook Time: 30 min

Total: 50 min

Cost Per Serving: $2.35

MACROS PER SERVING:
Calories: 285 | Protein: 24g |
Fat: 18g | Net Carbs: 5g

Instructions:

Make the meatballs:
1. In a bowl, combine ground beef, ground pork, egg, Parmesan, garlic, Italian seasoning, salt, and pepper. Mix gently with your hands.
2. Roll into small meatballs, about 1 inch in diameter (you should get about 30-35 meatballs).
3. Set aside on a plate.

Make the soup:
1. Heat olive oil in a large pot over medium heat.
2. Add onion and carrots. Cook for 5-6 minutes until starting to soften.
3. Add garlic and Italian seasoning. Cook for 1 minute.
4. Pour in chicken broth. Bring to a boil.
5. Gently drop meatballs into the boiling broth one at a time. Reduce heat to medium and simmer for 15 minutes until meatballs are cooked through.
6. Add diced zucchini. Simmer for 5 more minutes.
7. Stir in chopped spinach. Cook for 2-3 minutes until wilted.
8. Season with salt and pepper to taste.
9. Serve hot, topped with grated Parmesan and fresh parsley.

Tips:

Budget breakdown: Ground beef $3.50, ground pork $2.50, broth $3, vegetables $4, Parmesan and seasonings $2. Total: $15 for 8 servings.

Why no orzo: Traditional Italian wedding soup uses orzo pasta. We replace it with zucchini for volume and texture without the carbs.

Small meatballs: Keep them bite-sized (1 inch). They cook faster and are easier to eat with a spoon.

Ground turkey: Use all ground turkey instead of beef and pork for a leaner version. Add 1 tablespoon olive oil to the meatball mixture.

Storage: Refrigerate for up to 5 days or freeze for up to 3 months. The meatballs hold up beautifully.

Make ahead: Form meatballs in advance and refrigerate for up to 24 hours or freeze for up to 3 months. Drop frozen meatballs directly into boiling broth (add 5 minutes to cooking time).

Add more greens: Swap or add kale, escarole, or Swiss chard instead of all spinach for traditional flavor.

Instant Pot method: Sauté onions and carrots using sauté function. Add broth, meatballs, and seasonings. Pressure cook on high for 8 minutes with quick release. Stir in zucchini and spinach, simmer on sauté mode for 5 minutes.

Ingredients:

For the meatballs:
- 1 pound ground beef (80/20)
- ½ pound ground pork
- 1 large egg
- ¼ cup grated Parmesan cheese
- 2 cloves garlic, minced
- 1 teaspoon Italian seasoning
- ½ teaspoon salt
- ¼ teaspoon black pepper

For the soup:
- 8 cups chicken broth
- 4 cups fresh spinach, roughly chopped
- 2 medium zucchini, diced small
- 3 medium carrots, diced small
- 1 medium onion, diced
- 3 cloves garlic, minced
- 2 tablespoons olive oil
- 1 teaspoon Italian seasoning
- ½ teaspoon salt
- ¼ teaspoon black pepper
- ¼ cup grated Parmesan cheese (for serving)
- Fresh parsley for garnish

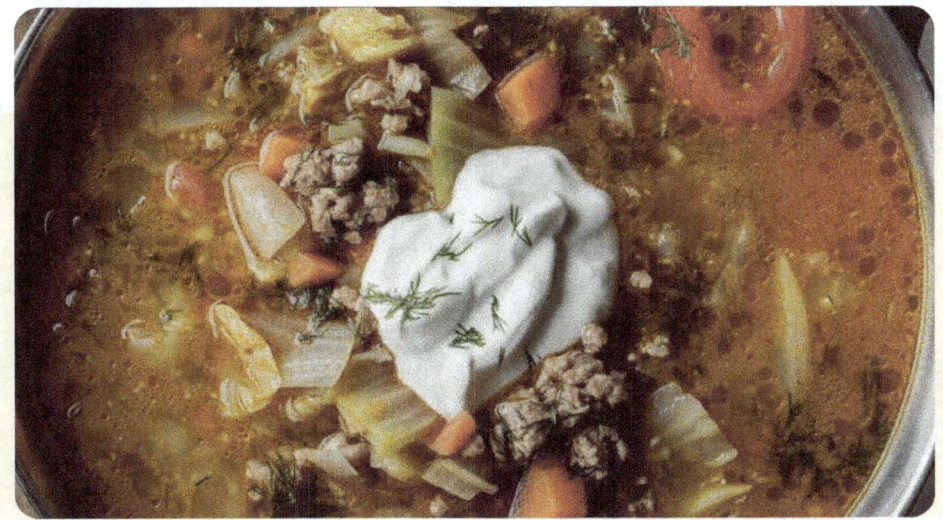

Pork & Cabbage Soup

Quick   One-Pan   Budget-Friendly

🍲 Serves: 8

🥗 Prep Time: 15 min

🍲 Cook Time: 30 min

🍲 Total: 45 min

💲 Cost Per Serving: $1.85

MACROS PER SERVING:

Calories: 265 | Protein: 22g | Fat: 16g | Net Carbs: 7g

Ingredients:

- 1½ pounds ground pork
- 8 cups chicken or beef broth
- 6 cups green cabbage, chopped
- 1 can (14.5 oz) diced tomatoes, undrained
- 1 medium onion, diced
- 3 carrots, diced
- 4 cloves garlic, minced
- 2 tablespoons tomato paste
- 2 teaspoons paprika
- 1 teaspoon caraway seeds (optional but traditional)
- 1 teaspoon dried thyme
- 1 teaspoon salt
- ½ teaspoon black pepper
- 2 bay leaves
- 2 tablespoons olive oil
- Sour cream for serving (optional)
- Fresh dill for garnish (optional)

Instructions:

1. Heat olive oil in a large pot over medium-high heat.
2. Add ground pork and cook, breaking it up, for 6-8 minutes until browned. Don't drain the fat.
3. Add onion and carrots. Cook for 5 minutes until starting to soften.
4. Add garlic, paprika, caraway seeds (if using), and thyme. Cook for 1 minute until fragrant.
5. Stir in tomato paste and cook for 1 minute.
6. Add broth, diced tomatoes (with juice), cabbage, bay leaves, salt, and pepper. Stir to combine.
7. Bring to a boil, then reduce heat to medium-low. Simmer for 20-25 minutes until cabbage is very tender and flavors have melded.
8. Remove bay leaves. Taste and adjust seasoning.
9. Serve hot with a dollop of sour cream and fresh dill if desired.

Tips:

Budget breakdown: Ground pork $5, broth $3, cabbage $2, vegetables and tomatoes $3, seasonings $1. Total: $14 for 8 servings.

Why this soup: It's inspired by Eastern European cabbage soup (kapusniak). Hearty, filling, and incredibly economical.

Ground beef: Works just as well as pork. Use whatever's cheaper.

Cabbage shrinks: Six cups of raw cabbage will cook down significantly. Don't worry if your pot looks overfilled at first.

Storage: Refrigerate for up to 5 days or freeze for up to 4 months. One of those soups that tastes even better the next day.

Add heat: Stir in ½ teaspoon red pepper flakes or serve with hot sauce.

Slow cooker method: Brown pork first, then transfer everything to slow cooker. Cook on low for 6-8 hours or high for 3-4 hours.

Make it creamy: Stir in ½ cup sour cream at the end for a richer soup (adds 2g fat per serving).

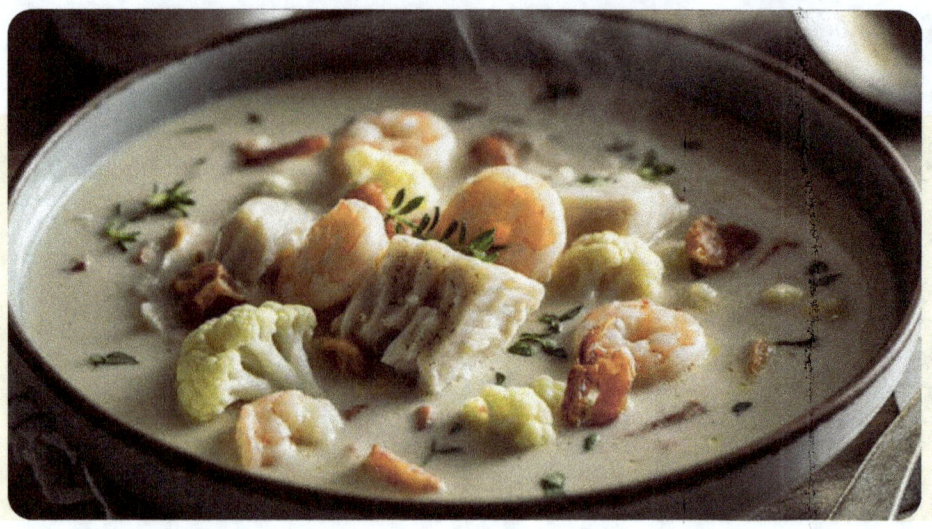

Seafood Chowder (No Potatoes)

Make-Ahead

🍽 Serves: 8

✂ Prep Time: 20 min

🍲 Cook Time: 30 min

🕐 Total: 50 min

💲 Cost Per Serving: $4.25

MACROS PER SERVING:

Calories: 335 | Protein: 26g |
Fat: 22g | Net Carbs: 8g

Instructions:

1. In a large pot, cook chopped bacon over medium heat until crispy, about 6-8 minutes. Transfer bacon to a paper towel-lined plate, leaving the fat in the pot.
2. Add butter, onion, and celery to the bacon fat. Cook for 5-6 minutes until softened.
3. Add garlic and thyme. Cook for 1 minute until fragrant.
4. Add cauliflower and broth. Bring to a boil, then reduce heat and simmer for 10-12 minutes until cauliflower is very tender.
5. Use an immersion blender to partially blend the soup, or mash some cauliflower against the side of the pot with a spoon. You want some chunks remaining, but the base should be creamy.
6. Stir in heavy cream, bay leaf, salt, pepper, and Old Bay (if using). Bring to a gentle simmer.
7. Add fish pieces. Simmer gently for 5 minutes.
8. Add shrimp (and clams if using). Simmer for 3-4 more minutes until shrimp are pink and cooked through.
9. Remove bay leaf. Taste and adjust seasoning.
10. Stir in half the cooked bacon. Reserve the rest for topping.

Ingredients:

- 1 pound firm white fish (cod, halibut, or mahi-mahi), cut into 1-inch pieces
- ½ pound shrimp, peeled and deveined
- 4 cups cauliflower florets, chopped small
- 4 cups chicken or seafood broth
- 2 cups heavy cream
- 4 strips bacon, chopped
- 1 medium onion, diced
- 3 celery stalks, diced
- 3 cloves garlic, minced
- 2 tablespoons butter
- 2 tablespoons fresh parsley, chopped
- 1 teaspoon dried thyme
- 1 bay leaf
- ¾ teaspoon salt
- ½ teaspoon black pepper
- ¼ teaspoon Old Bay seasoning (optional)
- Optional: ½ cup canned clams, drained

Tips:

Budget breakdown: Fish $8, shrimp $6, bacon $3, cream $3, cauliflower and other vegetables $4, broth $2. Total: $26 for 8 servings.

Buy frozen seafood: Much cheaper than fresh and works perfectly in soup. Thaw in the refrigerator overnight.

Potato substitute: Cauliflower provides the creamy, hearty texture of potatoes without the carbs. When partially blended, it thickens the soup beautifully.

Don't overcook seafood: Fish and shrimp cook quickly. Add them at the end and watch carefully. Overcooked seafood is tough and rubbery.

Storage: Refrigerate for up to 3 days. Don't freeze this one—cream and seafood don't freeze well together.

Make it cheaper: Use all cod or tilapia instead of mixed seafood. Still delicious.

Clam chowder variation: Use all clams (3-4 cans, drained) instead of fish and shrimp. Add juice from 1 can of clams to the broth for extra flavor.

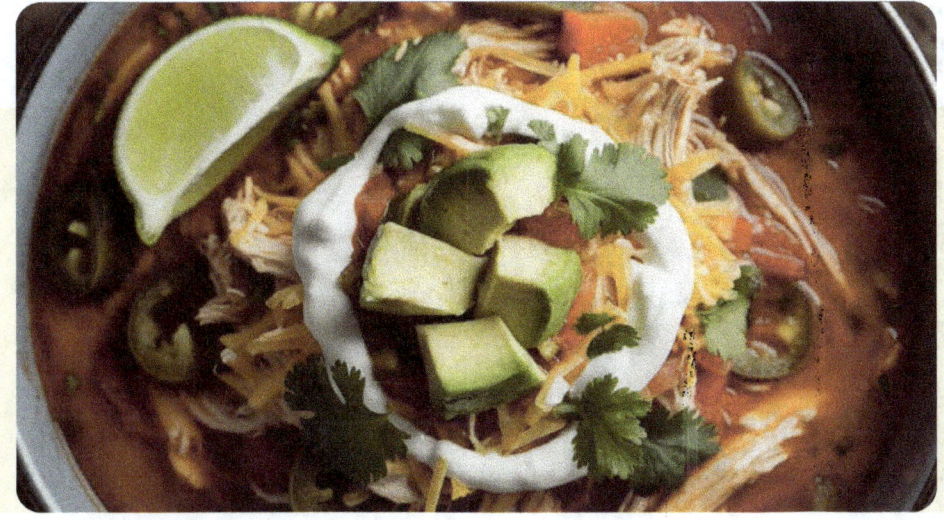

Chicken Tortilla Soup (No Tortillas)

Make-Ahead   Budget-Friendly

🍽 Serves: 8

✂ Prep Time: 15 min

🍲 Cook Time: 35 min

⏱ Total: 50 min

💲 Cost Per Serving: $2.35

MACROS PER SERVING:

Calories: 285 | Protein: 28g | Fat: 15g | Net Carbs: 8g

Instructions:

1. Heat olive oil in a large pot over medium-high heat.
2. Season chicken with salt and pepper. Add to pot and cook for 3-4 minutes per side until lightly browned. Transfer to a plate.
3. Add onion and bell peppers to the pot. Cook for 5-6 minutes until softened.
4. Add garlic, cumin, chili powder, paprika, and oregano. Cook for 1 minute until fragrant.
5. Stir in tomato paste and cook for 1 minute.
6. Add chicken broth, diced tomatoes (with juice), and green chiles. Bring to a boil.
7. Return chicken to the pot. Reduce heat to medium-low and simmer for 20-25 minutes until chicken is cooked through and tender.
8. Remove chicken from pot and shred with two forks. Return shredded chicken to the pot.
9. Stir in lime juice. Taste and adjust seasoning.

Tips:

Budget breakdown: Chicken $6, broth $3, tomatoes and chiles $2, vegetables $3, cheese and sour cream for topping $3. Total: $17 for 8 servings.

Tortilla substitute: The soup itself is filling enough without tortillas. If you want crunch, use crushed pork rinds or make cheese crisps (bake small piles of shredded cheese at 350°F for 5-7 minutes).

Rotisserie shortcut: Use a rotisserie chicken. Skip step 2. Add shredded chicken in step 8. Saves 30 minutes.

Spice level: This recipe is mild-medium. Add jalapeños or cayenne pepper for more heat.

Storage: Refrigerate for up to 5 days or freeze for up to 4 months.

Slow cooker method: Place raw chicken, all vegetables, broth, tomatoes, chiles, and seasonings in slow cooker. Cook on low for 6-8 hours or high for 3-4 hours. Shred chicken in the pot. Stir in lime juice before serving.

Instant Pot method: Sauté onions and peppers using sauté function. Add chicken, broth, tomatoes, chiles, and seasonings. Pressure cook on high for 15 minutes with quick release. Shred chicken in the pot.

Ingredients:

- 2 pounds boneless, skinless chicken breasts or thighs
- 8 cups chicken broth
- 1 can (14.5 oz) diced tomatoes, undrained
- 1 can (4 oz) diced green chiles
- 1 medium onion, diced
- 1 red bell pepper, diced
- 1 green bell pepper, diced
- 4 cloves garlic, minced
- 2 tablespoons tomato paste
- 2 tablespoons olive oil
- 2 teaspoons cumin
- 2 teaspoons chili powder
- 1 teaspoon paprika
- 1 teaspoon oregano
- 1 teaspoon salt
- ½ teaspoon black pepper
- Juice of 1 lime

For serving:
- 1 avocado, diced
- ½ cup shredded cheddar cheese
- ½ cup sour cream
- Fresh cilantro, chopped
- Lime wedges
- Optional: crushed pork rinds (tortilla chip substitute)

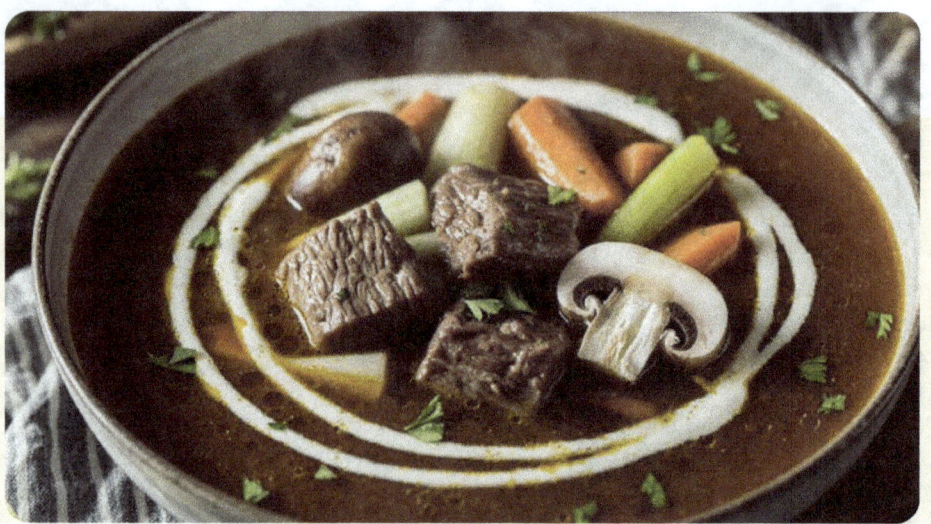

Beef & Mushroom Soup

Make-Ahead   Budget-Friendly

🔔 Serves: 8

⚙️ Prep Time: 15 min

🍲 Cook Time: 45 min

🕐 Total: 60 min

$ Cost Per Serving: $2.65

MACROS PER SERVING:

Calories: 295 | Protein: 26g |
Fat: 18g | Net Carbs: 6g

Instructions:

1. Pat beef cubes dry with paper towels. Season all sides with salt, pepper, and paprika.
2. Heat 1 tablespoon olive oil in a large pot over high heat.
3. Working in batches, sear beef cubes on all sides until browned, about 2-3 minutes per side. Transfer to a plate.
4. Add remaining tablespoon olive oil to the pot. Add mushrooms and cook over medium-high heat for 5-6 minutes until browned and liquid has evaporated.
5. Add onion, carrots, and celery. Cook for 5 minutes until starting to soften.
6. Add garlic and thyme. Cook for 1 minute.
7. Stir in tomato paste and cook for 1 minute.
8. Add beef broth, Worcestershire sauce, and bay leaves. Scrape up any browned bits from the bottom of the pot.
9. Return beef to the pot along with any accumulated juices. Bring to a boil.
10. Reduce heat to low, cover, and simmer for 45-50 minutes until beef is very tender.
11. If using heavy cream, stir it in at the end. Simmer for 2-3 minutes.
12. Remove bay leaves. Taste and adjust seasoning.

Tips:

Budget breakdown: Beef stew meat $9-10, broth $3, mushrooms $4, vegetables $3, other ingredients $2. Total: $21-22 for 8 servings.

Beef stroganoff-style: Add ½ cup sour cream instead of heavy cream at the end for tangy, creamy soup. Serve over cauliflower rice.

Storage: Refrigerate for up to 5 days or freeze for up to 4 months. The flavors deepen over time.

Slow cooker method: Sear beef and mushrooms first, then transfer everything to slow cooker. Cook on low for 7-8 hours or high for 4-5 hours.

Instant Pot method: Sear beef using sauté function. Add all ingredients except cream. Pressure cook on high for 25 minutes with natural release. Stir in cream before serving.

Ground beef version: Use ground beef instead of stew meat for a quicker, cheaper version. Brown beef first, then proceed with recipe. Ready in 30 minutes.

Ingredients:

- 1½ pounds beef stew meat, cut into ¾-inch cubes
- 8 cups beef broth
- 1 pound mushrooms (cremini or button), sliced
- 1 medium onion, diced
- 3 carrots, diced
- 3 celery stalks, diced
- 4 cloves garlic, minced
- 3 tablespoons tomato paste
- 2 tablespoons Worcestershire sauce
- 2 tablespoons olive oil
- 2 bay leaves
- 2 teaspoons dried thyme
- 1 teaspoon paprika
- 1 teaspoon salt
- ½ teaspoon black pepper
- ½ cup heavy cream (optional, for creamier soup)
- Fresh parsley for garnish

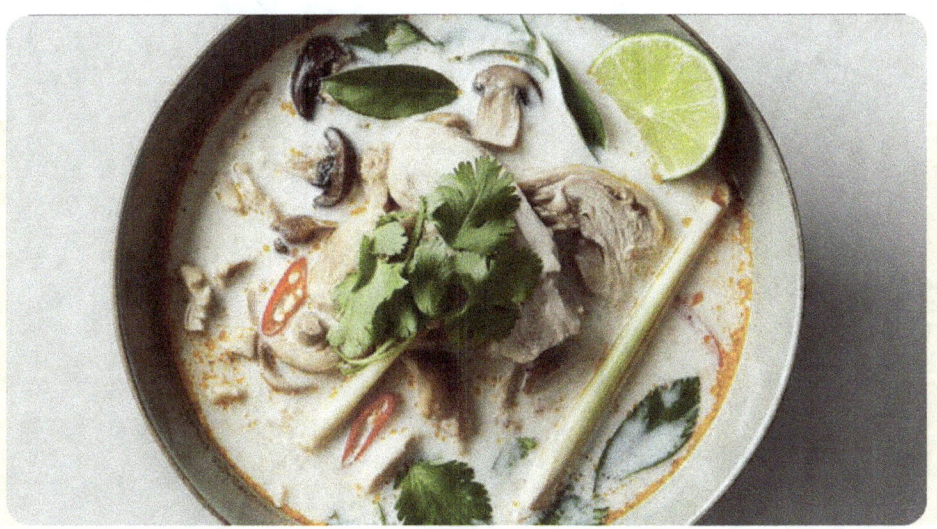

Tom Kha Gai
(Thai Coconut Chicken)

Make-Ahead

 Serves: 6

 Prep Time: 15 min

Cook Time: 25 min

Total: 40 min

 Cost Per Serving: $3.15

MACROS PER SERVING:
Calories: 365 | Protein: 28g | Fat: 26g | Net Carbs: 7g

Instructions:

1. Heat coconut oil in a large pot over medium-high heat.
2. Add chicken slices and cook for 3-4 minutes until lightly browned. Transfer to a plate.
3. In the same pot, add chicken broth, coconut milk, lemongrass, ginger, kaffir lime leaves (or lime zest), and Thai chiles. Bring to a boil.
4. Reduce heat to medium-low and simmer for 10 minutes to infuse flavors.
5. Add mushrooms and return chicken to the pot. Simmer for 8-10 minutes until chicken is cooked through and mushrooms are tender.
6. Stir in fish sauce, lime juice, sweetener (if using), and salt. Taste and adjust seasoning. The soup should be balanced between sour (lime), salty (fish sauce), and slightly sweet.
7. Remove lemongrass pieces before serving (they're not meant to be eaten, just for flavor).

Tips:

Budget breakdown: Chicken $5, coconut milk $3, broth $2, mushrooms $3, aromatics and seasonings $3. Total: $16 for 6 servings.

Authentic ingredients: Lemongrass, kaffir lime leaves, and fish sauce are available at Asian grocery stores. Regular grocery stores often carry lemongrass and fish sauce. In a pinch, use extra lime zest and juice if you can't find kaffir lime leaves.

Don't skip fish sauce: It's essential for authentic Thai flavor. It's not "fishy" in the final soup—it adds savory depth.

Lemongrass prep: Cut off the tough top portion. Use only the bottom 4 inches. Smash with the back of a knife to release oils, then cut into pieces.

Coconut milk: Use full-fat coconut milk, not lite. The fat is what makes this soup rich and satisfying.

Storage: Refrigerate for up to 4 days. The flavors actually improve overnight. Don't freeze this one—the coconut milk can separate.

Shrimp version: Use 1 pound shrimp instead of chicken. Add shrimp in the last 3-4 minutes of cooking.

Vegetarian version: Skip the chicken and use vegetable broth. Add extra mushrooms and some firm tofu for protein.

Ingredients:

- 1½ pounds boneless, skinless chicken breasts or thighs, thinly sliced
- 2 cans (14 oz each) full-fat coconut milk
- 4 cups chicken broth
- 8 oz mushrooms, sliced (shiitake or button)
- 3 tablespoons fresh lime juice
- 2 tablespoons fish sauce
- 2 tablespoons fresh ginger, sliced thin
- 3 stalks lemongrass (bottom 4 inches only), smashed and cut into 2-inch pieces
- 4 kaffir lime leaves (or zest of 1 lime)
- 3 Thai bird chiles, smashed (or ½ teaspoon red pepper flakes)
- 1 tablespoon coconut oil
- 2 teaspoons erythritol or monk fruit sweetener (optional, traditional recipes use palm sugar)
- ½ teaspoon salt
- Fresh cilantro for garnish
- Lime wedges for serving

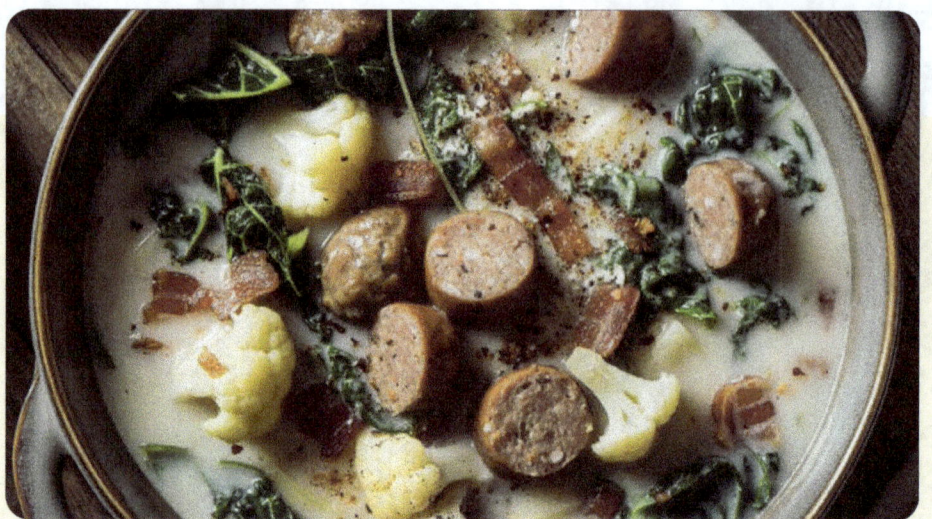

Zuppa Toscana (No Potatoes)

Make-Ahead   Budget-Friendly

Serves: 8

Prep Time: 15 min

Cook Time: 30 min

Total: 45 min

Cost Per Serving: $2.45

MACROS PER SERVING:
Calories: 385 | Protein: 22g |
Fat: 30g | Net Carbs: 6g

Ingredients:

- 1 pound Italian sausage (mild or hot), casings removed
- 6 strips bacon, chopped
- 6 cups cauliflower florets, cut into bite-sized pieces
- 6 cups chicken broth
- 2 cups heavy cream
- 4 cups fresh kale, stems removed, chopped
- 1 medium onion, diced
- 4 cloves garlic, minced
- ¾ teaspoon salt
- ½ teaspoon black pepper
- ½ teaspoon red pepper flakes (optional)
- Grated Parmesan cheese for serving

Instructions:

1. In a large pot, cook chopped bacon over medium heat until crispy, about 6-8 minutes. Transfer to a paper towel-lined plate, leaving the fat in the pot.
2. Add Italian sausage to the bacon fat. Cook, breaking it up with a spoon, for 6-8 minutes until browned and cooked through. Transfer to the plate with bacon.
3. Add onion to the pot and cook in the sausage fat for 5 minutes until softened.
4. Add garlic and red pepper flakes (if using). Cook for 1 minute.
5. Add chicken broth and cauliflower florets. Bring to a boil, then reduce heat and simmer for 10-12 minutes until cauliflower is tender.
6. Use a potato masher to break up some of the cauliflower (you want some chunks and some mashed for a creamy texture).
7. Stir in heavy cream, salt, and pepper. Bring to a gentle simmer.
8. Return bacon and sausage to the pot.
9. Add chopped kale. Stir and simmer for 3-4 minutes until kale is wilted and tender.
10. Taste and adjust seasoning.
11. Serve hot with grated Parmesan cheese on top.

Tips:

Budget breakdown: Italian sausage $4, bacon $3, cream $3, cauliflower $3, kale $2, broth $2, Parmesan $1. Total: $18 for 8 servings.

Copycat recipe: This is inspired by Olive Garden's Zuppa Toscana. We replace potatoes with cauliflower for the same hearty texture with fewer carbs.

Kale substitute: If you can't find kale or don't like it, use spinach. Add it at the very end and cook just until wilted (1-2 minutes).

Make it spicier: Use hot Italian sausage and increase red pepper flakes to 1 teaspoon.

Storage: Refrigerate for up to 5 days or freeze for up to 3 months. The cream may separate slightly when frozen, but whisking during reheating brings it back together.

Slow cooker method: Brown bacon and sausage first. Transfer all ingredients except cream and kale to slow cooker. Cook on low for 5-6 hours or high for 3 hours. Stir in cream and kale in the last 15 minutes.

Ground beef version: Use ground beef instead of Italian sausage to save money. Add 1 tablespoon Italian seasoning for flavor.

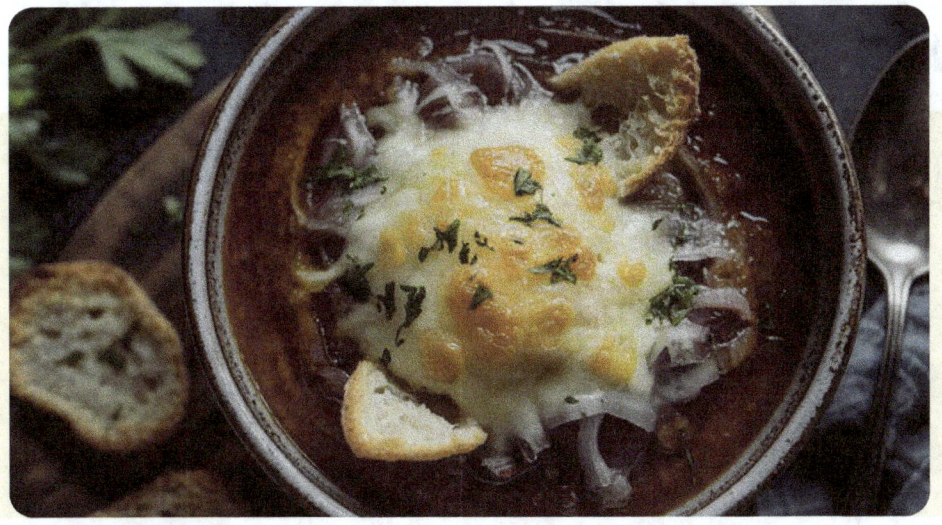

French Onion Soup (Low-Carb)

Make-Ahead

 Serves: 6

 Prep Time: 15 min

Cook Time: 55 min

Total: 70 min

 Cost Per Serving: $2.85

MACROS PER SERVING:
Calories: 295 | Protein: 16g |
Fat: 22g | Net Carbs: 8g

Instructions:

1. Heat butter and olive oil in a large pot or Dutch oven over medium heat.
2. Add sliced onions and a pinch of salt. Cook, stirring occasionally, for 30-40 minutes until onions are deeply caramelized and golden brown. Don't rush this step—it's where all the flavor comes from.
3. If onions start to stick or burn, add a splash of broth to deglaze the pot and continue cooking.
4. Add garlic and thyme. Cook for 1 minute.
5. Pour in wine (if using) and scrape up any browned bits from the bottom of the pot. Let wine simmer for 3-4 minutes to cook off the alcohol.
6. Add beef broth, bay leaves, Worcestershire sauce, salt, and pepper. Bring to a boil.
7. Reduce heat to low and simmer for 20 minutes to let flavors meld.

To serve:
1. Ladle soup into oven-safe bowls.
2. Top each bowl with a generous amount of shredded Gruyère and grated Parmesan.
3. Optional: Place a slice of provolone cheese on top for the "bread" element.
4. Place bowls on a baking sheet and broil for 2-3 minutes until cheese is melted, bubbly, and golden brown on top. Watch carefully—it can burn quickly.
5. Garnish with fresh parsley and serve immediately.

Ingredients:

- 4 large yellow onions, thinly sliced
- 8 cups beef broth
- 1 cup dry white wine (or additional broth)
- 4 tablespoons butter
- 2 tablespoons olive oil
- 4 cloves garlic, minced
- 2 bay leaves
- 2 teaspoons dried thyme
- 1 teaspoon Worcestershire sauce
- ¾ teaspoon salt
- ½ teaspoon black pepper
- 1½ cups shredded Gruyère cheese (or Swiss cheese)
- ½ cup grated Parmesan cheese
- Fresh parsley for garnish

For "croutons" (optional):
- 6 slices provolone cheese

Tips:

Budget breakdown: Onions $3, broth $3, cheese $7, wine $2, butter and seasonings $2. Total: $17 for 6 servings.

The caramelizing step: This takes time but it's essential. Properly caramelized onions are sweet, rich, and deeply flavorful. Low and slow is the key.

No croutons needed: The original has bread croutons under the cheese. We skip them—the cheese itself gets crispy and provides texture.

Cheese substitute: Gruyère is traditional and delicious, but Swiss or mozzarella work if that's what you have.

Storage: Refrigerate soup (without cheese topping) for up to 5 days. Don't freeze this one—the onions get mushy.

Reheating: Reheat soup on the stovetop, then portion into bowls, add cheese, and broil as directed.

Make ahead: Caramelize onions a day or two in advance. Store in the fridge. When ready to make soup, start at step 4.

CHAPTER 6 SUMMARY

You now have 12 soups and stews that will keep you warm, full, and satisfied without relying on noodles, potatoes, or rice. Here's how to make soup work for you:

The Soup Strategy:

Sunday Soup Routine: Make one large batch (8 servings) on Sunday. You now have:

- 4 lunches for the week
- 2 easy dinners
- 2 portions for the freezer

Total hands-on time: 20-30 minutes **Total cooking time:** 30 minutes to 2 hours (mostly hands-off)

My Favorite Soup Combinations:

For a cheap week:
- Monday: Pork & Cabbage Soup (makes 8 servings, $1.85/serving)
- Use leftovers for lunch Tuesday-Thursday
- Total cost: Under $15 for multiple meals

For meal prep:
- Make Beef Chili and Chicken Soup on Sunday
- Alternate lunches all week
- Never get bored

For variety:
- Make one soup per week
- By the end of the month, you've tried 4 different soups
- Freeze portions of each
- Now you have 4 different soup options in your freezer

Soup as a Weight Loss Tool:

Soup is one of the most effective foods for feeling full while eating fewer calories:

- High volume (lots of liquid)
- High protein (keeps you satisfied)
- Warm temperature (slows you down while eating)
- Rich flavors (satisfies cravings)

Studies show people who eat soup before meals consume fewer calories overall. But these soups are complete meals—you don't need anything else.

Freezer Soup Strategy:

Every time you make soup:

1. Eat 2-3 servings fresh
2. Refrigerate 2-3 servings for the week
3. Freeze the rest in portions

Label with:
- Name of soup
- Date made
- Reheating instructions if needed

Within a month, you'll have 4-5 different soups in the freezer. Instant dinner variety.

Soup Math:

Making soup yourself:
- Average cost per serving: $2-3
- Time investment: 20-30 min hands-on (rest is simmering)
- Servings per batch: 6-8

Buying soup at restaurants:
- Average cost per serving: $8-12
- Time investment: Driving, waiting, driving back
- Servings: 1

Savings: $5-10 per serving when you make it yourself

The Soups Everyone Should Try:

If you only make a few from this chapter, make these:

1. **Chicken Soup (Recipe 91):** Classic comfort food. Works when you're sick, tired, or just want something familiar.
2. **Beef Stew (Recipe 92):** Hearty, filling, economical. Tastes like you worked harder than you did.
3. **Creamy Broccoli Cheese Soup (Recipe 94):** When you want something rich and comforting. Tastes indulgent while hitting your protein goals.
4. **Beef Chili (Recipe 77 from Chapter 5):** I know it's from the previous chapter, but it's technically a soup/stew and it's perfect for meal prep.

Soup Serving Suggestions:

Most of these soups are complete meals on their own, but if you want sides:

Light soups (Egg Drop, Chicken Soup):
- Serve with a salad
- Add a hard-boiled egg or two
- Pair with cheese and deli meat

Hearty soups (Beef Stew, Seafood Chowder, Zuppa Toscana):
- These are complete meals
- Maybe add a small salad if you're still hungry
- That's it

Common Mistakes:
1. **Not seasoning enough.** Soup needs more salt than you think because of the volume of liquid. Taste before serving and adjust.
2. **Rushing the simmering.** Soup gets better the longer it cooks (within reason). Don't rush it.
3. **Boiling instead of simmering.** A gentle simmer extracts flavors. A rolling boil makes everything tough and cloudy.
4. **Adding dairy too early.** Always add cream, milk, or cheese toward the end. High heat makes dairy separate and curdle.
5. **Forgetting to taste before serving.** Flavors change as soup cooks and sits. Always taste and adjust seasoning before serving.

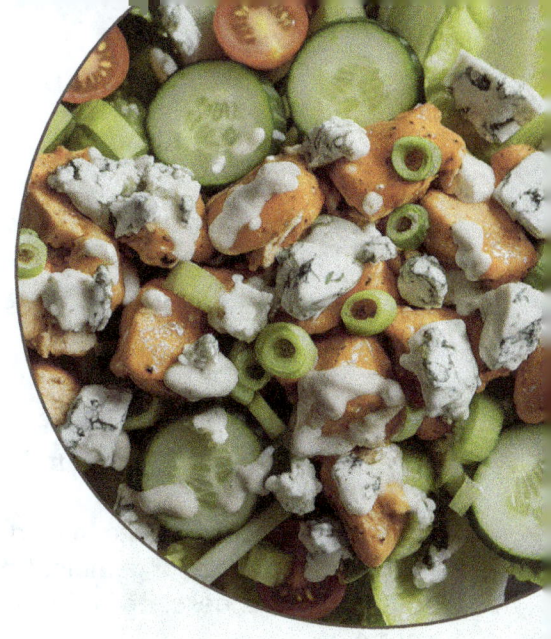

Let's address the elephant in the room: most people think salads are boring.

And you know what? They're right. A pile of iceberg lettuce with a sad tomato wedge and fat-free ranch dressing is boring. That's not a meal. That's rabbit food that leaves you hungry an hour later, raiding the pantry for something—anything—with actual substance.

But that's not what this chapter is about.

The salads and bowls in this chapter are complete, satisfying meals. They're protein-forward, flavor-packed, and substantial enough that you won't be thinking about food again for 4-5 hours. They're the kind of salads that make you actually look forward to lunch.

What Makes These Different:

Traditional salad:
- Base: Lettuce
- Protein: Maybe 2 oz of grilled chicken if you're lucky
- Dressing: Usually low-fat and tasteless
- Result: Hungry in an hour, 12g protein

Our salads:
- Base: Variety of vegetables (raw, cooked, or both)
- Protein: 6-8 oz of substantial protein (chicken, steak, eggs, tuna, shrimp)
- Dressing: Full-fat, flavorful, homemade
- Result: Satisfied for hours, 30-40g protein

The Bowl vs. Salad Question:
What's the difference between a salad and a bowl?

Salads: Usually cold, mostly raw vegetables, lighter proteins, typically eaten with a fork.

Bowls: Can be warm or cold, mix of raw and cooked ingredients, often include grains (in our case, cauliflower rice), heartier proteins, eaten with a fork or spoon.

Honestly, the distinction doesn't matter much. Both are complete meals in a bowl. Call them whatever you want.

Why These Work for High-Protein, Low-Carb:
1. **Protein is the star.** Vegetables are supporting cast. The meal is built around 30-40g of protein.
2. **Fats keep you full.** Full-fat dressings, avocado, nuts, cheese. These aren't optional—they're essential for satiety.

3. **Volume without carbs.** Leafy greens and non-starchy vegetables add volume and fiber without adding carbs.

4. **Endless variety.** Change the protein, swap the dressing, add different vegetables. Same format, completely different meal.

5. **Portable and practical.** Most of these pack well for lunch. Protein and vegetables in one container, dressing on the side.

The Formula for a Perfect Salad/Bowl:
Every recipe in this chapter follows this basic structure:

Base (2-4 cups): Lettuce, mixed greens, cauliflower rice, or combination **Protein (6-8 oz):** Chicken, steak, shrimp, tuna, eggs, or combination **Vegetables (1-2 cups):** Raw or cooked, your choice **Healthy Fat:** Avocado, nuts, olives, cheese, or fat in the dressing **Dressing (2-3 tablespoons):** Full-fat, flavorful, complements the protein

Total macros: 30-40g protein, 20-30g fat, 5-10g net carbs

Once you understand this formula, you can create infinite variations.

Meal Prep Strategy:
The secret to good salad meal prep is keeping things separate:

Sunday prep:
- Cook proteins (grill chicken, hard-boil eggs, etc.)
- Wash and chop vegetables
- Make dressings
- Store everything separately

Daily assembly: When you're ready to eat:
- Grab container of protein
- Grab container of vegetables
- Grab container of dressing
- Combine, toss, eat

Never pre-dress salads. They get soggy. Always dress right before eating.

Equipment:
- **Large mixing bowls:** For tossing salads
- **Sharp knife:** For chopping vegetables
- **Salad spinner (optional but nice):** Dries lettuce efficiently
- **Small jars with lids:** For dressings
- **Meal prep containers with compartments:** Keep components separate

Storage Tips:
Proteins: 3-4 days refrigerated **Washed/chopped vegetables:** 3-5 days refrigerated **Dressings:** 5-7 days refrigerated **Assembled salads:** Don't. Assemble fresh each time.

The Dressing Situation:

Chapter 9 has full dressing recipes, but here's the quick version:

Basic vinaigrette formula:
- 3 parts oil (olive, avocado)
- 1 part acid (lemon juice, vinegar)
- Salt, pepper, herbs
- Shake in a jar

Basic creamy dressing formula:
- Mayonnaise or sour cream base
- Acid (lemon juice, vinegar)
- Seasonings (garlic, herbs, spices)
- Thin with water or oil if needed

Store-bought dressings work too, but read labels. Many are loaded with sugar and seed oils. Look for dressings with clean ingredients and under 2g carbs per 2 tablespoons.

Common Salad Mistakes:
1. **Not enough protein.** If your salad doesn't have at least 6 oz of protein, it's a side salad, not a meal.
2. **Low-fat dressing.** Fat helps you absorb fat-soluble vitamins from vegetables and keeps you full. Use the real stuff.
3. **Too many toppings.** Croutons, dried fruit, candied nuts, sweetened dressing. Suddenly your "healthy" salad has 30g of carbs.
4. **All lettuce, no variety.** Mix raw and cooked vegetables. Add different textures and colors.
5. **Pre-dressing everything.** Soggy salad is sad salad. Always dress right before eating.

The Recipes:

Every salad and bowl in this chapter:

- Provides 30-40g protein per serving
- Stays under 10g net carbs
- Can be made ahead (with components stored separately)
- Actually tastes good enough to eat regularly
- Makes 1-2 servings (easy to scale up)

Some are classics (Cobb, Caesar). Some are inspired by restaurant favorites (Chipotle burrito bowl). Some are my own creations that I've been making for years.

All of them will change how you think about salad.

Let's cook.

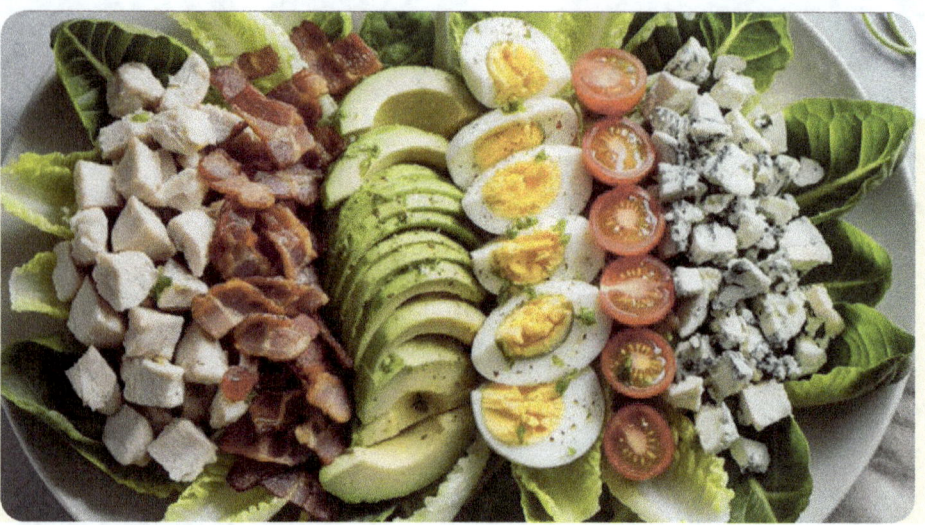

Cobb Salad

Quick   Make-Ahead (components)

Serves: 2

Prep Time: 15 min

Cook Time: 0 min (using precooked ingredients)

Total: 15 min

Cost Per Serving: $4.25

MACROS PER SERVING:

Calories: 485 | Protein: 38g | Fat: 34g | Net Carbs: 6g

Ingredients:

For the salad:
- 4 cups romaine lettuce, chopped
- 12 oz cooked chicken breast, diced
- 4 strips bacon, cooked and crumbled
- 2 hard-boiled eggs, chopped
- 1 medium avocado, diced
- ½ cup cherry tomatoes, halved
- ¼ cup blue cheese, crumbled
- 2 green onions, sliced

For the dressing:
- ¼ cup olive oil
- 2 tablespoons red wine vinegar
- 1 teaspoon Dijon mustard
- ½ teaspoon Worcestershire sauce
- 1 clove garlic, minced
- ¼ teaspoon salt
- ⅛ teaspoon black pepper

Instructions:

Make the dressing:
1. In a small jar or bowl, combine olive oil, red wine vinegar, Dijon mustard, Worcestershire sauce, garlic, salt, and pepper.
2. Shake or whisk until emulsified. Set aside.

Assemble the salad:
1. Divide chopped romaine between 2 large bowls or plates.
2. Arrange diced chicken, crumbled bacon, chopped eggs, avocado, tomatoes, and blue cheese in rows or sections on top of the lettuce (traditional Cobb presentation).
3. Sprinkle with sliced green onions.
4. Drizzle with dressing or serve dressing on the side.
5. Toss before eating or eat it in sections (I prefer tossing).

Tips:

Budget breakdown: Chicken $4, bacon $2, eggs $1, avocado $1.50, tomatoes $1, blue cheese $2, lettuce $1. Total: $12.50 for 2 servings. Still cheaper than restaurant Cobb salad ($12-15).

Meal prep: Cook chicken, bacon, and eggs on Sunday. Store separately. Assemble fresh salads throughout the week in 5 minutes.

Traditional presentation: Arrange ingredients in neat rows for visual appeal. It's prettier but takes longer.

Rotisserie shortcut: Use rotisserie chicken. Shred or dice it. Zero cooking required.

Blue cheese substitute: If you hate blue cheese (some people do), use feta, cheddar, or Parmesan.

Make it easier: Buy pre-cooked bacon, pre-washed lettuce, and use rotisserie chicken. Assembly time: 7 minutes.

Dressing variations: Ranch or blue cheese dressing also work perfectly here. Use what you prefer.

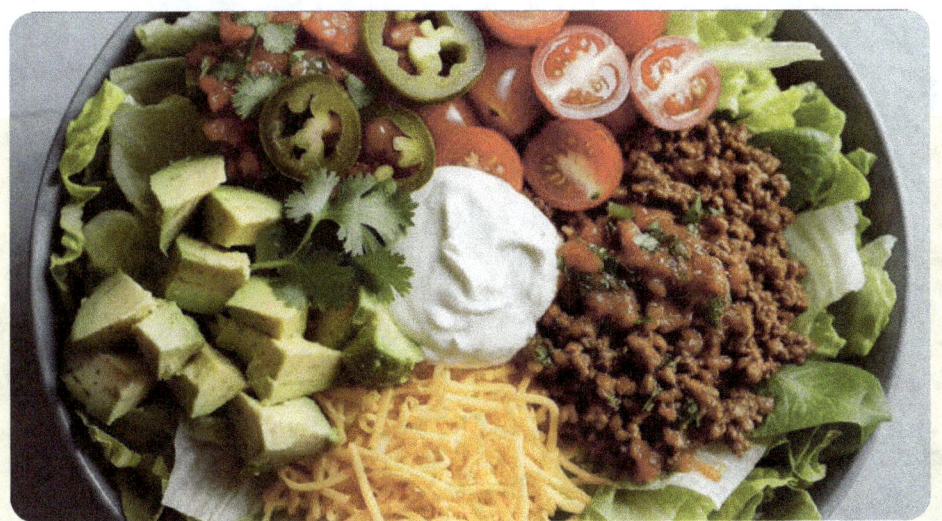

Taco Salad Bowl

Quick   Budget-Friendly   Make-Ahead (components)

🍽 Serves: 2

✂ Prep Time: 10 min

🍲 Cook Time: 10 min

🕐 Total: 20 min

💲 Cost Per Serving: $3.45

MACROS PER SERVING:

Calories: 495 | Protein: 36g | Fat: 34g | Net Carbs: 8g

Ingredients:

For the bowl:

- 12 oz ground beef (80/20)
- 2 tablespoons taco seasoning (homemade from Recipe 86 or store-bought)
- 4 cups romaine or iceberg lettuce, shredded
- 1 cup cherry tomatoes, halved
- 1 medium avocado, diced
- ½ cup shredded cheddar cheese
- ¼ cup sour cream
- ¼ cup salsa
- 2 tablespoons sliced jalapeños (optional)
- ¼ cup fresh cilantro, chopped
- Lime wedges for serving

Instructions:

1. Heat a large skillet over medium-high heat. Add ground beef and cook, breaking it up, for 6-8 minutes until browned.

2. Drain excess fat if there's more than 2 tablespoons.

3. Add taco seasoning and 3 tablespoons water. Stir and cook for 2 minutes until water evaporates and meat is well-coated.

4. Divide shredded lettuce between 2 large bowls.

5. Top each bowl with half the seasoned beef, tomatoes, avocado, cheese, sour cream, salsa, jalapeños (if using), and cilantro.

6. Serve with lime wedges. Squeeze lime over salad before eating.

Tips:

Budget breakdown: Ground beef $3.50, lettuce $1, tomatoes $1.50, avocado $1.50, cheese $1, other ingredients $1. Total: $9.50 for 2 servings.

Meal prep: Cook taco meat on Sunday (double or triple the batch). Store in the fridge. Assemble fresh salads daily with hot or cold meat.

Taco meat uses: This is the same taco meat from Recipe 86. Make a big batch and use it for multiple meals throughout the week.

Chip substitute: If you want crunch, crush some pork rinds and sprinkle on top. Or make cheese crisps (bake small piles of shredded cheese at 350°F for 5-7 minutes).

Ground turkey: Use ground turkey instead of beef for a leaner option. Add 1 tablespoon olive oil to keep it moist.

Make it a burrito bowl: Add ½ cup cauliflower rice per serving (warm or cold). Adds 2g net carbs.

Dressing: The salsa and sour cream act as dressing, but you can also add ranch or chipotle mayo.

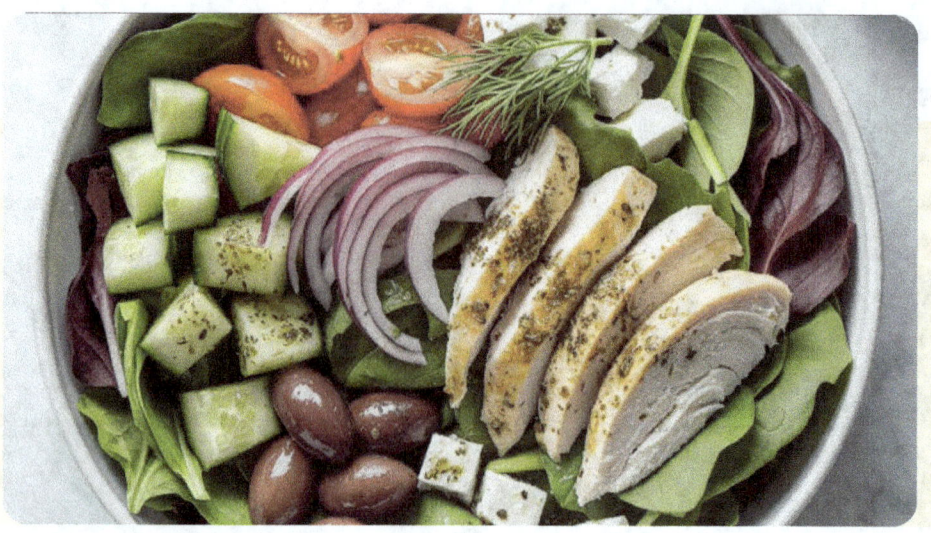

Greek Chicken Bowl

 Quick   Make-Ahead (components)

🍽 Serves: 2

🔪 Prep Time: 15 min

🍳 Cook Time: 0 min (using precooked chicken)

⏱ Total: 15 min

💲 Cost Per Serving: $4.15

MACROS PER SERVING:
Calories: 465 | Protein: 40g | Fat: 28g | Net Carbs: 8g

Instructions:

Make the vinaigrette:
1. Combine all dressing ingredients in a small jar. Shake vigorously until emulsified.

Assemble the bowls:
1. Divide mixed greens between 2 large bowls.
2. Top each with half the chicken, cucumber, tomatoes, red onion, olives, and feta cheese.
3. Sprinkle with fresh dill.
4. Drizzle with Greek vinaigrette or serve on the side.
5. Toss before eating.

Tips:

Budget breakdown: Chicken $4, greens $2, vegetables $3, feta $2, olives $2. Total: $13 for 2 servings.

Meal prep: Marinate and cook chicken using Recipe 87 (Marinated Chicken Thighs). Use throughout the week for multiple Greek bowls.

Tzatziki sauce: Make a quick tzatziki by mixing ½ cup Greek yogurt with ¼ cup diced cucumber, 1 minced garlic clove, 1 tablespoon lemon juice, and 1 tablespoon fresh dill. Adds creaminess and 3g protein per serving.

Warm or cold: This works with warm grilled chicken or cold meal-prepped chicken. Both are delicious.

Cauliflower rice option: Add 1 cup cooked cauliflower rice per serving for a heartier meal. Adds 2g net carbs.

Make it lamb: Use grilled lamb instead of chicken for authentic Greek flavor (more expensive but delicious).

Storage: Store all components separately. Assemble fresh bowls throughout the week.

Ingredients:

For the bowl:
- 12 oz cooked chicken breast or thighs, sliced or diced
- 4 cups mixed greens or romaine
- 1 cup cucumber, diced
- 1 cup cherry tomatoes, halved
- ½ red onion, thinly sliced
- ½ cup Kalamata olives, pitted
- ½ cup feta cheese, crumbled
- 2 tablespoons fresh dill, chopped (or 2 teaspoons dried)

For the Greek vinaigrette:
- ¼ cup olive oil
- 2 tablespoons lemon juice
- 1 tablespoon red wine vinegar
- 1 clove garlic, minced
- 1 teaspoon dried oregano
- ½ teaspoon Dijon mustard
- ¼ teaspoon salt
- ¼ teaspoon black pepper

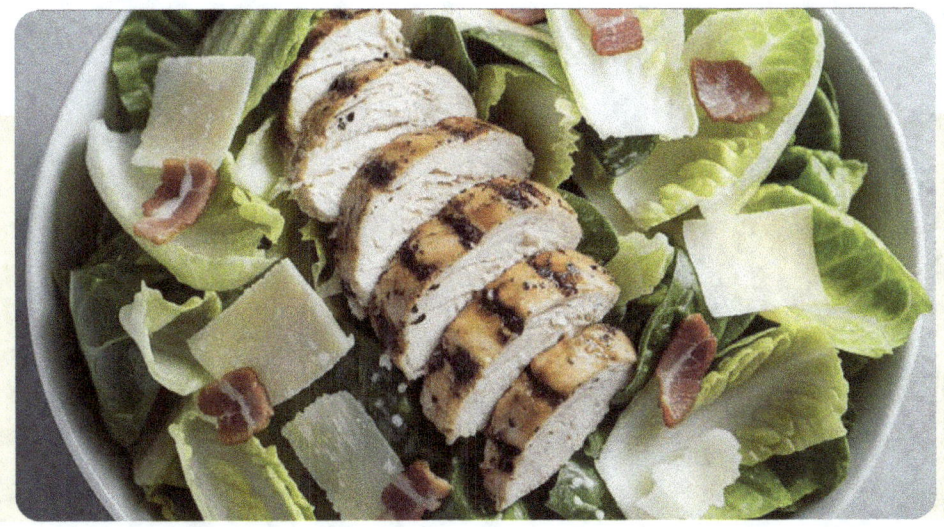

Caesar Salad
(with Grilled Chicken)

Quick   Make-Ahead (components)

🔔 Serves: 2

🕐 Prep Time: 10 min

🍲 Cook Time: 12 min (if cooking chicken fresh)

⏲ Total: 22 min

💲 Cost Per Serving: $3.85

MACROS PER SERVING:

Calories: 515 | Protein: 42g |
Fat: 36g | Net Carbs: 4g

Instructions:

Make the Caesar dressing:

1. In a bowl or jar, combine mayonnaise, lemon juice, Parmesan, Worcestershire sauce, garlic, Dijon mustard, anchovy paste (if using), salt, and pepper.

2. Whisk or shake until smooth. Add water 1 tablespoon at a time until dressing reaches desired consistency (should be thick but pourable).

3. Taste and adjust seasoning. Refrigerate until ready to use.

Grill the chicken (if not using precooked):

1. Season chicken breasts with salt, pepper, and a drizzle of olive oil.

2. Grill or pan-sear over medium-high heat for 6 minutes per side until internal temperature reaches 165°F.

3. Let rest for 5 minutes, then slice thin.

Assemble the salad:

1. Place chopped romaine in 2 large bowls.

2. Top each with sliced grilled chicken, Parmesan cheese, and bacon (if using).

3. Drizzle with Caesar dressing (about 3-4 tablespoons per serving).

4. Toss well before eating.

Tips:

Budget breakdown: Chicken $4, romaine $1.50, Parmesan $2, mayo and other dressing ingredients $2. Total: $9.50 for 2 servings.

Anchovy paste: Don't skip it if you have it. It adds authentic Caesar flavor without being fishy. If you don't have it, the dressing is still good.

Make extra dressing: This recipe makes about ¾ cup dressing (enough for 3-4 salads). Store leftovers in the fridge for up to 1 week.

Crouton substitute: Make Parmesan crisps. Bake small piles of shredded Parmesan at 350°F for 5-7 minutes until golden and crispy. Break into pieces and use as "croutons."

Rotisserie chicken: Use rotisserie chicken for zero-cook assembly. Warm or cold.

Restaurant copycat: This tastes better than most restaurant Caesar salads and costs half as much.

Make it a wrap: Use large romaine or butter lettuce leaves as wraps. Fill with chicken and Caesar dressing for lettuce wrap Caesars.

Ingredients:

For the salad:

- 12 oz chicken breast, grilled and sliced
- 6 cups romaine lettuce, chopped
- ½ cup Parmesan cheese, shaved or grated
- Optional: 6 strips bacon, cooked and crumbled

For Caesar dressing:

- ½ cup mayonnaise
- 2 tablespoons lemon juice
- 2 tablespoons grated Parmesan cheese
- 1 tablespoon Worcestershire sauce
- 2 cloves garlic, minced
- 1 teaspoon Dijon mustard
- 1 teaspoon anchovy paste (optional but traditional)
- ¼ teaspoon salt
- ¼ teaspoon black pepper
- 2-3 tablespoons water (to thin if needed)

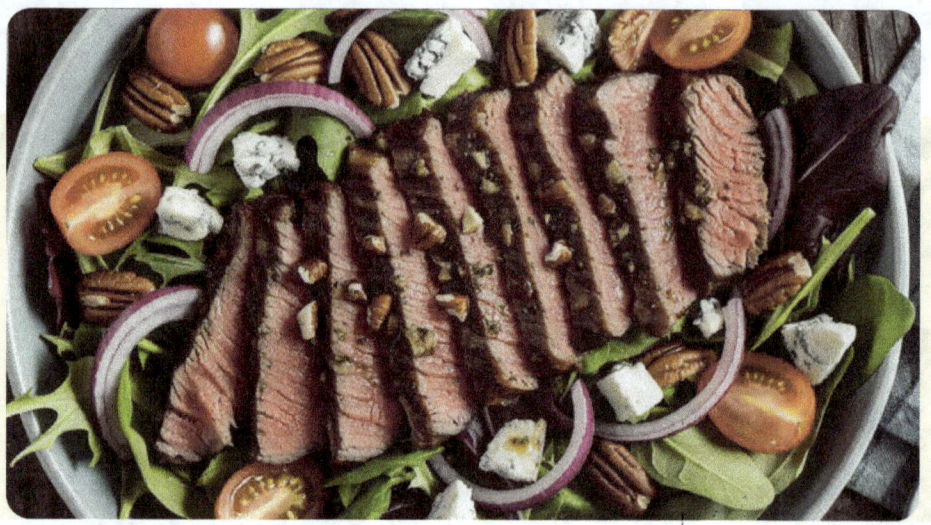

Quick

 Serves: 2

Prep Time: 10 min

 Cook Time: 12 min

 Total: 22 min

Cost Per Serving: $6.50

MACROS PER SERVING:
Calories: 545 | Protein: 42g |
Fat: 39g | Net Carbs: 6g

Ingredients:

For the salad:
- 12 oz sirloin or ribeye steak
- 6 cups mixed greens (spring mix, arugula, spinach)
- 1 cup cherry tomatoes, halved
- ½ red onion, thinly sliced
- ½ cup blue cheese, crumbled
- ¼ cup pecans or walnuts, chopped
- 1 tablespoon olive oil (for cooking steak)
- Salt and pepper for steak

For the dressing:
- 3 tablespoons olive oil
- 1 tablespoon balsamic vinegar
- 1 teaspoon Dijon mustard
- ½ teaspoon salt
- ¼ teaspoon black pepper

Instructions:

Cook the steak:
1. Pat steak dry with paper towels. Season generously on both sides with salt and pepper.
2. Heat olive oil in a cast-iron skillet or heavy pan over high heat until just smoking.
3. Add steak and cook for 4-5 minutes per side for medium-rare (130-135°F internal temperature), or adjust time for your preferred doneness.
4. Transfer to a cutting board and let rest for 5-10 minutes. Slice thin against the grain.

Make the dressing:
1. Whisk together olive oil, balsamic vinegar, Dijon mustard, salt, and pepper in a small bowl.

Assemble the salad:
1. Divide mixed greens between 2 large bowls or plates.
2. Top with cherry tomatoes, red onion, blue cheese, and nuts.
3. Arrange sliced steak on top.
4. Drizzle with balsamic vinaigrette.
5. Serve immediately.

Tips:

Budget breakdown: Steak $10-12, greens $2, tomatoes $1.50, blue cheese $2, nuts $1.50. Total: $17-19 for 2 servings. This is a splurge meal.

Cheaper cuts: Flank steak, skirt steak, or flat iron work great and cost less. Slice them thin against the grain after cooking.

Blue cheese substitute: Feta, goat cheese, or Gorgonzola all work. Or skip cheese entirely and use more nuts.

Let it rest: Don't skip the resting step. Slicing immediately causes all the juices to run out, leaving dry steak.

Warm or cold: This is great with warm steak, but also works with cold leftover steak the next day.

Add avocado: Half an avocado per serving adds creaminess and healthy fats. Adds 4g fat, 2g net carbs.

Make it a meal prep: Grill 2 pounds of steak on Sunday. Slice and store. Use for steak salads, steak and eggs, or just eat with vegetables.

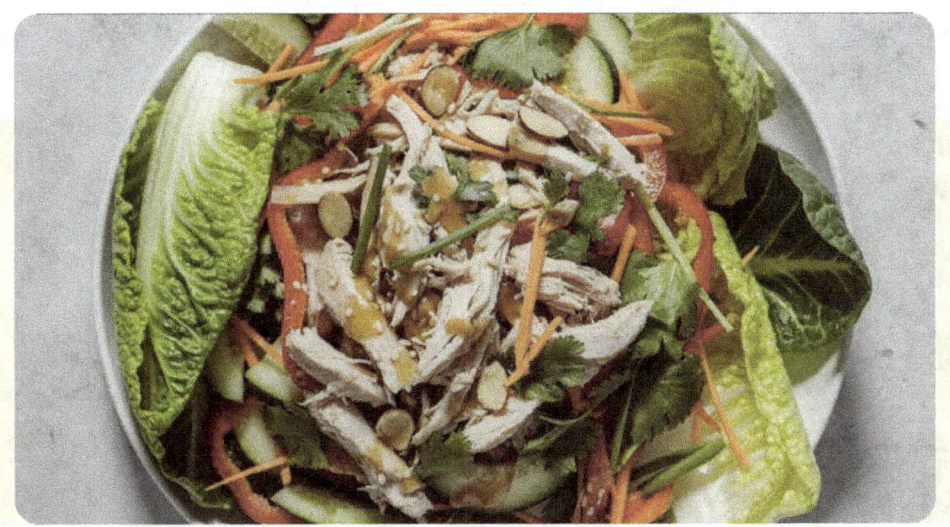

Asian Chicken Salad

Quick Make-Ahead (components)

Serves: 2

Prep Time: 15 min

Cook Time: 0 min (using precooked chicken)

Total: 15 min

Cost Per Serving: $3.95

MACROS PER SERVING:
Calories: 445 | Protein: 38g | Fat: 28g | Net Carbs: 9g

Instructions:

Make the dressing:
1. Combine all dressing ingredients in a small jar. Shake vigorously until emulsified.
2. Taste and adjust seasoning. Set aside.

Assemble the salad:
1. In 2 large bowls, combine shredded cabbage, romaine, bell pepper, carrots, and cucumber.
2. Top each bowl with half the chicken.
3. Sprinkle with green onions, cilantro, and almonds or sesame seeds.
4. Drizzle with Asian vinaigrette or serve on the side.
5. Toss well before eating.

Tips:

Budget breakdown: Chicken $4, cabbage $1.50, vegetables $3, sesame oil and seasonings $2. Total: $10.50 for 2 servings.

Coleslaw mix: Buy pre-shredded coleslaw mix to save time. Swap out half the cabbage for it.

Rotisserie chicken: Shred a rotisserie chicken. Use for this and other salads throughout the week.

Make it crunchier: Add ¼ cup crushed pork rinds or make wonton crisps from cheese (bake small squares of provolone or cheddar until crispy).

Meal prep: All components store separately for 3-4 days. Assemble fresh salads throughout the week.

Mandarin oranges: Traditional Asian chicken salad has mandarin oranges. If you have carb room, add ¼ cup per serving (adds 5g net carbs).

Shrimp version: Use 12 oz cooked shrimp instead of chicken. Same dressing, same vegetables, different protein.

Ingredients:

For the salad:
- 12 oz cooked chicken breast or thighs, shredded or diced
- 4 cups Napa cabbage or green cabbage, shredded
- 2 cups romaine lettuce, chopped
- 1 cup red bell pepper, thinly sliced
- ½ cup shredded carrots
- ½ cup cucumber, julienned or diced
- 3 green onions, sliced
- ¼ cup cilantro, chopped
- 2 tablespoons sliced almonds or sesame seeds

For the Asian vinaigrette:
- 3 tablespoons sesame oil
- 2 tablespoons rice vinegar
- 1 tablespoon soy sauce (or coconut aminos)
- 1 tablespoon lime juice
- 1 teaspoon fresh ginger, grated
- 1 clove garlic, minced
- 1 teaspoon erythritol or 3-4 drops liquid stevia (optional)
- ¼ teaspoon red pepper flakes

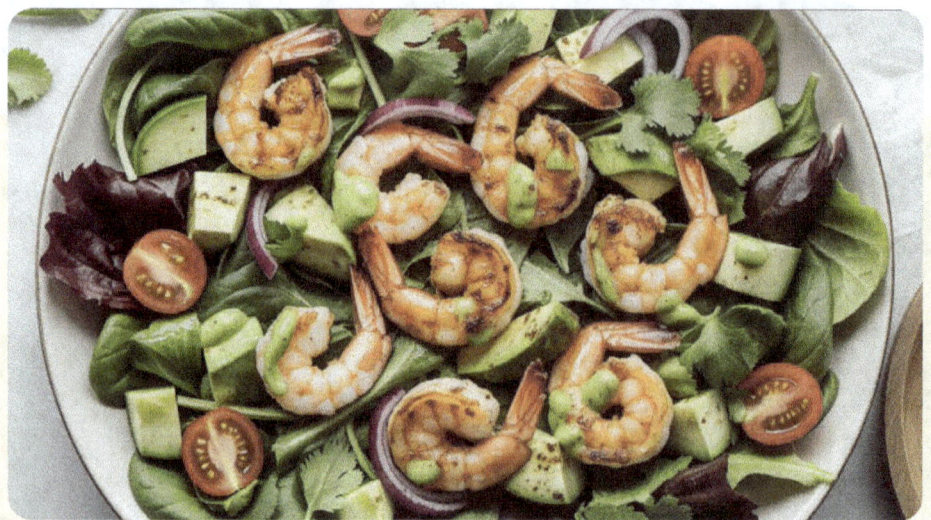

Shrimp Avocado Salad

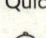
Quick

🔔 Serves: 2

Prep Time: 15 min

Cook Time: 5 min

Total: 20 min

$ Cost Per Serving: $5.25

MACROS PER SERVING:
Calories: 425 | Protein: 32g |
Fat: 30g | Net Carbs: 7g

Instructions:

Cook the shrimp:
1. Pat shrimp dry with paper towels. Season with paprika, salt, and pepper.
2. Heat olive oil in a large skillet over high heat.
3. Add shrimp in a single layer (work in batches if needed). Cook for 2 minutes per side until pink and cooked through.
4. Transfer to a plate.

Make the dressing:
1. Whisk together all dressing ingredients in a small bowl. Set aside.

Assemble the salad:
1. Divide mixed greens between 2 bowls.
2. Top each with half the shrimp (warm or let cool), avocado, tomatoes, cucumber, and red onion.
3. Sprinkle with fresh cilantro.
4. Drizzle with cilantro-lime dressing.
5. Serve immediately.

Tips:

Budget breakdown: Shrimp $8-9, avocado $1.50, vegetables $3, greens $2. Total: $14.50 for 2 servings. This is a treat-yourself meal.

Frozen shrimp: Buy frozen, thaw under cold running water for 5 minutes. Just as good as fresh and often cheaper.

Don't overcook: Shrimp cook fast. Overcooked shrimp are tough and rubbery. They're done when they turn pink and curl into a "C" shape.

Make it a meal prep: Cook shrimp on Sunday. Store in the fridge. Assemble salads with cold shrimp throughout the week.

Warm or cold: This works with warm just-cooked shrimp or cold meal-prepped shrimp.

Add heat: Dice a jalapeño and add to the salad, or add hot sauce to the dressing.

Grilled version: Thread shrimp on skewers and grill instead of pan-searing. Same cooking time.

Ingredients:

For the salad:
- 12 oz large shrimp, peeled and deveined
- 1 tablespoon olive oil
- 1 teaspoon paprika
- ½ teaspoon salt
- ¼ teaspoon black pepper
- 4 cups mixed greens or butter lettuce
- 1 large avocado, diced
- 1 cup cherry tomatoes, halved
- ½ cup cucumber, diced
- ¼ red onion, thinly sliced
- 2 tablespoons fresh cilantro, chopped

For the cilantro-lime dressing:
- 3 tablespoons olive oil
- 2 tablespoons lime juice
- 1 tablespoon fresh cilantro, chopped
- 1 clove garlic, minced
- ½ teaspoon cumin
- ¼ teaspoon salt
- ⅛ teaspoon black pepper

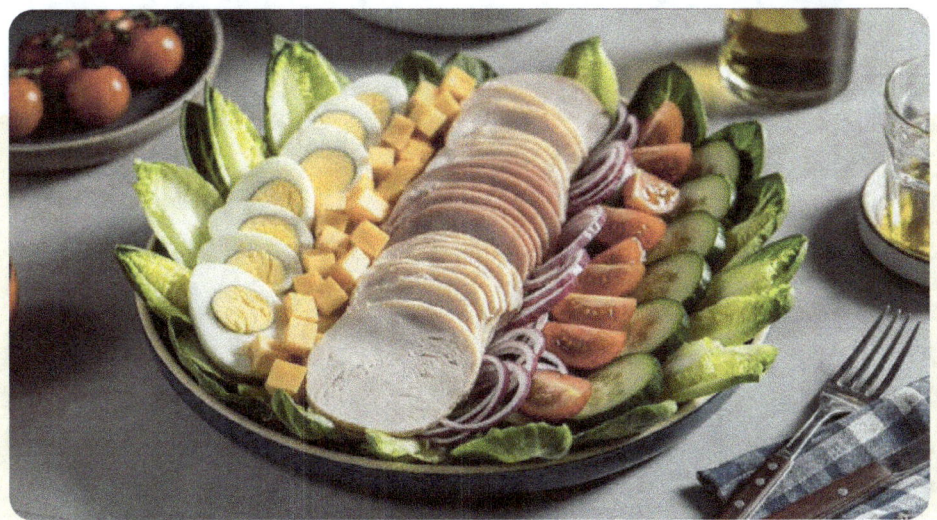

Chef Salad

Quick   Budget-Friendly   Make-Ahead (components)

🍽️ Serves: 2

✂️ Prep Time: 15 min

🍲 Cook Time: 0 min

⏲️ Total: 15 min

💲 Cost Per Serving: $3.25

MACROS PER SERVING:

Calories: 465 | Protein: 35g |
Fat: 32g | Net Carbs: 6g

Ingredients:

For the salad:
- 6 cups romaine or iceberg lettuce, chopped
- 6 oz deli turkey, rolled and sliced
- 6 oz deli ham, rolled and sliced
- 4 oz cheddar cheese, cubed or sliced
- 2 hard-boiled eggs, sliced
- 1 cup cherry tomatoes, halved
- ½ cup cucumber, sliced
- ¼ red onion, thinly sliced

For the dressing (choose one):
- Ranch dressing (store-bought or Recipe 119)
- Blue cheese dressing
- Thousand Island (mix 3 tablespoons mayo, 1 tablespoon sugar-free ketchup, 1 teaspoon pickle relish)

Instructions:

1. Divide chopped lettuce between 2 large bowls or plates.
2. Arrange turkey, ham, cheese, and sliced eggs in sections or rows on top of lettuce.
3. Add tomatoes, cucumber, and red onion.
4. Serve with dressing of choice on the side.
5. Toss before eating or eat in sections.

Tips:

Budget breakdown: Deli meat $4, cheese $2, eggs $1, lettuce $1, vegetables $2. Total: $10 for 2 servings. One of the most economical salads.

Deli meat quality: Read labels. Look for meats without added sugars or fillers. Boar's Head and similar brands are good quality.

Roll and slice: Rolling deli meat before slicing makes it easier to eat and looks nicer.

Add bacon: Crumble 4 strips of cooked bacon on top for extra flavor and fat.

Meal prep: Prep all components on Sunday. Store separately. Assemble fresh salads in 5 minutes throughout the week.

Kid-friendly: Most kids will eat this. It's familiar ingredients arranged on lettuce.

Restaurant classic: This is a diner staple for good reason. Simple, satisfying, affordable.

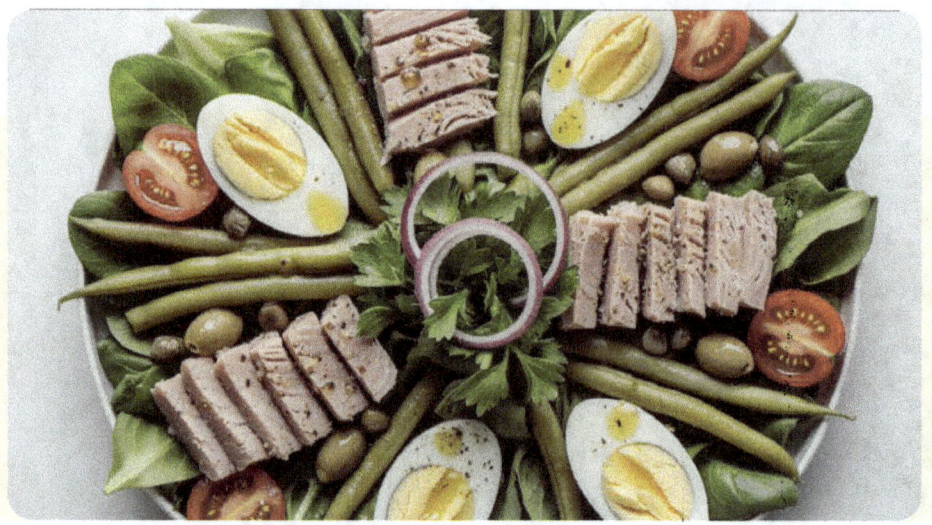

Niçoise Salad (No Potatoes)

Quick

 Serves: 2

Prep Time: 20 min

Cook Time: 0 min (using precooked components)

Total: 20 min

Cost Per Serving: $4.85

MACROS PER SERVING:
Calories: 485 | Protein: 34g | Fat: 35g | Net Carbs: 7g

Instructions:

Blanch the green beans (if not using pre-blanched):
1. Bring a pot of salted water to boil. Add green beans and cook for 3-4 minutes until tender-crisp.
2. Drain and immediately transfer to a bowl of ice water to stop cooking. Drain again and pat dry.

Make the vinaigrette:
1. Whisk together all dressing ingredients in a small bowl. Set aside.

Assemble the salad:
1. Divide mixed greens between 2 large plates.
2. Arrange tuna, green beans, egg halves, tomatoes, olives, red onion, and capers in sections on top of the greens (traditional Niçoise presentation is arranged, not tossed).
3. Sprinkle with fresh parsley.
4. Drizzle with Dijon vinaigrette or serve on the side.

Tips:

Budget breakdown: Canned tuna $3, eggs $1.50, green beans $2, olives $2, tomatoes $1.50, greens $2. Total: $12 for 2 servings.

Traditional Niçoise: Uses fresh seared tuna instead of canned. If you want to splurge, sear 12 oz tuna steaks for 2 minutes per side (keep them rare in the center).

Potato substitute: Traditional Niçoise has potatoes. We use extra green beans and eggs for substance without carbs.

Anchovy option: Add 4-6 anchovy fillets for authentic flavor. They're salty and briny, not fishy.

Meal prep: Hard-boil eggs and blanch green beans on Sunday. Store separately. Assembly takes 10 minutes.

Tuna quality: Use good quality tuna. Solid white albacore in olive oil tastes better than chunk light in water.

French bistro: This is a classic French composed salad. Each ingredient is carefully placed rather than tossed together.

Ingredients:

For the salad:
- 2 cans (5 oz each) tuna in olive oil or water, drained
- 4 cups mixed greens or butter lettuce
- 2 cups green beans, blanched and cooled
- 4 hard-boiled eggs, halved
- 1 cup cherry tomatoes, halved
- ½ cup Kalamata olives
- ½ red onion, thinly sliced
- 2 tablespoons capers
- 2 tablespoons fresh parsley, chopped

For the Dijon vinaigrette:
- ¼ cup olive oil
- 2 tablespoons lemon juice
- 1 tablespoon Dijon mustard
- 1 clove garlic, minced
- ¼ teaspoon salt
- ¼ teaspoon black pepper

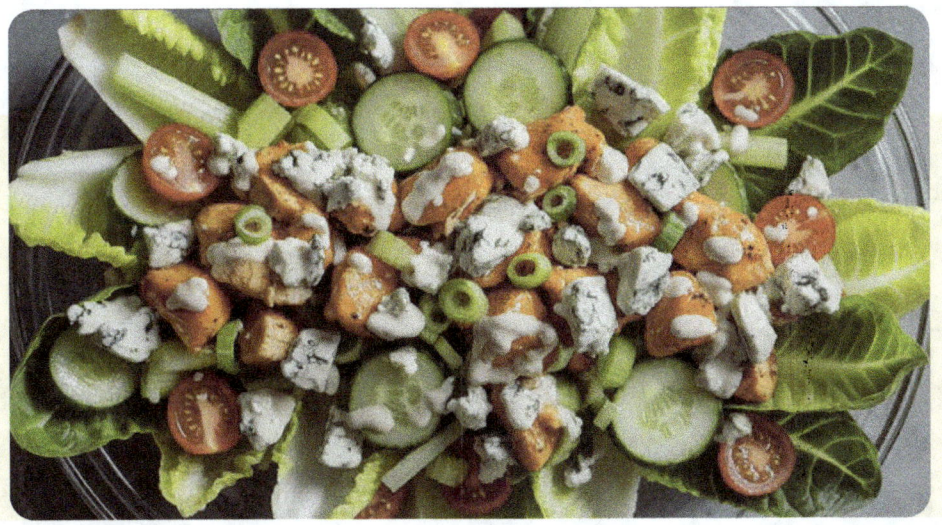

Buffalo Chicken Salad

Quick   Make-Ahead (components)

🔔 Serves: 2

Prep Time: 10 min

Cook Time: 0 min (using precooked chicken)

Total: 10 min

Cost Per Serving: $3.75

MACROS PER SERVING:

Calories: 485 | Protein: 40g |
Fat: 32g | Net Carbs: 6g

Instructions:

Make buffalo chicken:

1. In a bowl, mix diced chicken with hot sauce and melted butter until well coated. Set aside.

Make the dressing:

1. In a small bowl, combine mayonnaise, sour cream, blue cheese, lemon juice, garlic, salt, and pepper. Whisk until mostly smooth (some blue cheese chunks are good).

2. Add water 1 tablespoon at a time until dressing reaches desired consistency.

Assemble the salad:

1. Divide chopped romaine between 2 large bowls.

2. Top each with half the buffalo chicken, tomatoes, cucumber, celery, blue cheese, and green onions.

3. Drizzle with blue cheese dressing.

4. Toss before eating.

Tips:

Budget breakdown: Chicken $4, hot sauce and butter $1, lettuce $1.50, vegetables $2, blue cheese $2, mayo and sour cream $1. Total: $11.50 for 2 servings.

Rotisserie shortcut: Use rotisserie chicken. Toss with hot sauce and butter. Done.

Warm or cold: Use warm just-cooked chicken or cold meal-prepped chicken. Both work.

Spice level: Frank's RedHot is medium heat. Use less for mild, more for spicy, or add cayenne pepper.

Ranch substitute: If you hate blue cheese, use ranch dressing instead.

Make extra buffalo chicken: Double the chicken. Use for salads, lettuce wraps, or eat it straight.

Meal prep: Make buffalo chicken on Sunday. Store in the fridge. Assemble fresh salads throughout the week in 5 minutes.

Ingredients:

For the salad:

- 12 oz cooked chicken breast or thighs, diced
- ¼ cup Frank's RedHot sauce
- 2 tablespoons butter, melted
- 6 cups romaine lettuce, chopped
- 1 cup cherry tomatoes, halved
- ½ cup cucumber, diced
- ½ cup celery, sliced
- ½ cup blue cheese, crumbled
- 2 green onions, sliced

For the blue cheese dressing:

- ¼ cup mayonnaise
- ¼ cup sour cream
- ¼ cup blue cheese, crumbled
- 1 tablespoon lemon juice
- 1 clove garlic, minced
- ¼ teaspoon salt
- ⅛ teaspoon black pepper
- 2 tablespoons water (to thin)

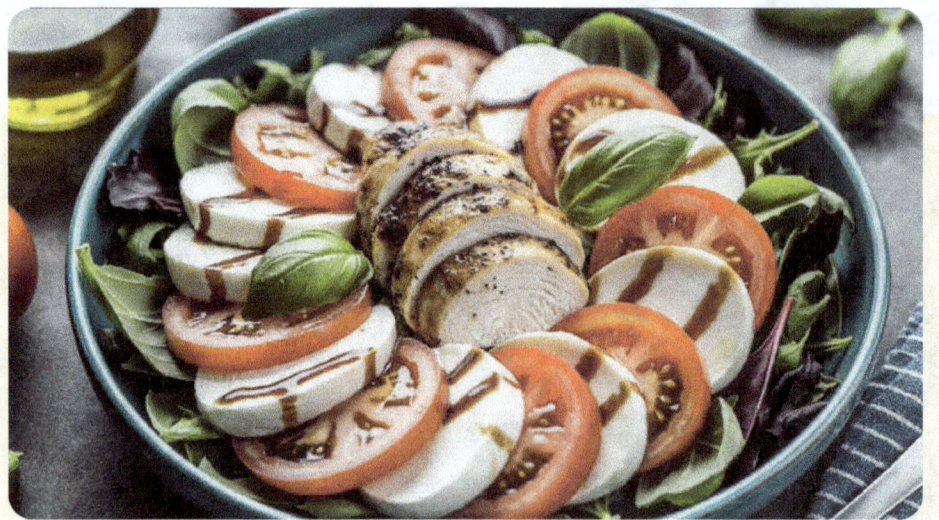

Caprese Chicken Bowl

Quick

🔔 Serves: 2

✂️ Prep Time: 10 min

🍲 Cook Time: 12 min (if cooking chicken fresh)

⏲️ Total: 22 min

💲 Cost Per Serving: $4.65

MACROS PER SERVING:
Calories: 495 | Protein: 42g | Fat: 32g | Net Carbs: 6g

Instructions:

Cook the chicken (if not using precooked):
1. Season chicken breasts with salt and pepper.
2. Grill or pan-sear over medium-high heat for 6 minutes per side until internal temperature reaches 165°F.
3. Let rest for 5 minutes, then slice.

Reduce balsamic vinegar (optional but recommended):
1. Pour balsamic vinegar into a small saucepan. Simmer over medium heat for 5-7 minutes until reduced by half and syrupy. Let cool.

Assemble the bowls:
1. Divide greens between 2 bowls or plates.
2. Arrange sliced chicken, mozzarella, and tomatoes on top.
3. Scatter fresh basil leaves over everything.
4. Drizzle with olive oil and reduced balsamic vinegar (or regular balsamic if not reducing).
5. Season with salt and pepper.
6. Serve immediately.

Ingredients:

For the bowl:
- 12 oz chicken breast, grilled and sliced
- 4 cups mixed greens or arugula
- 8 oz fresh mozzarella, sliced
- 2 medium tomatoes, sliced
- ¼ cup fresh basil leaves
- 2 tablespoons balsamic vinegar (reduced, if possible)
- 3 tablespoons olive oil
- Salt and pepper to taste

Tips:

Budget breakdown: Chicken $4, mozzarella $3.50, tomatoes $2, greens $2, basil $2, olive oil and vinegar $1.50. Total: $15 for 2 servings.

Fresh mozzarella: This is worth buying. It's creamy and mild, completely different from shredded mozzarella. Look for it in the deli or cheese section, packed in water or whey.

Tomato season: This salad is best in summer when tomatoes are ripe and flavorful. Winter tomatoes don't have the same impact.

Balsamic reduction: Reducing balsamic makes it sweeter and thicker, more like a glaze. It's worth the extra 5 minutes.

Make it simpler: Skip reducing the balsamic. Use regular balsamic vinegar. Still delicious.

Warm or cold: Traditionally served with room temperature or cold ingredients, but warm grilled chicken works too.

Add avocado: Half an avocado per serving adds creaminess and healthy fats.

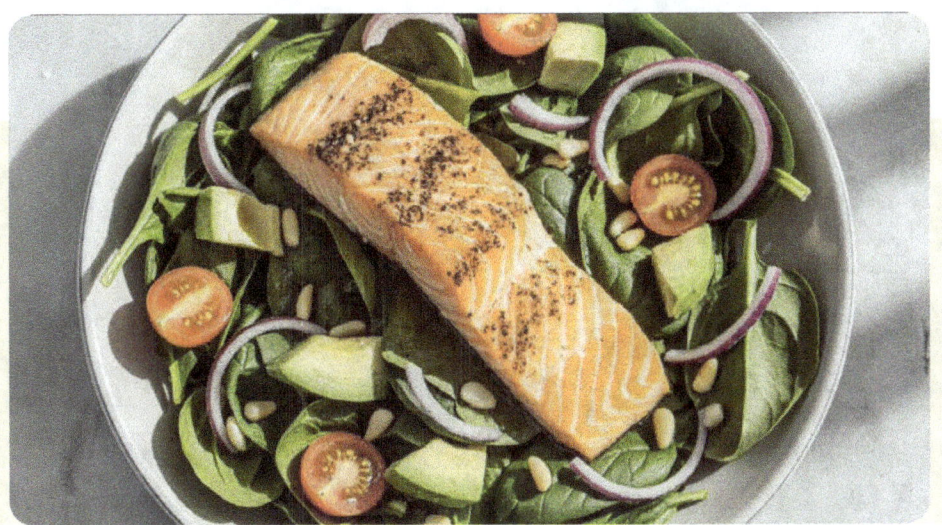

Salmon & Spinach Salad

Quick

🔔 Serves: 2

✂️ Prep Time: 10 min

🍲 Cook Time: 12 min

🍳 Total: 22 min

💲 Cost Per Serving: $5.75

MACROS PER SERVING:
Calories: 485 | Protein: 38g |
Fat: 34g | Net Carbs: 5g

Instructions:

Cook the salmon:
1. Pat salmon dry with paper towels. Season both sides with salt and pepper.
2. Heat olive oil in a large skillet over medium-high heat.
3. Add salmon skin-side up (if skin-on) and cook for 5-6 minutes until golden.
4. Flip and cook for another 4-5 minutes until salmon flakes easily with a fork and internal temperature reaches 145°F.
5. Transfer to a plate. You can leave it in one piece or flake it apart.

Make the vinaigrette:
1. Whisk together all dressing ingredients in a small bowl.

Assemble the salad:
1. Divide spinach between 2 bowls.
2. Top each with half the salmon (warm or let cool), avocado, tomatoes, red onion, and pine nuts.
3. Drizzle with lemon vinaigrette.
4. Serve immediately.

Ingredients:

For the salad:
- 12 oz salmon fillets
- 6 cups fresh spinach
- 1 avocado, diced
- ½ cup cherry tomatoes, halved
- ¼ red onion, thinly sliced
- 2 tablespoons pine nuts or sliced almonds
- 1 tablespoon olive oil (for cooking salmon)
- Salt and pepper for salmon

For the lemon vinaigrette:
- 3 tablespoons olive oil
- 2 tablespoons lemon juice
- 1 teaspoon Dijon mustard
- 1 clove garlic, minced
- ¼ teaspoon salt
- ¼ teaspoon black pepper

Tips:

Budget breakdown: Salmon $9-10 (when on sale), spinach $2, avocado $1.50, nuts $1.50, other ingredients $2. Total: $16-17 for 2 servings. This is a splurge meal.

Buy salmon on sale: Stock up when it's under $8/pound. Freeze in portions.

Skin or no skin: Either works. If skin-on, the skin gets crispy when cooked properly. If you don't like eating it, it peels off easily after cooking.

Meal prep: Cook salmon on Sunday. Store in the fridge. Use cold salmon for salads throughout the week.

Warm or cold: Both work beautifully.

Canned salmon: In a pinch, use 2 cans (6 oz each) of salmon. Not as good as fresh, but works for meal prep.

Add extras: Hard-boiled eggs, cucumber, bell peppers all work well here.

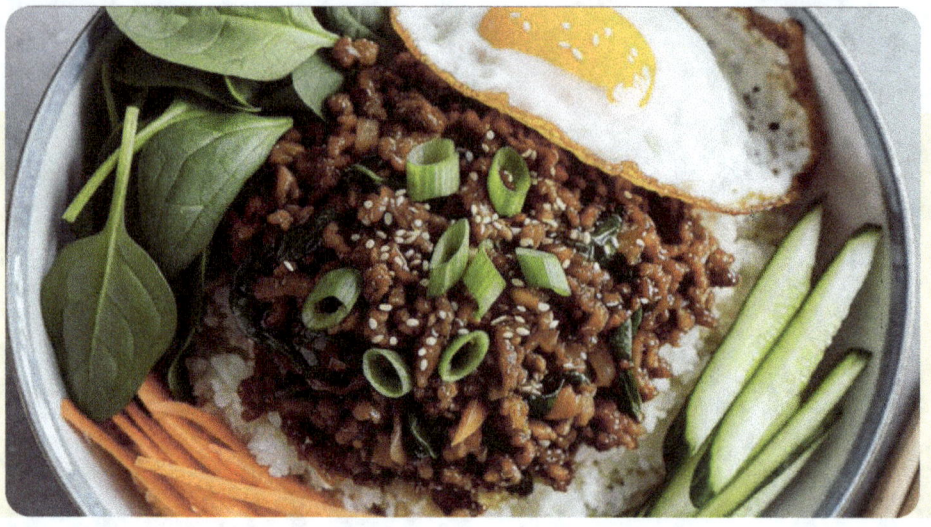

Korean Beef Bowl

Quick   Budget-Friendly

Serves: 2

Prep Time: 10 min

Cook Time: 12 min

Total: 22 min

Cost Per Serving: $3.85

MACROS PER SERVING:
Calories: 465 | Protein: 34g |
Fat: 30g | Net Carbs: 9g

Instructions:

Make the sauce:
1. Whisk together all sauce ingredients in a small bowl. Set aside.

Cook the beef:
1. Heat 1 tablespoon sesame oil in a large skillet over high heat.
2. Add ground beef and cook, breaking it up, for 6-8 minutes until browned.
3. Add garlic and ginger. Cook for 1 minute.
4. Pour in Korean sauce and stir to coat. Cook for 1-2 minutes. Remove from heat.

Cook the cauliflower rice:
1. In another skillet, heat remaining tablespoon sesame oil over medium-high heat.
2. Add cauliflower rice and cook for 5-6 minutes until tender and any excess moisture evaporates.

Assemble the bowls:
1. Divide cauliflower rice between 2 bowls.
2. Top each with half the Korean beef, spinach or greens, carrots, and cucumber.
3. Sprinkle with green onions and sesame seeds.
4. If using, top each bowl with a fried egg.
5. Serve immediately.

Tips:

Budget breakdown: Ground beef $3.50, cauliflower rice $2, vegetables $2.50, sauces and seasonings $2. Total: $10 for 2 servings.

Traditional bibimbap: This is inspired by Korean bibimbap. Traditional versions have multiple vegetables, each cooked separately. This is a simplified weeknight version.

The egg: Topping with a fried egg (runny yolk) is traditional and adds richness. Highly recommended.

Gochujang: If you have Korean chili paste (gochujang), add 1 tablespoon to the sauce for authentic flavor. Check the label for sugar content.

Kimchi: Add ¼ cup kimchi per serving for authentic Korean flavor and probiotics. Adds 2g net carbs.

Meal prep: Make Korean beef on Sunday. Store separately from cauliflower rice and vegetables. Assemble fresh bowls throughout the week.

Ground turkey: Works great if it's cheaper than ground beef.

Ingredients:

For the bowl:
- 12 oz ground beef (80/20)
- 2 cups cauliflower rice
- 2 cups spinach or mixed greens
- ½ cup shredded carrots
- ½ cucumber, sliced thin
- 2 cloves garlic, minced
- 1 teaspoon fresh ginger, grated
- 2 tablespoons sesame oil, divided
- 2 green onions, sliced
- 1 tablespoon sesame seeds
- Optional: 1 fried egg per serving

For the Korean sauce:
- 3 tablespoons soy sauce (or coconut aminos)
- 1 tablespoon rice vinegar
- 1 tablespoon erythritol or monk fruit sweetener
- 1 teaspoon sesame oil
- ¼ teaspoon red pepper flakes

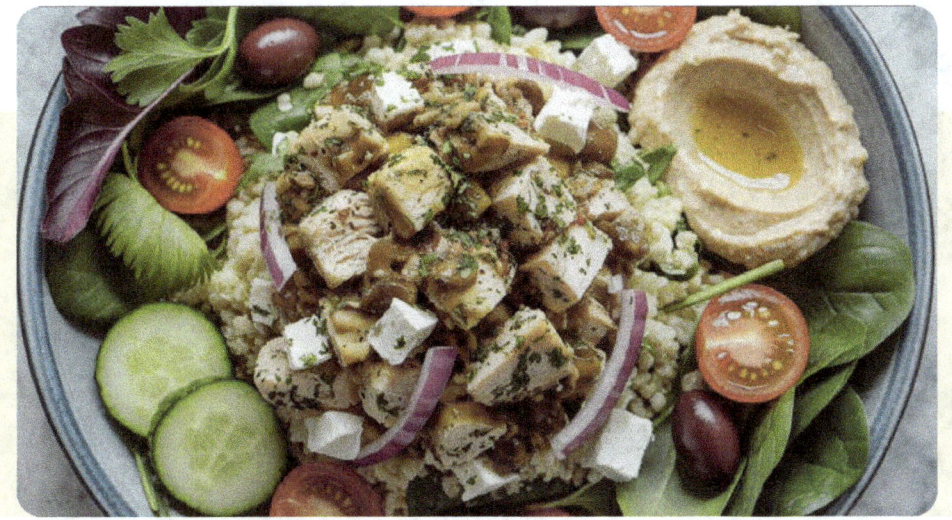

Mediterranean Bowl

Quick   Make-Ahead (components)

Serves: 2

Prep Time: 15 min

Cook Time: 0 min (using precooked chicken)

Total: 15 min

Cost Per Serving: $4.45

MACROS PER SERVING:
Calories: 495 | Protein: 38g | Fat: 34g | Net Carbs: 8g

Instructions:

Make the tahini dressing:
1. Whisk together tahini, lemon juice, water, garlic, cumin, salt, and pepper in a small bowl. Add more water if needed to reach desired consistency (should be thick but pourable).

Assemble the bowls:
1. Divide cauliflower rice between 2 bowls. Top with mixed greens.
2. Arrange chicken, tomatoes, cucumber, olives, red onion, and feta cheese on top.
3. Add a dollop of hummus if using.
4. Drizzle with tahini dressing.
5. Sprinkle with fresh parsley.
6. Mix everything together before eating.

Tips:

Budget breakdown: Chicken $4, cauliflower rice $2, vegetables $3, feta $2, olives $2, tahini $1.50. Total: $14.50 for 2 servings.

Tahini: Made from sesame seeds. Find it in the international aisle or near peanut butter. It separates in the jar, so stir well before using.

Warm or cold: This works with warm cauliflower rice and chicken, or all cold components. Both are good.

Lamb version: Use grilled lamb instead of chicken for authentic Mediterranean flavor.

Meal prep: Cook chicken and cauliflower rice on Sunday. Store all components separately. Assemble fresh bowls throughout the week.

Add protein: Add 2 hard-boiled eggs per serving for extra protein and richness.

Falafel-style: Make "falafel" from seasoned ground beef or turkey. Form into balls, bake at 400°F for 15 minutes. Use instead of diced chicken.

Ingredients:

For the bowl:
- 12 oz cooked chicken breast or thighs, diced
- 2 cups cauliflower rice, cooked
- 2 cups mixed greens
- ½ cup cherry tomatoes, halved
- ½ cup cucumber, diced
- ¼ cup Kalamata olives, pitted
- ¼ cup red onion, diced
- ½ cup feta cheese, crumbled
- 2 tablespoons hummus (optional, adds 3g net carbs)
- 2 tablespoons fresh parsley, chopped

For the tahini dressing:
- 3 tablespoons tahini
- 2 tablespoons lemon juice
- 2 tablespoons water
- 1 clove garlic, minced
- ¼ teaspoon cumin
- ¼ teaspoon salt
- ⅛ teaspoon black pepper

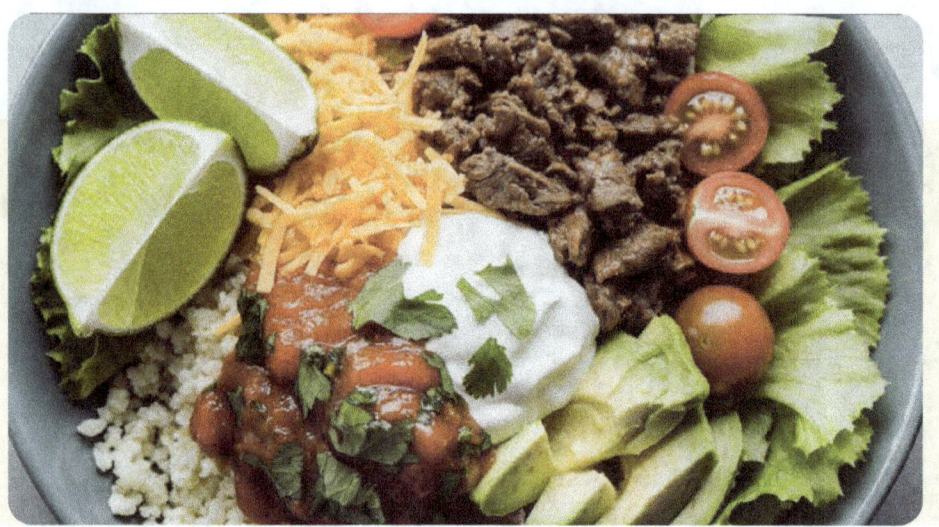

Burrito Bowl (No Rice or Beans)

Quick   Budget-Friendly   Make-Ahead (components)

🍲 Serves: 2

✂️ Prep Time: 10 min

🍳 Cook Time: 12 min

⏱️ Total: 22 min

💲 Cost Per Serving: $3.95

MACROS PER SERVING:
Calories: 525 | Protein: 38g | Fat: 36g | Net Carbs: 9g

Ingredients:

For the bowl:
- 12 oz ground beef or chicken
- 2 tablespoons taco seasoning
- 2 cups cauliflower rice, cooked
- 2 cups romaine lettuce, shredded
- 1 cup cherry tomatoes, halved
- 1 avocado, diced
- ½ cup shredded cheddar cheese
- ½ cup sour cream
- ¼ cup salsa
- 2 tablespoons fresh cilantro, chopped
- Lime wedges for serving
- Optional: jalapeños, hot sauce

Instructions:

Cook the meat:
1. Heat a large skillet over medium-high heat.
2. Add ground beef or chicken and cook, breaking it up, for 8-10 minutes until browned and cooked through.
3. Drain excess fat if needed.
4. Add taco seasoning and 3 tablespoons water. Stir and cook for 2 minutes until water evaporates.

Assemble the bowls:
1. Divide cauliflower rice between 2 bowls. Top with shredded lettuce.
2. Add seasoned meat, tomatoes, avocado, cheese, sour cream, and salsa.
3. Sprinkle with cilantro.
4. Serve with lime wedges. Squeeze lime over bowl before eating.
5. Add jalapeños or hot sauce if desired.
6. Mix everything together before eating.

Tips:

Budget breakdown: Ground beef $3.50, cauliflower rice $2, lettuce $1, avocado $1.50, cheese $1, other ingredients $2. Total: $11 for 2 servings.

Chipotle copycat: This is basically a Chipotle burrito bowl without the rice and beans. Just as satisfying, half the carbs.

Meal prep: Make taco meat and cauliflower rice on Sunday. Store separately. Assemble fresh bowls throughout the week in 5 minutes.

Carnitas version: Use pulled pork from Recipe 84 instead of ground meat.

Add black beans: If you have carb room, add ¼ cup black beans per serving. Adds 5g net carbs but makes it feel more like the "real thing."

Make it bigger: Add a fried egg on top for extra protein and richness.

Warm or cold: Traditionally the meat and cauliflower rice are warm, toppings are cold. But this works as a cold meal prep bowl too.

CHAPTER 7 SUMMARY

You now have 15 salads and bowls that prove vegetables don't have to be boring. Here's how to make them work in your life:

The Weekly Salad Strategy:

Monday-Friday Lunches:
- Sunday: Prep 2-3 proteins (chicken, taco meat, hard-boiled eggs)
- Sunday: Wash and chop vegetables, store in containers
- Sunday: Make 2 dressings
- Daily: Assemble fresh salads in 5 minutes each morning

Total Sunday time: 60-90 minutes **Total daily time:** 5 minutes **Result:** 5 perfect lunches with zero weekday stress

My Favorite Combinations:

For maximum protein:
- Cobb Salad (38g protein)
- Caesar Salad with Grilled Chicken (42g protein)
- Steak Salad (42g protein)

For budget-friendly:
- Taco Salad Bowl ($3.45/serving)
- Chef Salad ($3.25/serving)
- Korean Beef Bowl ($3.85/serving)

For meal prep:
- Greek Chicken Bowl (all components store separately)
- Buffalo Chicken Salad (buffalo chicken lasts all week)
- Asian Chicken Salad (shredded chicken is versatile)

The Build-Your-Own Formula:
Once you understand the structure, create infinite variations:

Base (pick 1):
- Romaine, iceberg, mixed greens, spinach, arugula, butter lettuce, or cauliflower rice

Protein (6-8 oz, pick 1):
- Grilled chicken, steak, shrimp, tuna, salmon, ground beef, deli meat, hard-boiled eggs

Vegetables (1-2 cups, pick 2-3):
- Tomatoes, cucumber, bell peppers, onions, carrots, celery, avocado, olives

Healthy Fat (pick 1-2):
- Full-fat dressing, cheese, nuts, avocado, olives

Flavor boost (optional):
- Fresh herbs, bacon, pickles, peppers, citrus

Mix and match = hundreds of combinations.

Dressing Math:
Store-bought: $4-6 per bottle, lasts 2-3 weeks **Homemade:** $2-3 in ingredients, makes 1 cup, lasts 1 week

Savings: About $10-15 per month making your own

Plus you control the ingredients and avoid seed oils, sugar, and preservatives.

Salad as a Fat Loss Tool:

When you build salads correctly:
- High protein (keeps you full 4-5 hours)
- High volume (stretches your stomach, signals fullness)
- Nutrient-dense (vitamins, minerals, fiber)
- Moderate calories (400-500 calories)

Result: You can eat until you're genuinely full and still be in a calorie deficit if that's your goal.

The Lunch Box Reality:

Salad done right:
- Costs $3-5 per meal
- Takes 5 minutes to assemble
- Provides 30-40g protein
- Keeps you full until dinner
- No post-lunch crash

Typical lunch out:
- Costs $10-15
- Takes 30-45 minutes (including travel/waiting)
- Often high in carbs, low in protein
- Leaves you hungry by 3 PM
- Post-lunch food coma

The math is obvious.

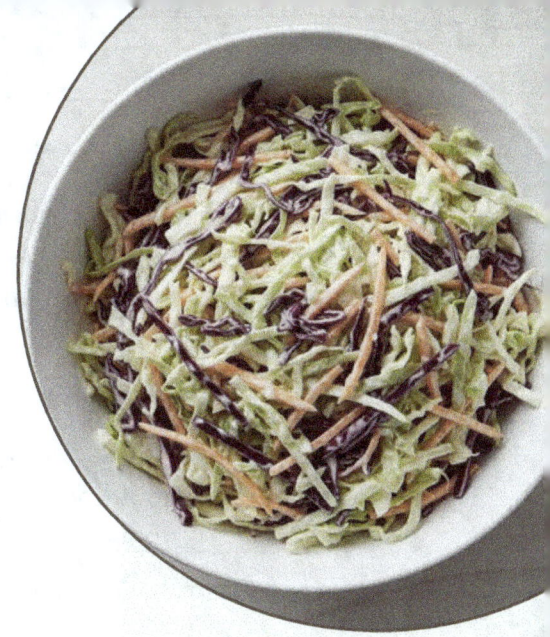

We need to talk about the side dish problem.

For most of your life, side dishes were probably potatoes, rice, pasta, or bread. They filled up your plate, stretched the meal, and made everything feel complete. When you remove those, you're left staring at a plate that looks... empty. Just protein and maybe some vegetables. It doesn't feel like a "real meal."

I get it. I struggled with this too.

But here's what I learned: you don't need carb-heavy sides to make a meal feel complete. You need vegetables that taste good, provide volume, and complement your protein. Once you find 5-6 vegetable sides you actually enjoy, this stops being a problem.

And snacks? Most "healthy snacks" are just carbs in disguise. Granola bars, fruit, crackers, pretzels—they're all sugar spikes waiting to happen. Real snacks should provide protein and fat to actually tide you over between meals, not create a blood sugar rollercoaster.

This chapter solves both problems.

What Makes a Good Side Dish:

A good side dish should:
1. **Complement the protein.** Roasted Brussels sprouts pair well with steak. Zucchini noodles work with marinara and meatballs.
2. **Add different textures.** If your protein is soft, add something crispy. If it's dry, add something with sauce.
3. **Be easy to make.** You're already cooking protein. The side shouldn't require complex techniques or timing.
4. **Reheat well.** Meal prep only works if sides stay good for 3-4 days.
5. **Actually taste good.** You're not a child. You don't have to suffer through steamed plain broccoli.

The Vegetable Hierarchy:
Not all vegetables are created equal for low-carb eating. Here's what you need to know:

Lowest carb (0-3g net carbs per cup):
- Spinach, lettuce, arugula, leafy greens (basically fiber and water)
- Celery, cucumber (mostly water)
- Mushrooms (great for volume)

Low carb (3-5g net carbs per cup):
- Broccoli, cauliflower, cabbage (cruciferous vegetables—your best friends)
- Zucchini, summer squash (versatile and neutral-tasting)
- Asparagus, green beans (great roasted)

- Bell peppers (raw or cooked)

Moderate carb (6-10g net carbs per cup):
- Tomatoes (technically a fruit, but we use them as vegetables)
- Brussels sprouts (higher than you'd think, but so good)
- Carrots (use sparingly)
- Onions (use for flavoring, not as a main vegetable)

Higher carb (avoid or use very sparingly):
- Potatoes, sweet potatoes (15-25g net carbs per cup)
- Corn, peas (15-20g net carbs per cup)
- Winter squash (10-15g net carbs per cup)

Focus on the first two categories. That's where most of these recipes live.

Cooking Methods That Make Vegetables Taste Good:

Roasting (400-450°F, 20-30 minutes):
- Brings out natural sweetness through caramelization
- Creates crispy edges
- Works for: broccoli, cauliflower, Brussels sprouts, asparagus, zucchini
- Method: Toss with oil and salt, spread on baking sheet, roast until tender and browned

Sautéing (medium-high heat, 5-10 minutes):
- Quick and easy
- Adds flavor from fat (butter, olive oil, bacon grease)
- Works for: spinach, mushrooms, zucchini, peppers, green beans
- Method: Heat fat, add vegetables, cook until tender, season

Grilling (high heat, 5-15 minutes):
- Adds smoky char flavor
- Creates grill marks that make vegetables look appealing
- Works for: asparagus, zucchini, bell peppers, mushrooms
- Method: Oil vegetables, grill until tender and charred

Steaming (5-10 minutes):
- Preserves nutrients
- Quick and hands-off
- Works for: broccoli, cauliflower, green beans, asparagus
- Method: Steam until tender-crisp, then season generously

The secret: Vegetables need fat and salt to taste good. Don't be afraid of butter, olive oil, bacon grease, and generous seasoning.

About Snacks:
Real talk: if you're eating enough protein and fat at meals, you shouldn't need snacks constantly. When I first went low-carb, I was shocked at how long I could go between meals without getting hungry.

But sometimes you do need something:
- Between lunch and dinner (if it's 6+ hours)
- After a workout
- On long travel days
- When a meal gets delayed

That's what the snack section is for. These aren't "100-calorie packs" or diet foods. They're actual food that provides protein and fat to hold you over.

Good Snacks Provide:
- Protein: 5-15g minimum
- Fat: Enough to keep you satisfied
- Low carbs: Under 5g net carbs
- Portability: Easy to grab and go

Examples:
- Hard-boiled eggs (6g protein, 0g carbs, $0.30)
- String cheese (6g protein, 1g carbs, $0.50)
- Deli meat rollups (10-15g protein, 1g carbs, $1)
- Nuts (in moderation—easy to overeat)
- Pork rinds (8g protein per serving, 0g carbs)

The Recipes:
This chapter is divided into two sections:

Vegetable Sides (10 recipes): Things to serve alongside your protein. All under 5g net carbs per serving.

Snacks (10 recipes): Things to eat between meals or as appetizers. All high-protein, low-carb, portable.

Every recipe is:
- Simple to make
- Uses common ingredients
- Reheats well or doesn't need reheating
- Actually tastes good

Let's start with vegetables.

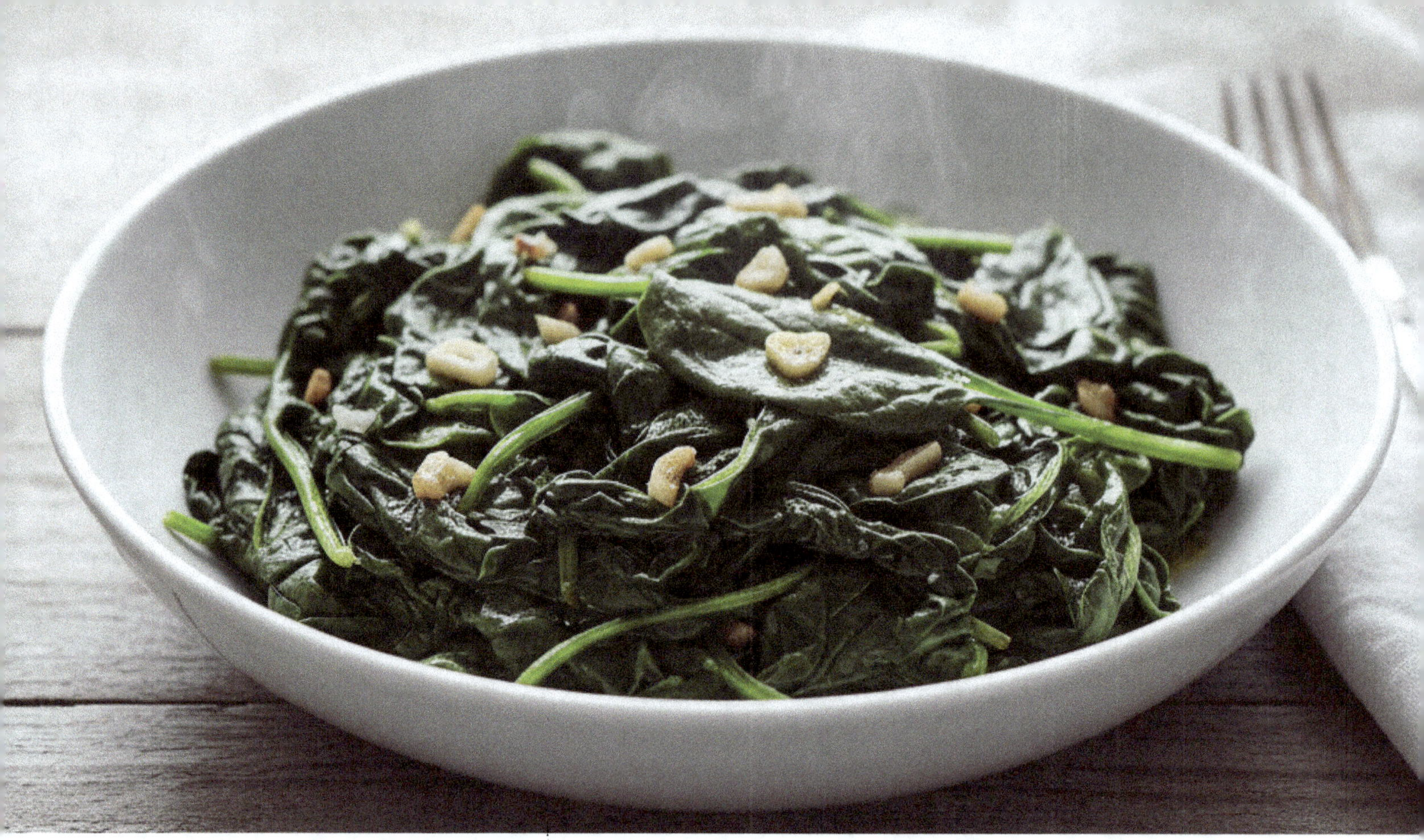

VEGETABLE SIDES

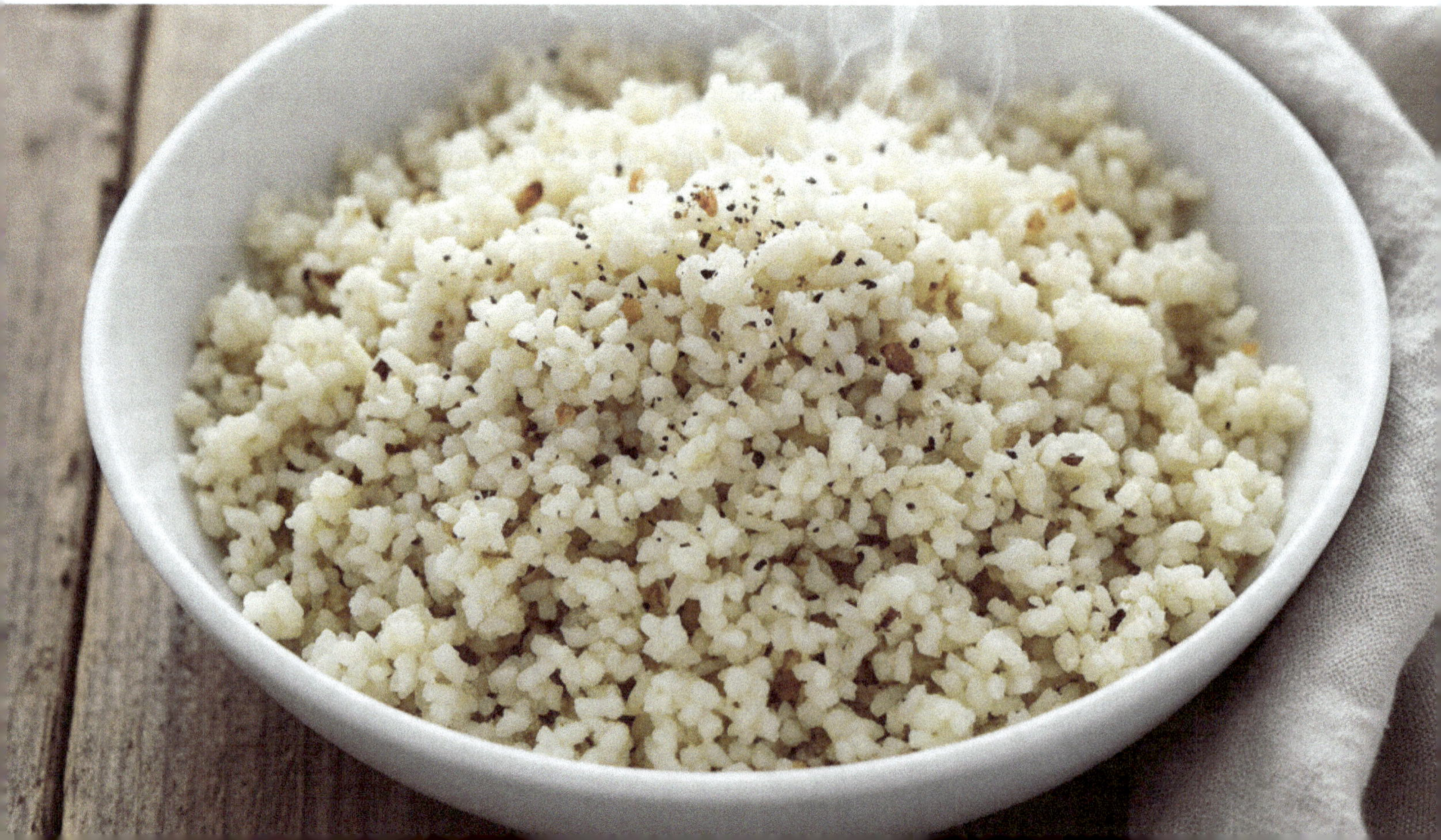

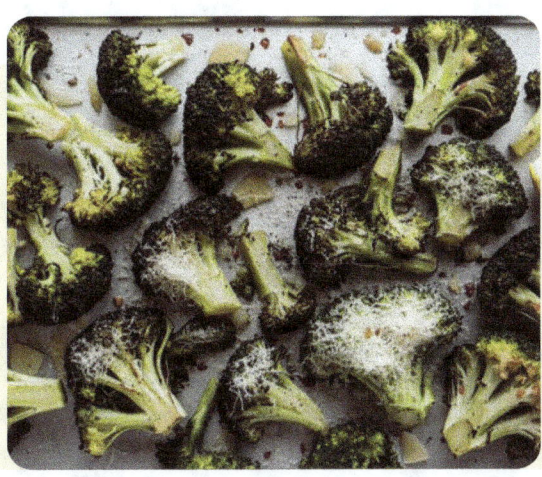

Roasted Broccoli with Parmesan

Quick   One-Pan   Budget-Friendly

🍲 Serves: 4
🎛 Prep Time: 5 min
🍳 Cook Time: 20 min
⏱ Total: 25 min
💲 Cost Per Serving: $1.25

MACROS PER SERVING:

Calories: 115 | Protein: 6g |
Fat: 8g | Net Carbs: 4g

Ingredients:

- 6 cups broccoli florets (about 2 large heads)
- 3 tablespoons olive oil
- 3 cloves garlic, minced
- ½ teaspoon salt
- ¼ teaspoon black pepper
- ¼ teaspoon red pepper flakes (optional)
- ½ cup grated Parmesan cheese
- Lemon wedges for serving

Instructions:

1. Preheat oven to 425°F. Line a large baking sheet with parchment paper.
2. In a large bowl, toss broccoli florets with olive oil, garlic, salt, pepper, and red pepper flakes (if using).
3. Spread broccoli in a single layer on the baking sheet. Don't overcrowd—use two sheets if needed.
4. Roast for 18-20 minutes, flipping halfway through, until broccoli is tender and edges are crispy and slightly charred.
5. Remove from oven and immediately sprinkle with Parmesan cheese while still hot.
6. Transfer to a serving dish. Serve with lemon wedges for squeezing.

Tips:

Budget breakdown: Broccoli $3, Parmesan $1, olive oil and garlic $1. Total: $5 for 4 servings.

Dry the broccoli: Pat florets completely dry before tossing with oil. Wet broccoli steams instead of roasts.

Don't skip the char: Those crispy, almost-burnt edges are where the flavor is. Don't pull it out too early.

Storage: Refrigerate for up to 4 days. Reheat in a 425°F oven for 5-7 minutes to restore crispiness (microwave makes it soggy).

Variations: Try with lemon zest, balsamic vinegar drizzle, or swap Parmesan for nutritional yeast.

Pairs with: Everything. Chicken, steak, pork, fish, eggs. This is the most versatile side dish.

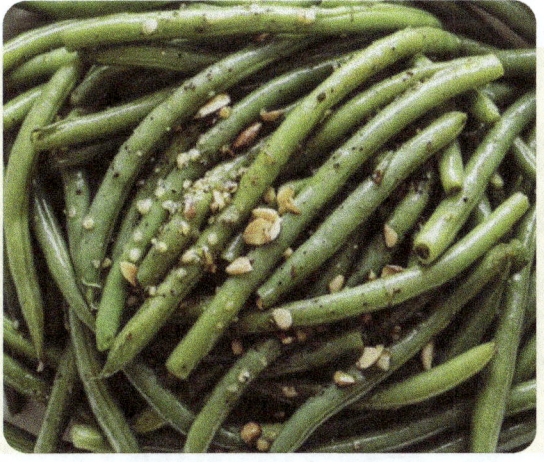

Garlic Green Beans

Quick   One-Pan   Budget-Friendly

🍲 Serves: 6
🎛 Prep Time: 5 min
🍳 Cook Time: 12 min
⏱ Total: 17 min
💲 Cost Per Serving: $1.15

MACROS PER SERVING:

Calories: 340 | Protein: 24g |
Fat: 24g | Net Carbs: 6g

Ingredients:

- 1½ pounds fresh green beans, trimmed
- 3 tablespoons butter
- 4 cloves garlic, minced
- ½ teaspoon salt
- ¼ teaspoon black pepper
- 2 tablespoons sliced almonds (optional)
- Lemon juice for serving (optional)

Instructions:

1. Bring a large pot of salted water to boil.
2. Add green beans and blanch for 3-4 minutes until bright green and tender-crisp.
3. Drain and immediately transfer to a bowl of ice water to stop cooking. Drain again and pat dry.
4. Heat butter in a large skillet over medium heat.
5. Add garlic and cook for 1 minute until fragrant (don't let it burn).
6. Add green beans, salt, and pepper. Toss to coat and cook for 3-4 minutes until heated through and coated in garlic butter.
7. If using almonds, toast them in a dry skillet for 2-3 minutes until golden, then sprinkle over beans.
8. Transfer to a serving dish. Drizzle with lemon juice if desired.

Tips:

Budget breakdown: Green beans $3, butter $1, almonds $0.50. Total: $4.50 for 4 servings.

Skip the blanching: If you're short on time, skip steps 1-3. Just add raw green beans to the skillet in step 6 and cook for 6-8 minutes with a splash of water, covered, until tender.

Frozen green beans: Work great. Skip blanching. Just add frozen beans to the garlic butter and cook until heated through.

Storage: Refrigerate for up to 4 days. Reheat in skillet or microwave.

Bacon version: Cook 3 strips of chopped bacon first, remove, use bacon fat instead of butter, add garlic, then beans. Top with bacon bits.

Pairs with: Pork chops, chicken, steak, salmon. Classic steakhouse side dish.

Cauliflower Mash

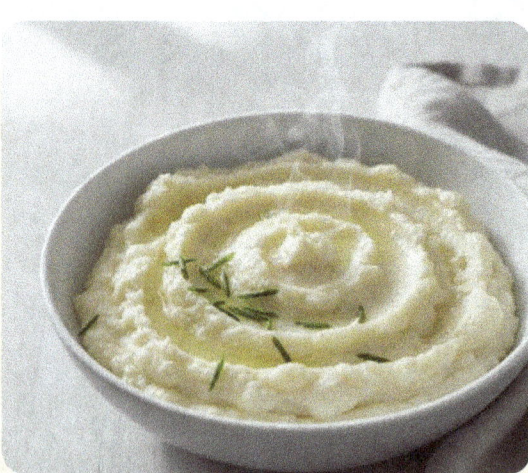

 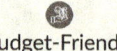
Quick   Budget-Friendly

 Serves: 6

Prep Time: 10 min

Cook Time: 15 min

Total: 25 min

Cost Per Serving: $0.95

MACROS PER SERVING:
Calories: 95 | Protein: 3g | Fat: 7g | Net Carbs: 4g

Ingredients:

- 1 large head cauliflower, cut into florets (about 8 cups)
- 4 tablespoons butter
- ¼ cup heavy cream
- 2 cloves garlic, minced
- ¾ teaspoon salt
- ¼ teaspoon black pepper
- ¼ cup grated Parmesan cheese (optional)
- 2 tablespoons fresh chives, chopped (optional)

Instructions:

1. Bring a large pot of salted water to boil.
2. Add cauliflower florets and boil for 10-12 minutes until very tender (a fork should slide through easily).
3. Drain cauliflower well. Let sit in the colander for 2-3 minutes to release excess moisture.
4. Transfer cauliflower to a food processor. Add butter, heavy cream, garlic, salt, and pepper.
5. Process until smooth and creamy, 1-2 minutes. Scrape down sides as needed.
6. Taste and adjust seasoning. If too thick, add more cream. If too thin, add Parmesan cheese (which also thickens and adds flavor).
7. Transfer to a serving bowl. Top with chives if using.

Tips:

Budget breakdown: Cauliflower $3, butter $1, cream $1, Parmesan $0.50. Total: $5.50 for 6 servings.
Get it smooth: The key is cooking the cauliflower until very tender and processing it thoroughly. Don't undercook or it'll be lumpy.
Moisture matters: Cauliflower holds a lot of water. Let it drain well after cooking or your mash will be watery.
No food processor: Use a potato masher or immersion blender. Won't be quite as smooth, but still delicious.
Storage: Refrigerate for up to 5 days. Reheat in microwave or on stovetop with a splash of cream.
Flavor variations: Add roasted garlic, sour cream, cream cheese, different cheeses, or fresh herbs.
Potato replacement: Use this anywhere you'd use mashed potatoes. Under gravy, next to meatloaf, as a shepherd's pie topping.

Sautéed Spinach

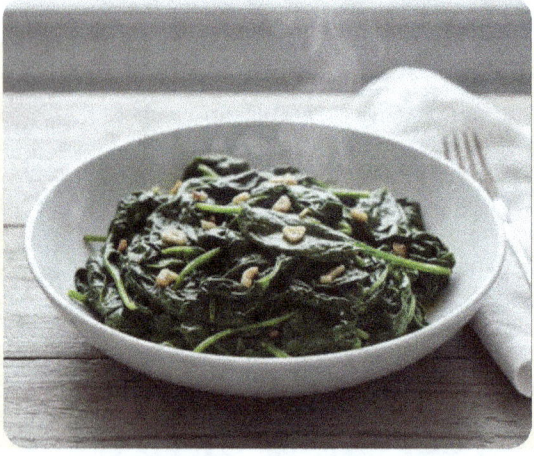

Quick   One-Pan   Budget-Friendly

 Serves: 4

Prep Time: 2 min

Cook Time: 5 min

Total: 7 min

Cost Per Serving: $0.85

MACROS PER SERVING:
Calories: 75 | Protein: 3g | Fat: 6g | Net Carbs: 2g

Ingredients:

- 1 pound fresh spinach (about 12 cups)
- 2 tablespoons butter or olive oil
- 3 cloves garlic, minced
- ½ teaspoon salt
- ¼ teaspoon black pepper
- ¼ teaspoon nutmeg (optional but recommended)
- 1 tablespoon lemon juice (optional)

Instructions:

1. Heat butter or olive oil in a large skillet over medium-high heat.
2. Add garlic and cook for 30 seconds until fragrant.
3. Add half the spinach. It will seem like too much, but it wilts down dramatically.
4. As first batch wilts (about 1 minute), add remaining spinach.
5. Cook, stirring frequently, for 2-3 minutes until all spinach is wilted and most liquid has evaporated.
6. Season with salt, pepper, and nutmeg (if using).
7. Drizzle with lemon juice if desired.
8. Serve immediately.

Tips:

Budget breakdown: Spinach $3, garlic and butter $0.50. Total: $3.50 for 4 servings.
Volume reduction: 12 cups raw spinach = about 1½ cups cooked. Don't be alarmed.
Remove excess liquid: If there's a lot of liquid in the pan, drain it off before serving.
Frozen spinach: Use 2 packages (10 oz each) frozen spinach. Thaw, squeeze out all water, then sauté with garlic and seasonings for 3-4 minutes.
Storage: Refrigerate for up to 3 days. Reheats well.
Creamed spinach: Add ¼ cup heavy cream and 2 oz cream cheese in step 6. Simmer until creamy. Increases calories to 135, fat to 11g per serving.
Pairs with: Everything, but especially good with eggs, steak, salmon, or any Italian dish.

Roasted Brussels Sprouts with Bacon

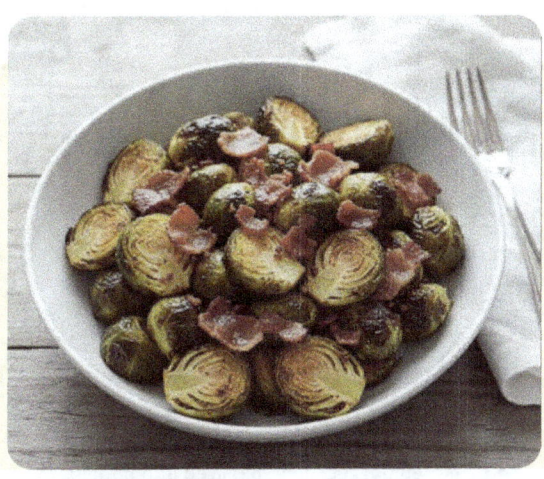

Quick   One-Pan

🍲 Serves: 4

✂️ Prep Time: 10 min

🍲 Cook Time: 25 min

🕐 Total: 35 min

💲 Cost Per Serving: $2.15

MACROS PER SERVING:
Calories: 165 | Protein: 7g |
Fat: 12g | Net Carbs: 6g

Ingredients:

- 1½ pounds Brussels sprouts, trimmed and halved
- 6 strips bacon, chopped
- 2 tablespoons olive oil
- 3 cloves garlic, minced
- ½ teaspoon salt
- ¼ teaspoon black pepper
- 2 tablespoons balsamic vinegar (optional)

Instructions:

1. Preheat oven to 425°F. Line a large baking sheet with parchment paper.
2. In a large bowl, toss Brussels sprouts with olive oil, salt, and pepper.
3. Spread Brussels sprouts cut-side down on the baking sheet. Scatter chopped bacon around them.
4. Roast for 20-25 minutes, stirring halfway through, until Brussels sprouts are tender and caramelized and bacon is crispy.
5. Remove from oven. Sprinkle with minced garlic and toss (the residual heat will cook the garlic slightly).
6. If using balsamic vinegar, drizzle over everything and toss.
7. Transfer to a serving dish.

Tips:

Budget breakdown: Brussels sprouts $4, bacon $2.50, olive oil and garlic $1. Total: $7.50 for 4 servings.

Cut-side down: Placing them cut-side down creates maximum caramelization and crispy edges.

Bacon fat: The bacon renders fat as it cooks, which bastes the Brussels sprouts. Don't drain it.

Storage: Refrigerate for up to 4 days. Reheat in a 425°F oven for 5-7 minutes to restore crispiness.

No bacon version: Use 3 tablespoons olive oil total. Still delicious, just not as bacony.

Balsamic glaze: For extra fancy, reduce balsamic vinegar in a small pan until syrupy, then drizzle over.

Pairs with: Pork chops, roasted chicken, steak, or holiday meals.

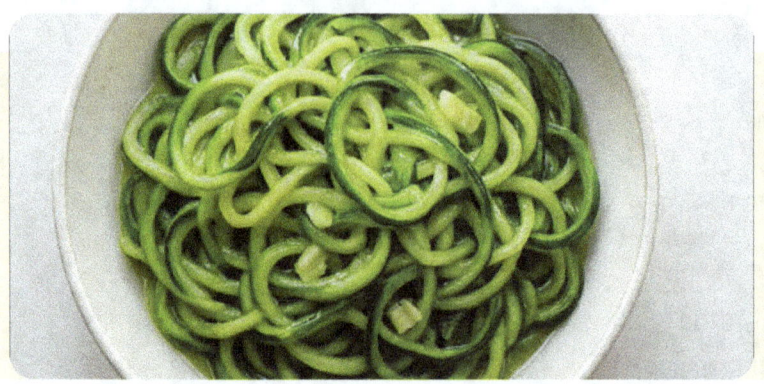

Zucchini Noodles (3 Ways)

Quick   Budget-Friendly

🛎 Serves: 4   📋 Prep Time: 10 min

🍲 Cook Time: 5 min   ⏱ Total: 15 min

💲 COST PER SERVING: $1.25

MACROS PER SERVING (base recipe):
Calories: 65 | Protein: 2g | Fat: 5g | Net Carbs: 3g

Base Instructions:

1. Spiralize zucchini into noodles. If you don't have a spiralizer, use a vegetable peeler to make ribbons.
2. Place zucchini noodles in a colander and sprinkle with ½ teaspoon salt. Let sit for 10 minutes (this draws out excess moisture).
3. Pat zucchini noodles dry with paper towels or a clean kitchen towel.
4. Heat olive oil or butter in a large skillet over medium-high heat.
5. Add garlic and cook for 30 seconds.
6. Add zucchini noodles and cook, tossing frequently, for 2-3 minutes until just tender but still has a slight bite. Don't overcook or they'll get mushy.
7. Season with salt and pepper. Serve immediately.

Base Ingredients:

- 4 medium zucchini, spiralized into noodles
- 2 tablespoons olive oil or butter
- 2 cloves garlic, minced
- ½ teaspoon salt
- ¼ teaspoon black pepper

VARIATION 1:
Garlic Butter Zucchini Noodles

Add to base recipe:

- 2 extra tablespoons butter
- ¼ cup grated Parmesan cheese
- Fresh parsley

Additional macros: +60 calories, +6g fat, +2g protein

VARIATION 2:
Pesto Zucchini Noodles

Add to base recipe:

- ¼ cup pesto (store-bought or homemade)
- 2 tablespoons pine nuts, toasted
- Cherry tomatoes, halved

Additional macros: +85 calories, +8g fat, +2g protein, +2g carbs

VARIATION 3: Italian Zucchini Noodles

Add to base recipe:

- 1 cup marinara sauce
- ¼ cup grated Parmesan

- Fresh basil
- Optional: meatballs or Italian sausage on top

Additional macros: +45 calories, +3g fat, +2g protein, +4g carbs

Tips:

Budget breakdown: Zucchini $3, olive oil and garlic $1. Total: $4 for 4 servings.

Salt and drain: This step is crucial. Zucchini is mostly water. If you don't remove some, your noodles will be watery and sad.

Don't overcook: 2-3 minutes max. You want them tender but with texture, not mushy.

No spiralizer: Use a julienne peeler, regular vegetable peeler (for ribbons), or buy pre-spiralized zucchini at the store.

Storage: Best eaten fresh. Cooked zucchini noodles get watery when stored. If you must store, keep unseasoned and reheat gently.

Meal prep: Spiralize raw zucchini noodles on Sunday. Store in the fridge. Cook fresh each day (takes 3 minutes).

Pairs with: Any dish where you'd use pasta. Meatballs, bolognese, shrimp scampi, chicken parmesan, etc.

Cauliflower Rice (Basic & Flavored)

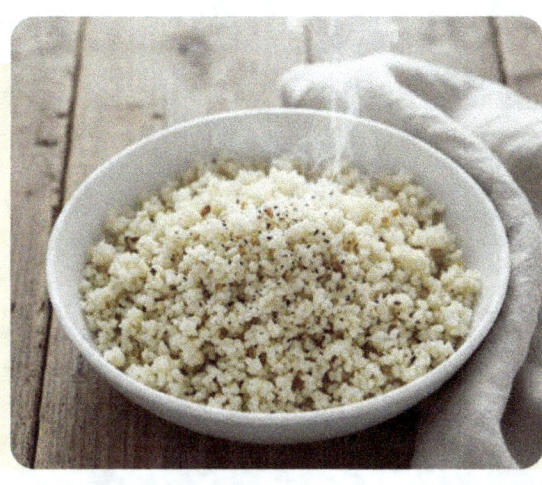

 Quick   Budget-Friendly   Make-Ahead

 Serves: 6 (1 cup per serving)

 Prep Time: 10 min

 Cook Time: 8 min

 Total: 18 min

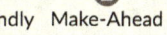 Cost Per Serving: $0.75

MACROS PER SERVING (basic):
Calories: 50 | Protein: 2g | Fat: 4g | Net Carbs: 2g

Base Ingredients:
- 1 large head cauliflower (or 6 cups pre-riced cauliflower)
- 2 tablespoons butter or olive oil
- ½ teaspoon salt
- ¼ teaspoon black pepper

Base Instructions:

If making from scratch:
1. Cut cauliflower into florets. Working in batches, pulse in food processor until rice-sized (don't over-process or it becomes mushy).
2. Heat butter or oil in a large skillet over medium-high heat.
3. Add cauliflower rice, salt, and pepper. Cook for 6-8 minutes, stirring occasionally, until tender and any excess moisture has evaporated.
4. Serve immediately or let cool for meal prep.

If using frozen:
1. Don't thaw frozen cauliflower rice.
2. Heat butter or oil in skillet over medium-high heat.
3. Add frozen cauliflower rice. Cook for 8-10 minutes, stirring occasionally, until tender and moisture evaporates.

Flavor Variations:

Cilantro Lime (Mexican style): Add: juice of 1 lime, zest of 1 lime, ¼ cup cilantro, 1 minced garlic clove.

Garlic Herb (Italian style): Add: 4 cloves minced garlic, 1 tablespoon Italian seasoning, ¼ cup Parmesan.

Fried "Rice" Style (Asian style): Add: 2 beaten eggs (scramble in the pan first), 2 tablespoons soy sauce, 1 teaspoon sesame oil, green onions.

Tips:

Budget breakdown: Cauliflower $3, butter $1. Total: $4 for 6 servings.

Buy it pre-riced: Saves time. Costs about $1 more but worth it for convenience.

Moisture is the enemy: Cook cauliflower rice over medium-high heat without a lid. You want moisture to evaporate, not steam.

Storage: Refrigerate for up to 5 days. Reheat in skillet or microwave.

Meal prep: Make a big batch on Sunday. Use as a base for bowls, stir-fries, or sides all week.

Pairs with: Everything. Use anywhere you'd use regular rice.

Make it special: Toast in butter until slightly crispy for extra flavor and texture.

Asparagus with Hollandaise

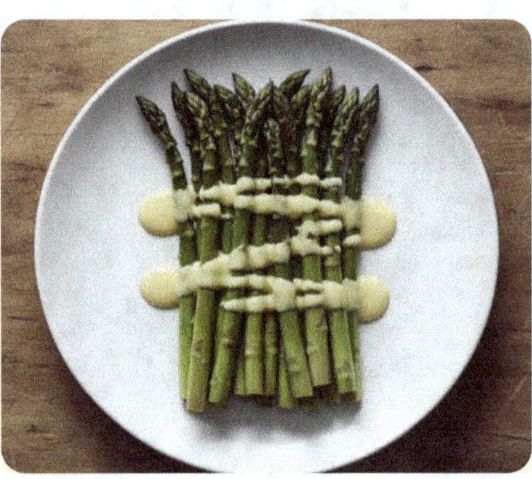

Quick

🍽 Serves: 4

⏱ Prep Time: 5 min

🍳 Cook Time: 12 min

⏰ Total: 17 min

💲 Cost Per Serving: $2.45

MACROS PER SERVING:

Calories: 185 | Protein: 4g |
Fat: 17g | Net Carbs: 4g

Ingredients:

For the asparagus:
- 1½ pounds asparagus, trimmed
- 1 tablespoon olive oil
- ½ teaspoon salt
- ¼ teaspoon black pepper

For the hollandaise:
- 3 egg yolks
- 1 tablespoon lemon juice
- ½ teaspoon Dijon mustard
- ½ cup (1 stick) butter, melted and hot
- Pinch of cayenne pepper
- Salt to taste

Instructions:

Roast the asparagus:
1. Preheat oven to 425°F.
2. Toss asparagus with olive oil, salt, and pepper. Arrange on a baking sheet in a single layer.
3. Roast for 10-12 minutes until tender and slightly charred.

Make the hollandaise (while asparagus roasts):
1. In a blender, combine egg yolks, lemon juice, and Dijon mustard. Blend for 10 seconds.
2. With blender running on low, slowly drizzle in hot melted butter in a thin stream. The sauce will thicken as you add the butter.
3. Add cayenne pepper and salt to taste. Blend briefly.
4. If sauce is too thick, add 1 teaspoon of warm water at a time until desired consistency.

Serve:
1. Arrange roasted asparagus on a serving platter. Drizzle with hollandaise sauce or serve sauce on the side.

Tips:

Budget breakdown: Asparagus $5, butter $2, eggs $1, lemon $1. Total: $9 for 4 servings. This is a special occasion side.

Hot butter is key: The hot butter cooks the egg yolks and creates an emulsion. If butter isn't hot enough, sauce won't thicken.

Broken sauce: If hollandaise breaks (looks curdled), start with a new egg yolk in the blender, then slowly blend in the broken sauce.

Storage: Hollandaise is best fresh. If you must store it, keep at room temperature for up to 2 hours. Don't refrigerate (it solidifies) or keep hot for long (eggs cook).

Blender method: Much easier than the traditional double-boiler method and just as good.

Asparagus alternatives: This hollandaise is also great on eggs Benedict (without the English muffin), salmon, or broccoli.

Pairs with: Steak, salmon, eggs. Classic brunch or fancy dinner side.

Creamed Spinach

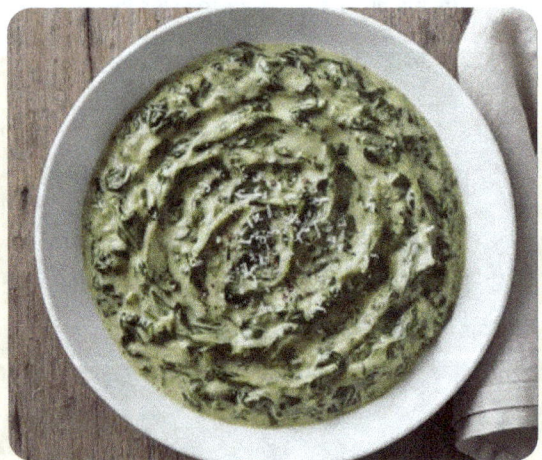

Quick

🍽 Serves: 6

⏱ Prep Time: 5 min

🍳 Cook Time: 15 min

⏰ Total: 20 min

💲 Cost Per Serving: $1.35

MACROS PER SERVING:

Calories: 145 | Protein: 5g |
Fat: 12g | Net Carbs: 4g

Ingredients:

- 2 packages (10 oz each) frozen spinach, thawed
- 4 tablespoons butter
- 1 small onion, diced fine
- 4 cloves garlic, minced
- 4 oz cream cheese, softened
- ½ cup heavy cream
- ½ cup grated Parmesan cheese
- ¼ teaspoon nutmeg
- ½ teaspoon salt
- ¼ teaspoon black pepper

Instructions:

1. Thaw frozen spinach and squeeze out as much water as possible (use a clean kitchen towel or press between paper towels).
2. Melt butter in a large skillet over medium heat.
3. Add onion and cook for 3-4 minutes until softened.
4. Add garlic and cook for 1 minute.
5. Add cream cheese and heavy cream. Stir until cream cheese melts and mixture is smooth.
6. Add spinach, Parmesan, nutmeg, salt, and pepper. Stir to combine.
7. Simmer for 5-7 minutes, stirring occasionally, until heated through and creamy.
8. Taste and adjust seasoning.
9. Serve hot.

Tips:

Budget breakdown: Frozen spinach $3, cream cheese $2, heavy cream $1, Parmesan $1.50, butter and onion $1. Total: $8.50 for 6 servings.

Squeeze the spinach: This is crucial. Frozen spinach holds a ton of water. If you don't remove it, your creamed spinach will be watery.

Fresh spinach: Use 2 pounds fresh spinach. Sauté until wilted, then drain and chop before adding to cream sauce.

Storage: Refrigerate for up to 5 days. Reheats beautifully.

Make ahead: This actually improves when made a day ahead. Make it, refrigerate, reheat when ready to serve.

Restaurant classic: This is a steakhouse staple. Now you can make it at home for a fraction of the price.

Pairs with: Steak, prime rib, roasted chicken, or any dish that needs a rich, decadent side.

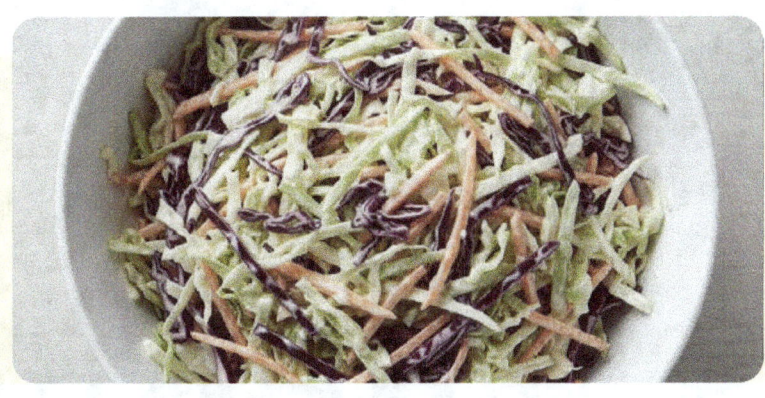

Cabbage Slaw (Multiple Versions)

Quick   Budget-Friendly   Make-Ahead

Serves: 8   Prep Time: 15 min

Cook Time: 0 min   Total: 15 min

COST PER SERVING: $0.65

MACROS PER SERVING (basic coleslaw):
Calories: 95 | Protein: 1g | Fat: 8g | Net Carbs: 4g

Base Ingredients:

- 6 cups green cabbage, shredded
- 2 cups red cabbage, shredded (or use all green)
- 1 cup carrots, shredded

VARIATION 1: Classic Coleslaw

Instructions:

1. Combine shredded cabbage and carrots in a large bowl.
2. Whisk together all dressing ingredients.
3. Pour dressing over vegetables and toss well.
4. Refrigerate for at least 30 minutes before serving (improves flavor).

Dressing:

- ½ cup mayonnaise
- 2 tablespoons apple cider vinegar
- 1 tablespoon Dijon mustard
- 1 tablespoon erythritol or monk fruit sweetener
- ½ teaspoon celery seed
- ½ teaspoon salt
- ¼ teaspoon black pepper

VARIATION 2: Asian Slaw

Dressing:

- ¼ cup rice vinegar
- 3 tablespoons sesame oil
- 2 tablespoons soy sauce
- 1 tablespoon fresh ginger, grated
- 1 clove garlic, minced
- 1 teaspoon erythritol or sweetener

Add to vegetables:

- 3 green onions, sliced
- ¼ cup cilantro, chopped
- 2 tablespoons sesame seeds

VARIATION 3: Creamy Cilantro Lime Slaw

Dressing:

- ½ cup mayonnaise
- ¼ cup sour cream
- Juice of 2 limes
- ¼ cup cilantro, chopped

- 1 jalapeño, minced (optional)
- ½ teaspoon cumin
- ½ teaspoon salt

Tips:

Budget breakdown: Cabbage $2, carrots $1, mayo and other dressing ingredients $2. Total: $5 for 8 servings.

Buy pre-shredded: Coleslaw mix saves time. Just add your dressing.

Storage: Dressed slaw keeps for 3-4 days in the fridge. Gets more flavorful over time but cabbage softens.

Meal prep: Make a big batch on Sunday. Serve as a side all week.

Pairs with: Pulled pork, BBQ anything, fried chicken, fish tacos, burgers.

Volume: Cabbage is mostly water and fiber. You can eat a ton for very few calories and carbs.

SNACKS

Deviled Eggs (3 Variations)

Quick   Budget-Friendly   Make-Ahead

Makes: 24 deviled egg halves   **Prep Time:** 15 min   **Cook Time:** 12 min   **Total:** 27 min

COST PER SERVING (2 halves): $0.60   **MACROS PER SERVING (2 halves, classic):** Calories: 155 | Protein: 12g | Fat: 11g | Net Carbs: 1g

Base Instructions:

1. Hard-boil eggs using your preferred method (see Recipe 81 for detailed instructions).
2. Cut eggs in half lengthwise. Remove yolks to a bowl.
3. Mash yolks with a fork until crumbly.
4. Add mayonnaise, mustard, vinegar, salt, and pepper. Mix until smooth and creamy.
5. Spoon or pipe mixture back into egg white halves (a piping bag makes them pretty, but a spoon works fine).
6. Sprinkle with paprika.
7. Refrigerate until ready to serve.

Base Ingredients:

- 12 large eggs, hard-boiled and peeled
- ½ cup mayonnaise
- 2 teaspoons Dijon mustard
- 1 teaspoon white vinegar or lemon juice
- ¼ teaspoon salt
- ⅛ teaspoon black pepper
- Paprika for garnish

VARIATION 1: Bacon Ranch Deviled Eggs

Add to yolk mixture:

- 2 tablespoons ranch dressing (replace some mayo)
- 4 strips bacon, cooked and crumbled
- 2 tablespoons chives, chopped

Top each with a bacon crumble

VARIATION 2: Buffalo Deviled Eggs

Add to yolk mixture:

- 2 tablespoons Frank's RedHot sauce
- 2 tablespoons blue cheese, crumbled
- Reduce mayo to ⅓ cup

Top with extra blue cheese crumbles and a dash of hot sauce

VARIATION 3: Avocado Deviled Eggs

Add to yolk mixture:

- ½ ripe avocado, mashed
- 1 tablespoon lime juice
- ¼ teaspoon cumin
- Reduce mayo to ¼ cup

Top with cilantro and a lime wedge

Tips:

Budget breakdown: Eggs $3, mayo $1, bacon for variations $1. Total: $5 for 12 servings.

Storage: Refrigerate for up to 3 days in an airtight container.

Make ahead: Perfect for meal prep. Make on Sunday, grab 2 halves for a quick snack.

Transport: Use an egg carrier or place in a container with paper towels between layers.

Protein snack: 2 deviled egg halves = 12g protein. Perfect between meals or post-workout.

Party favorite: Always disappear first at gatherings.

Quick   Budget-Friendly

🍽 Makes: 16 crisps

✂ Prep Time: 5 min

🍲 Cook Time: 7 min

🍮 Total: 12 min

💲 COST PER SERVING (4 crisps): $1.25

MACROS PER SERVING (4 crisps):

Calories: 115 | Protein: 8g |
Fat: 9g | Net Carbs: 1g

Egg Roll in a Bowl

Ingredients:

- 2 cups shredded cheddar cheese (or Parmesan, mozzarella, or a mix)
- Optional seasonings: garlic powder, paprika, Italian seasoning, everything bagel seasoning

Instructions:

Oven method:
1. Preheat oven to 350°F. Line a baking sheet with parchment paper or a silicone mat.
2. Place small mounds of shredded cheese (about 2 tablespoons each) on the baking sheet, spacing them 2 inches apart. Flatten slightly.
3. Sprinkle with desired seasonings if using.
4. Bake for 5-7 minutes until cheese is melted, bubbly, and golden brown around the edges.
5. Let cool on the baking sheet for 2-3 minutes (they'll crisp up as they cool).
6. Transfer to a wire rack to cool completely.

Microwave method:
1. Place parchment paper on a microwave-safe plate.
2. Place small mounds of cheese (2 tablespoons each) on the parchment, spacing them apart.
3. Microwave on high for 60-90 seconds until cheese is melted and starting to brown.
4. Let cool for 1-2 minutes, then peel off parchment.

Tips:

Budget breakdown: Cheese $5. Total: $5 for 4 servings.

Don't skip the cooling: They need to cool to crisp up. If you try to move them too soon, they'll be floppy.

Storage: Store in an airtight container at room temperature for up to 3 days. They'll lose some crispness over time.

Make ahead: Make a big batch. Use as "crackers" for dips, crumble over salads, or eat as chips.

Flavor variations: Try different cheeses. Parmesan makes very crispy, nutty crisps. Cheddar is classic. Pepper jack is spicy.

Use for: Chip substitute, salad topper, soup dipper, or snack straight from the jar.

Pepperoni Chips

Ingredients:

- 4 oz pepperoni slices (about 60 slices)

 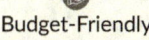
Quick   Budget-Friendly

🍽 Serves: 4

✂ Prep Time: 2 min

🍲 Cook Time: 8 min

🍮 Total: 10 min

💲 COST PER SERVING: $1.15

MACROS PER SERVING:

Calories: 135 | Protein: 6g |
Fat: 12g | Net Carbs: 0g

Instructions:

Oven method:
1. Preheat oven to 425°F. Line a baking sheet with parchment paper.
2. Arrange pepperoni slices in a single layer on the baking sheet (they can touch slightly).
3. Bake for 6-8 minutes until pepperoni is crispy and fat has rendered. Watch carefully—they can burn quickly.
4. Transfer to a paper towel-lined plate to drain excess grease.
5. Let cool for 2-3 minutes (they'll crisp up more as they cool).

Microwave method:
1. Place pepperoni slices in a single layer on a microwave-safe plate lined with paper towels.
2. Cover with another paper towel.
3. Microwave on high for 45-60 seconds until crispy.
4. Let cool briefly.

Tips:

Budget breakdown: Pepperoni $4.50. Total: $4.50 for 4 servings.

Storage: Store in an airtight container at room temperature for up to 3 days.

Use the grease: Save the rendered pepperoni fat. It's excellent for cooking eggs or vegetables.

Flavor variations: Try salami, prosciutto, or other cured meats using the same method.

Use for: Snacking, salad topper, pizza topping (on cauliflower crust), or crushed as a "breadcrumb" coating.

Kid-friendly: Most kids love these. They're like meat chips.

Bacon-Wrapped Jalapeños

Make-Ahead

- Makes: 12 pieces
- Prep Time: 15 min
- Cook Time: 25 min
- Total: 40 min
- COST PER SERVING (2 pieces): $1.85

MACROS PER SERVING (2 pieces):

Calories: 185 | Protein: 10g | Fat: 15g | Net Carbs: 2g

Ingredients:

- 6 large jalapeños
- 4 oz cream cheese, softened
- ½ cup shredded cheddar cheese
- 12 strips bacon

Instructions:

1. Preheat oven to 400°F. Line a baking sheet with parchment paper or foil.
2. Cut jalapeños in half lengthwise. Use a spoon to scoop out seeds and membranes (this reduces heat—leave some seeds if you want it spicier).
3. In a bowl, mix cream cheese and cheddar cheese until combined.
4. Fill each jalapeño half with cheese mixture (about 1 tablespoon per half).
5. Wrap each stuffed jalapeño with 1 strip of bacon, securing with a toothpick if needed.
6. Place on prepared baking sheet.
7. Bake for 20-25 minutes until bacon is crispy and jalapeños are tender.
8. Let cool for 5 minutes before serving (cheese will be molten hot).

Tips:

Budget breakdown: Jalapeños $2, cream cheese $2, cheddar $1.50, bacon $3.50. Total: $9 for 6 servings.

Wear gloves: When handling jalapeños, wear gloves or wash hands immediately. Don't touch your eyes.

Make ahead: Assemble stuffed jalapeños in advance. Refrigerate for up to 24 hours before baking.

Freezer-friendly: Freeze assembled (unbaked) jalapeños for up to 2 months. Bake from frozen, adding 5-10 minutes to cooking time.

Storage: Refrigerate leftovers for up to 3 days. Reheat in 400°F oven for 5-7 minutes.

Party food: These are always a hit. Make a double batch—they disappear fast.

Use for: Appetizer, game day snack, or a protein-rich treat.

Deli Meat Roll-Ups

Ingredients:

- 12 slices deli turkey or ham
- 6 oz cream cheese, softened
- 12 pickle spears (dill pickles work best)
- Optional: mustard, everything bagel seasoning

Instructions:

1. Lay out deli meat slices on a cutting board.
2. Spread about 1½ tablespoons cream cheese on each slice.
3. If using mustard, add a thin line of mustard.
4. Sprinkle with everything bagel seasoning if using.
5. Place a pickle spear at one end of each slice.
6. Roll up tightly.
7. Secure with a toothpick if needed.
8. Serve immediately or refrigerate.

Quick   **Budget-Friendly**

- Serves: 4 (3 roll-ups per serving)
- Prep Time: 10 min
- Cook Time: 0 min
- Total: 10 min
- COST PER SERVING: $1.85

MACROS PER SERVING (3 roll-ups):

Calories: 245 | Protein: 18g | Fat: 18g | Net Carbs: 2g

Tips:

Budget breakdown: Deli meat $4, cream cheese $2, pickles $1.50. Total: $7.50 for 4 servings.

Quality matters: Buy decent deli meat without added sugars or fillers.

Variations:
- Use different deli meats (roast beef, salami, pepperoni)
- Swap pickles for pepperoncini, jalapeños, or asparagus spears
- Add lettuce, tomato, or avocado
- Use different spreads (pesto, olive tapenade, herbed cream cheese)

Storage: Refrigerate for up to 3 days. Best within 24 hours.

Portable: Pack for lunch or snacks. They travel well.

Make ahead: Prep a batch on Sunday for grab-and-go snacks all week.

Makes: 12 muffings

Prep Time: 10 min

Cook Time: 20 min

Total: 30 min

COST PER SERVING (2 muffins): $1.45

MACROS PER SERVING (2 muffins):

Calories: 190 | Protein: 14g | Fat: 13g | Net Carbs: 2g

Egg Muffins (Portable)

Ingredients:

- 8 large eggs
- ¼ cup heavy cream
- 1 cup diced ham, cooked sausage, or cooked bacon
- 1 cup shredded cheese (cheddar, mozzarella, or Swiss)
- ½ cup diced bell pepper
- ¼ cup diced onion
- ½ teaspoon salt
- ¼ teaspoon black pepper
- Cooking spray

Instructions:

1. Preheat oven to 350°F. Spray a 12-cup muffin tin generously with cooking spray.
2. In a large bowl, whisk together eggs, heavy cream, salt, and pepper.
3. Divide ham, cheese, bell pepper, and onion evenly among the 12 muffin cups.
4. Pour egg mixture over the fillings, filling each cup about three-quarters full.
5. Stir each cup gently with a fork to distribute ingredients.
6. Bake for 18-20 minutes until eggs are set and tops are lightly golden.
7. Let cool in the pan for 5 minutes, then run a butter knife around edges and pop them out.

Tips:

Budget breakdown: Eggs $2, ham $2, cheese $2, vegetables $1.50. Total: $7.50 for 6 servings (12 muffins).

Storage: Refrigerate for up to 5 days or freeze for up to 2 months.

Reheating: From fridge, microwave 2 muffins for 45-60 seconds. From frozen, microwave for 90 seconds.

Endless variations: Use any protein, cheese, and vegetable combination you like.

Portable protein: Perfect for busy mornings, road trips, or desk snacks.

Make a double batch: These freeze beautifully. Make 24 at once.

Buffalo Chicken Dip

Ingredients:

- 2 cups cooked chicken, shredded
- 8 oz cream cheese, softened
- ½ cup Frank's RedHot sauce
- ½ cup ranch or blue cheese dressing
- 1 cup shredded mozzarella cheese, divided
- ½ cup shredded cheddar cheese
- Optional: blue cheese crumbles, green onions for topping

For serving: celery sticks, bell pepper slices, cucumber rounds, pork rinds, or cheese crisps

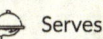

Serves: 8

Prep Time: 10 min

Cook Time: 25 min

Total: 35 min

COST PER SERVING: $1.85

MACROS PER SERVING:

Calories: 245 | Protein: 18g | Fat: 18g | Net Carbs: 2g

Instructions:

1. Preheat oven to 375°F.
2. In a large bowl, mix cream cheese, hot sauce, and ranch dressing until smooth.
3. Stir in shredded chicken, ½ cup mozzarella, and all the cheddar cheese.
4. Transfer to an 8x8-inch baking dish or small cast-iron skillet.
5. Top with remaining ½ cup mozzarella and blue cheese crumbles if using.
6. Bake for 20-25 minutes until bubbly and cheese is melted.
7. Top with sliced green onions if desired.
8. Serve hot with vegetables or pork rinds for dipping.

Tips:

Budget breakdown: Chicken $3 (use rotisserie), cream cheese $2, cheeses $3, hot sauce and ranch $2. Total: $10 for 8 servings.

Rotisserie shortcut: Use a rotisserie chicken. Shred the meat. Zero cooking required.

Slow cooker: Combine all ingredients in slow cooker. Cook on low for 2 hours, stirring occasionally. Keep warm on low for serving.

Storage: Refrigerate for up to 5 days. Reheat in microwave or oven.

Party favorite: This is always a hit. Make a double batch—it disappears fast.

Serve with: Celery, bell peppers, cucumber, pork rinds, or cheese crisps. Skip the tortilla chips.

Tuna Salad Cucumber Bites

Quick **Budget-Friendly**

🍽️ Serves: 4 (6 bites per serving)

⏱️ Prep Time: 15 min

🍳 Cook Time: 0 min

⏲️ Total: 15 min

💲 COST PER SERVING: $1.65

MACROS PER SERVING (6 bites):

Calories: 185 | Protein: 16g | Fat: 12g | Net Carbs: 2g

Ingredients:

- 2 cans (5 oz each) tuna in water, drained
- ¼ cup mayonnaise
- 1 tablespoon Dijon mustard
- 2 tablespoons diced celery
- 1 tablespoon diced red onion
- 1 tablespoon lemon juice
- ¼ teaspoon salt
- ⅛ teaspoon black pepper
- 2 large cucumbers
- Paprika for garnish
- Optional: fresh dill

Instructions:

1. In a bowl, combine drained tuna, mayonnaise, Dijon mustard, celery, red onion, lemon juice, salt, and pepper. Mix well.
2. Slice cucumbers into ½-inch thick rounds (you'll need about 24 rounds).
3. Use a small spoon to scoop out a shallow well in each cucumber round (optional, but helps hold more tuna).
4. Top each cucumber round with about 1 tablespoon of tuna salad.
5. Sprinkle with paprika and garnish with fresh dill if using.
6. Serve immediately or refrigerate for up to 2 hours.

Tips:

Budget breakdown: Canned tuna $3, cucumber $1.50, mayo and other ingredients $1.50. Total: $6 for 4 servings.

Make ahead: Prepare tuna salad and slice cucumbers separately. Assemble just before serving to prevent cucumbers from getting soggy.

Storage: Tuna salad keeps for 3-4 days. Cucumber rounds are best fresh.

Variations: Use chicken salad, egg salad, or salmon salad instead.

Portable: Pack tuna salad and cucumber rounds separately. Assemble when ready to eat.

Low-effort protein: Perfect afternoon snack or light lunch.

Beef Jerky (Homemade)

Ingredients:

- 2 pounds lean beef (top round, bottom round, or sirloin tip), sliced ⅛-¼ inch thick
- ½ cup soy sauce (or coconut aminos)
- 2 tablespoons Worcestershire sauce
- 2 tablespoons apple cider vinegar
- 1 tablespoon erythritol or monk fruit sweetener
- 2 teaspoons liquid smoke
- 1 teaspoon black pepper
- 1 teaspoon garlic powder
- 1 teaspoon onion powder
- ½ teaspoon red pepper flakes (optional)

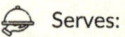

Make-Ahead

🍽️ Serves: 8

⏱️ Prep Time: 15 min (plus marinating)

🍳 Cook Time: 3-4 hours

⏲️ Total: 4+ hours

💲 COST PER SERVING: $2.25

MACROS PER SERVING (1 oz):

Calories: 85 | Protein: 15g | Fat: 2g | Net Carbs: 2g

Instructions:

Prep the meat:
1. Freeze beef for 1-2 hours until firm but not solid (easier to slice thin).
2. Slice beef against the grain into ⅛-¼ inch thick strips. Trim all visible fat (fat goes rancid and shortens shelf life).

Marinate:
3. In a large bowl or zip-top bag, combine soy sauce, Worcestershire sauce, vinegar, sweetener, liquid smoke, pepper, garlic powder, onion powder, and red pepper flakes (if using).
4. Add beef strips and turn to coat. Marinate in the refrigerator for 4-24 hours (longer = more flavor).

Dehydrate:
Oven method:
5. Preheat oven to 175°F (or lowest setting).
6. Line baking sheets with foil and place wire racks on top.
7. Arrange beef strips on racks in a single layer, not touching.
8. Dry in oven for 3-4 hours, flipping halfway through, until beef is dry and leathery but still flexible.
9. Let cool completely before storing.

Dehydrator method:
10. Arrange strips on dehydrator trays in a single layer.
11. Dehydrate at 160°F for 4-6 hours until dry and leathery.

Tips:

Budget breakdown: Beef $12-15 (buy on sale), soy sauce and seasonings $3. Total: $15-18 for 8 servings. Cheaper than store-bought jerky ($2-3 per oz).

Slice it thin: The thinner you slice, the faster it dries and the more tender the final product.

Against the grain: Slicing against the grain makes jerky more tender and easier to chew.

Storage: Store in an airtight container or zip-top bags for up to 2 weeks at room temperature, 1 month in the fridge, or 6 months in the freezer.

Perfect for: Road trips, hiking, travel, desk snacks, post-workout protein.

No dehydrator needed: The oven method works perfectly fine.

Quick

Serves: 4

Prep Time: 15 min

Cook Time: 0 min

Total: 15 min

COST PER SERVING: $4.50

MACROS PER SERVING (approximate):

Calories: 385 | Protein: 22g | Fat: 32g | Net Carbs: 4g

Cheese & Charcuterie Plate Guide

How to Build a Keto Charcuterie Plate:

Proteins (choose 2-3):
- Salami slices
- Prosciutto
- Pepperoni
- Hard-boiled eggs
- Rolled deli meats

Cheeses (choose 2-3):
- Hard cheeses (cheddar, Gouda, aged Parmesan)
- Soft cheeses (brie, goat cheese, blue cheese)
- Semi-soft cheeses (Havarti, Muenster)

Vegetables (choose 2-3):
- Cherry tomatoes
- Cucumber slices
- Bell pepper strips
- Celery sticks
- Radishes
- Olives
- Pickles

Nuts (small portions, high carb):
- Almonds (¼ cup per plate)
- Pecans
- Macadamias

Optional Additions:
- Mustard (for dipping)
- Sugar-free jam (in very small amounts)
- Pork rinds (as "crackers")
- Cheese crisps

Assembly Tips:

1. **Choose variety:** Different colors, textures, and flavors.
2. **Portion proteins:** About 4-6 oz total meat per person.
3. **Portion cheese:** About 2-3 oz per person.
4. **Arrange aesthetically:** Group similar items together. Create height and dimension.
5. **Leave space:** Don't overcrowd. White space makes it look elegant.
6. **Serve at room temperature:** Take cheese out of fridge 30 minutes before serving for best flavor.

Tips:

Budget breakdown: Cured meats $8, cheeses $8, vegetables $3, nuts $3. Total: $22 for 4 servings. This is a splurge meal or party option.

Scale it: Easy to double or triple for parties.

Make ahead: Assemble everything except cheese 1 hour ahead. Add cheese 30 minutes before serving.

Portable: Pack components separately for picnics or travel.

Use for: Appetizers, light dinners, wine nights, parties, or when you don't feel like cooking.

No cooking required: Perfect for lazy evenings.

CHAPTER 8 SUMMARY

You now have 20 sides and snacks that make low-carb eating easier and more sustainable. Here's how to use them:

The Side Dish Strategy:
Master 3-4 vegetable sides you actually like.

That's all you need. Rotate them with your proteins:
- Monday: Chicken + Roasted Broccoli
- Tuesday: Steak + Garlic Green Beans
- Wednesday: Pork Chops + Cauliflower Mash
- Thursday: Salmon + Sautéed Spinach
- Friday: Burgers + Cabbage Slaw

Same proteins you'd make anyway. Now they feel like complete meals.

My Weekly Veggie Rotation:

I keep it simple:
- Roasted vegetables (broccoli, Brussels sprouts, asparagus) - 2-3 times per week
- Sautéed greens (spinach, kale) - 2-3 times per week
- Cauliflower rice or mash - 1-2 times per week
- Cabbage slaw - 1 time per week

That's it. Four types of sides, infinite combinations with different proteins.

The Snack Strategy:
Most days, you shouldn't need snacks. When you eat enough protein and fat at meals, you stay full for hours.

But when you do need snacks:

Always in the house:
- Hard-boiled eggs (make a dozen every Sunday)
- String cheese or cheese cubes
- Deli meat
- Nuts (portion controlled—easy to overeat)

Batch on Sunday:
- Deviled eggs
- Egg muffins
- Cheese crisps

Total prep time: 45 minutes gets you snacks for the week.

Emergency Snacks (no prep):
- String cheese + pepperoni
- Hard-boiled eggs + mustard
- Deli meat roll-ups
- Pork rinds
- Olives
- Pickles

Snack vs. Meal:
If you're eating "snacks" every 2 hours, you're not eating enough at meals.

Good meal timing:
- Breakfast: 7 AM
- Lunch: 12 PM (5 hours later - no snack needed)
- Dinner: 6 PM (6 hours later - no snack needed)

If you need a snack:
- Mid-morning (if breakfast was light)
- Mid-afternoon (if lunch was light or dinner is delayed)
- Post-workout
- Evening (if dinner was early and you're hungry before bed)

Otherwise, skip the snacks and eat bigger meals.

Budget Reality:

Sides:
- Most vegetable sides cost $0.75-$2 per serving
- Much cheaper than carb-heavy sides (pasta, potatoes, rice)
- Last 4-5 days in the fridge

Snacks:
- Homemade always cheaper than store-bought
- Hard-boiled eggs: $0.30 each
- Deviled eggs: $0.60 for 2
- Store-bought keto snacks: $2-4 per serving

Make your own. Save your money.

Common Mistakes:
1. **Eating plain steamed vegetables.** No wonder you hate them. Add fat and salt. Roast them. Sauté them. Make them taste good.
2. **Skipping sides entirely.** Just eating protein gets boring. Vegetables add volume, nutrients, and variety.
3. **Relying on "keto snacks."** Most packaged keto snacks are expensive and not very filling. Real food is better.
4. **Constant grazing.** If you're snacking every hour, you're not eating enough at meals. Eat more protein and fat at mealtime.

Not meal prepping sides. Roast a big batch of vegetables on Sunday. Reheat portions all week.

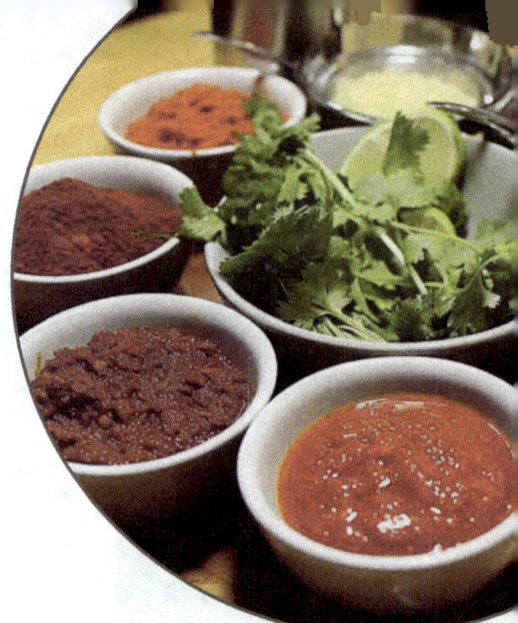

Here's the truth about cooking: technique matters less than you think. Seasoning matters more than you realize.

You can cook a perfect medium-rare steak using flawless technique, but if all you add is salt, it's going to be boring by the third time you eat it. You can grill chicken breasts to exactly 165°F, but without proper seasoning, they'll taste like cardboard.

This is where most people fail at eating high-protein, low-carb. They master cooking the protein. They learn to roast vegetables. But they forget about flavor. After two weeks of "grilled chicken and broccoli," they're so bored they order pizza and declare that healthy eating is unsustainable.

The problem isn't the chicken. It's that you're eating the same underseasoned chicken every time.

This chapter solves that problem.

The recipes here are the difference between "I guess I'll eat chicken again" and "I'm genuinely excited about dinner." They're the secret weapons that make the same basic proteins taste completely different every night of the week.

CHAPTER 9: SAUCES & SEASONINGS

Garlic Butter

Ingredients:

- ½ cup (1 stick) butter, softened to room temperature
- 4 cloves garlic, minced (or 1 teaspoon garlic powder)
- 2 tablespoons fresh parsley, finely chopped (or 2 teaspoons dried)
- ¼ teaspoon salt
- ⅛ teaspoon black pepper
- Optional: ½ teaspoon lemon zest, ¼ teaspoon red pepper flakes

Instructions:

1. Place softened butter in a bowl.
2. Add minced garlic, parsley, salt, pepper, and any optional ingredients.
3. Mix thoroughly with a fork or spoon until all ingredients are evenly distributed.
4. Taste and adjust seasoning if needed.
5. Transfer to a small container or roll into a log using plastic wrap or parchment paper (makes slicing easier).
6. Refrigerate for at least 30 minutes to let flavors meld and butter firm up.

Tips:

Budget breakdown: Butter $2, garlic and parsley $1.50. Total: $3.50 for 12 servings.

Room temperature butter: Must be soft to mix properly. Leave out for 30-60 minutes or microwave for 5-10 seconds.

Storage: Refrigerate for up to 2 weeks or freeze for up to 3 months.

Make a log: Roll into a log, freeze, then slice off rounds as needed. Perfect for topping steaks or fish.

Fresh vs. dried garlic: Fresh garlic tastes better. Garlic powder works if that's what you have.

Uses:

- Top grilled steaks, chicken, pork chops, or fish
- Toss with roasted vegetables
- Melt over cooked shrimp
- Stir into scrambled eggs
- Spread on low-carb bread
- Mix into cauliflower mash

Flavor variations:

Herb butter: Add thyme, rosemary, or basil instead of parsley

Lemon butter: Add 1 tablespoon lemon juice and 1 teaspoon lemon zest

Cajun butter: Add 1 tablespoon Cajun seasoning

Blue cheese butter: Add 2 tablespoons crumbled blue cheese

Blue Cheese Dressing

Ingredients:

- ½ cup mayonnaise
- ½ cup sour cream
- ⅓ cup buttermilk (or heavy cream thinned with 1 tablespoon lemon juice)
- ¾ cup blue cheese, crumbled (divided)
- 1 tablespoon lemon juice
- 1 teaspoon Worcestershire sauce
- 1 clove garlic, minced
- ¼ teaspoon salt
- ¼ teaspoon black pepper

Instructions:

1. In a bowl, whisk together mayonnaise, sour cream, and buttermilk until smooth.
2. Add lemon juice, Worcestershire sauce, garlic, salt, and pepper. Whisk to combine.
3. Crumble half the blue cheese into very small pieces. Add to dressing and stir.
4. Add remaining blue cheese in larger chunks (for texture).
5. Taste and adjust seasoning. If too thick, add 1 tablespoon buttermilk at a time until desired consistency.
6. Refrigerate for at least 30 minutes before serving (flavors meld and improve).

Tips:

Budget breakdown: Mayo $1.50, sour cream $1.50, blue cheese $3, buttermilk $1.50. Total: $7.50 for 12 servings.

Blue cheese quality: Good blue cheese makes better dressing. Look for Gorgonzola, Roquefort, or quality domestic blue cheese.

Storage: Refrigerate in an airtight container for up to 1 week.

Consistency: This dressing thickens in the fridge. Thin with buttermilk or water before serving if needed.

Make it chunkier: Add more blue cheese chunks for texture and stronger flavor.

Uses:

- Buffalo chicken salad or wings
- Steak salad
- Cobb salad
- Vegetable dip (celery, carrots, bell peppers)
- Drizzle over roasted Brussels sprouts
- Burger topping

Don't like blue cheese? Use the ranch recipe below instead. Same uses, different flavor.

Quick Budget-Friendly Make-Ahead

Ranch Dressing (From Scratch)

Makes: About 1½ cups
(12 servings, 2 tablespoons each)

Prep Time: 5 min

Cook Time: 0 min

Total: 5 min

COST PER SERVING: $0.45

MACROS PER SERVING (2 tablespoons):

Calories: 115 | Protein: 1g |
Fat: 12g | Net Carbs: 1g

Ingredients:

- ¾ cup mayonnaise
- ½ cup sour cream
- ¼ cup heavy cream (or buttermilk)
- 2 tablespoons fresh parsley, finely chopped (or 2 teaspoons dried)
- 1 tablespoon fresh dill, finely chopped (or 1 teaspoon dried)

- 1 tablespoon fresh chives, finely chopped (or 1 teaspoon dried)
- 2 cloves garlic, minced
- 1 teaspoon onion powder
- ½ teaspoon salt
- ¼ teaspoon black pepper
- 1 tablespoon lemon juice or white vinegar

Instructions:

1. In a bowl, whisk together mayonnaise, sour cream, and heavy cream until smooth.
2. Add parsley, dill, chives, garlic, onion powder, salt, pepper, and lemon juice.
3. Whisk until well combined.
4. Taste and adjust seasoning. Add more salt, herbs, or acid as needed.
5. If too thick, add 1 tablespoon heavy cream or water at a time until desired consistency.
6. Refrigerate for at least 1 hour before serving (flavors improve dramatically with time).

Tips:

Budget breakdown: Mayo $1.50, sour cream $1.50, heavy cream $0.50, herbs $2. Total: $5.50 for 12 servings.
Fresh vs. dried herbs: Fresh tastes better. Dried works fine. Use 1/3 the amount of dried compared to fresh.
Storage: Refrigerate in an airtight container for up to 1 week. Flavors improve over first 24 hours.
Make it ahead: This actually needs to sit. Make it the night before for best flavor.
Dry ranch seasoning: Want to make your own packets? Mix: 1 tablespoon dried parsley, 1 teaspoon dried dill, 1 teaspoon garlic powder, 1 teaspoon onion powder, ½ teaspoon salt, ¼ teaspoon pepper. Store in jar. Add 2 tablespoons of this mix to mayo and sour cream base.

Uses:
- Salad dressing (any salad, but especially Cobb or chicken)
- Vegetable dip
- Buffalo chicken topping
- Drizzle over roasted vegetables
- Mix with shredded chicken for chicken salad
- Burger or sandwich spread
- Pizza sauce alternative (on cauliflower crust)

Flavor variations:
- **Spicy ranch:** Add ½ teaspoon cayenne pepper or 1 tablespoon hot sauce
- **Bacon ranch:** Crumble 4 strips cooked bacon into finished dressing
- **Jalapeño ranch:** Add 1 minced jalapeño or 1 tablespoon diced pickled jalapeños

---

Caesar Dressing

Ingredients:

- ¾ cup mayonnaise
- ¼ cup grated Parmesan cheese
- 2 tablespoons lemon juice
- 1 tablespoon Worcestershire sauce
- 2 cloves garlic, minced
- 1 teaspoon Dijon mustard

- 1 teaspoon anchovy paste (optional but traditional)
- ¼ teaspoon salt
- ¼ teaspoon black pepper
- 2-3 tablespoons water (to thin if needed)

Quick   Make-Ahead

Makes: About 1 cup (8 servings, 2 tablespoons each)

Prep Time: 5 min

Cook Time: 0 min

Total: 5 min

COST PER SERVING: $0.55

MACROS PER SERVING (2 tablespoons):

Calories: 135 | Protein: 2g |
Fat: 14g | Net Carbs: 1g

Instructions:

1. In a bowl or jar, combine mayonnaise, Parmesan cheese, lemon juice, Worcestershire sauce, garlic, Dijon mustard, and anchovy paste (if using).
2. Whisk or shake vigorously until smooth and well combined.
3. Add salt and pepper. Taste and adjust seasoning.
4. If too thick, add water 1 tablespoon at a time until desired consistency (should be thick but pourable).
5. Refrigerate for at least 30 minutes before serving (flavors meld and improve).

Tips:

Budget breakdown: Mayo $1.50, Parmesan $1.50, lemon $0.50, anchovy paste $1. Total: $4.50 for 8 servings.
Anchovy paste: Don't skip it if you want authentic Caesar flavor. It adds umami depth without tasting fishy. Find it in the canned fish aisle or near the tomato paste.
No anchovy paste: Substitute with 2 additional teaspoons Worcestershire sauce. Won't be traditional, but still good.
Storage: Refrigerate in an airtight container for up to 1 week.
Blender method: Combine all ingredients in a blender for ultra-smooth dressing. Add water to thin.

Uses:
- Caesar salad (obviously)
- Chicken Caesar wraps (lettuce wraps)
- Drizzle over grilled chicken or fish
- Vegetable dip
- Marinade for chicken before grilling
- Mix with shredded chicken for Caesar chicken salad

Make it creamier: Replace 2 tablespoons mayo with sour cream or Greek yogurt.

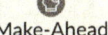
Budget-Friendly   Make-Ahead

Makes: About 1½ cups
(12 servings, 2 tablespoons each)

Prep Time: 5 min

Cook Time: 20 min

Total: 25 min

COST PER SERVING: $0.35

MACROS PER SERVING (2 tablespoons):

Calories: 15 | Protein: 0g |
Fat: 0g | Net Carbs: 2g

Sugar-Free BBQ Sauce

Ingredients:

- 1 can (15 oz) tomato sauce
- 3 tablespoons tomato paste
- 3 tablespoons apple cider vinegar
- 2 tablespoons Worcestershire sauce
- 2 tablespoons erythritol or monk fruit sweetener
- 1 tablespoon Dijon mustard
- 1 teaspoon liquid smoke

- 1 teaspoon garlic powder
- 1 teaspoon onion powder
- 1 teaspoon paprika
- ½ teaspoon salt
- ½ teaspoon black pepper
- ¼ teaspoon cayenne pepper (optional)

Instructions:

1. In a medium saucepan, combine all ingredients.
2. Whisk until smooth and well combined.
3. Bring to a simmer over medium heat.
4. Reduce heat to low and simmer, stirring occasionally, for 15-20 minutes until sauce thickens to desired consistency.
5. Taste and adjust seasoning. Add more sweetener for sweeter sauce, more vinegar for tangier, more cayenne for spicier.
6. Let cool completely before storing.

Tips:

Budget breakdown: Tomato sauce $1, tomato paste $1, vinegar $0.50, sweetener $1, spices $1. Total: $4.50 for 12 servings.
Storage: Refrigerate in an airtight container for up to 2 weeks or freeze for up to 3 months.
Sweetener options: Erythritol, monk fruit, or allulose all work. Don't use stevia alone (too much has bitter aftertaste).
Thicker sauce: Simmer longer to reduce further. Or add 1 teaspoon xanthan gum while whisking continuously.
Thinner sauce: Add 2-3 tablespoons water.
Store-bought alternative: G Hughes, Primal Kitchen, and Lillie's Q make good sugar-free BBQ sauces if you don't want to make your own.

Uses:
- Grilled chicken or pork
- Ribs
- Pulled pork or chicken
- Meatloaf glaze
- Burger topping
- Mix with ground beef for sloppy joes
- Dipping sauce for chicken wings or tenders

Flavor variations:
- **Smoky:** Double the liquid smoke
- **Spicy:** Add 1 teaspoon cayenne or hot sauce
- **Tangy:** Add extra vinegar and mustard
- **Sweet:** Add extra sweetener (increases carbs slightly)

Hollandaise Sauce

Ingredients:

- 3 large egg yolks
- 1 tablespoon lemon juice
- ½ teaspoon Dijon mustard

- ½ cup (1 stick) butter, melted and hot
- Pinch of cayenne pepper
- Salt to taste

Quick

Makes: About ¾ cup
(6 servings, 2 tablespoons each)

Prep Time: 2 min

Cook Time: 3 min

Total: 5 min

COST PER SERVING: $0.75

MACROS PER SERVING (2 tablespoons):

Calories: 165 | Protein: 2g |
Fat: 18g | Net Carbs: 0g

Instructions:

Blender method (easiest):
1. Melt butter in microwave or on stovetop until hot and bubbling (about 1 minute).
2. While butter melts, add egg yolks, lemon juice, and Dijon mustard to blender.
3. Blend on low for 10 seconds to combine.
4. With blender running on low, slowly drizzle hot melted butter through the top in a thin, steady stream (should take about 30 seconds).
5. As you add the butter, the sauce will emulsify and thicken.
6. Add cayenne pepper and salt to taste. Blend briefly to combine.
7. If sauce is too thick, add 1 teaspoon warm water at a time while blending until desired consistency.
8. Serve immediately.

Stovetop method (traditional):
1. Create a double boiler: Fill a pot with 2 inches of water and bring to a simmer. Place a metal bowl on top (bowl shouldn't touch water).
2. In the bowl, whisk egg yolks, lemon juice, and mustard until smooth.
3. While whisking constantly, slowly drizzle in melted butter.
4. Continue whisking over simmering water until sauce thickens, 2-3 minutes.
5. Remove from heat. Add cayenne and salt. Serve immediately.

Tips:

Budget breakdown: Eggs $1, butter $2, lemon $0.50. Total: $3.50 for 6 servings.
Blender is easier: The blender method is foolproof and much easier than the traditional double-boiler method.
Hot butter is key: The hot butter cooks the egg yolks and creates the emulsion. If butter isn't hot enough, sauce won't thicken.
Broken sauce fix: If sauce breaks (looks curdled), start with a new egg yolk in the blender. Slowly blend in the broken sauce. It will come back together.
Serve immediately: Hollandaise is best fresh. Don't refrigerate (it solidifies). Keep at room temperature for up to 2 hours if needed.
Reheating: If it gets cold, warm gently in a double boiler while whisking. Don't microwave (it will break).

Uses:
- Eggs Benedict (without the English muffin)
- Asparagus or broccoli
- Grilled fish, especially salmon
- Steak (Béarnaise variation)
- Poached eggs over vegetables

Béarnaise variation: Add 1 tablespoon fresh tarragon and 1 tablespoon white wine vinegar. Serve with steak.

Quick   Budget-Friendly

Makes: About 2 cups (8 servings, ¼ cup each)

Prep Time: 2 min

Cook Time: 8 min

Total: 10 min

COST PER SERVING: $0.85

MACROS PER SERVING (¼ cup):

Calories: 185 | Protein: 4g |
Fat: 18g | Net Carbs: 2g

Alfredo Sauce

Ingredients:

- 4 tablespoons butter
- 2 cloves garlic, minced
- 1½ cups heavy cream
- 1 cup grated Parmesan cheese
- ½ teaspoon salt
- ¼ teaspoon black pepper
- ¼ teaspoon nutmeg (optional but recommended)

Instructions:

1. Melt butter in a medium saucepan over medium heat.
2. Add garlic and cook for 1 minute until fragrant (don't let it brown).
3. Pour in heavy cream. Bring to a gentle simmer.
4. Reduce heat to low and simmer for 3-4 minutes, stirring occasionally, until cream thickens slightly.
5. Add Parmesan cheese, salt, pepper, and nutmeg (if using).
6. Stir constantly until cheese melts and sauce is smooth and creamy, about 2 minutes.
7. Remove from heat. Sauce will continue to thicken as it cools.
8. If too thick, add 1-2 tablespoons heavy cream or pasta water (if serving over zucchini noodles) to thin.
9. Serve immediately.

Tips:

Budget breakdown: Butter $2, heavy cream $2.50, Parmesan $2. Total: $6.50 for 8 servings.

Don't boil: High heat causes cream to break and separate. Keep it at a gentle simmer.

Fresh Parmesan: Use freshly grated Parmesan, not the pre-grated stuff. It melts better and tastes better.

Storage: Refrigerate for up to 4 days. Reheat gently on stovetop over low heat, whisking constantly. Add cream to thin if needed.

Make it thicker: Simmer longer to reduce further, or add more Parmesan.

Uses:
- Zucchini noodles or shirataki noodles
- Over grilled chicken or shrimp
- Mix with cooked vegetables (broccoli, cauliflower)
- As a dipping sauce for vegetables
- Base for creamy soups
- Mix with cooked ground beef for a quick casserole

Flavor variations:
- **Garlic Alfredo:** Double the garlic
- **Herb Alfredo:** Add 1 tablespoon fresh basil or parsley
- **Sun-dried tomato Alfredo:** Add ¼ cup chopped sun-dried tomatoes
- **Spinach Alfredo:** Add 2 cups fresh spinach in step 6, cook until wilted

Quick   Budget-Friendly   Make-Ahead

🍽 Makes: About ⅓ cup
(enough for 5-6 pounds of meat)

✂ Prep Time: 5 min

🍲 Cook Time: 0 min

⏰ Total: 5 min

$ COST PER BATCH: $2.50

MACROS PER SERVING (2 tablespoons):

Calories: 20 | Protein: 1g |
Fat: 0g | Net Carbs: 2g

Taco Seasoning (Homemade Blend)

Ingredients:

- 3 tablespoons chili powder
- 2 tablespoons ground cumin
- 2 tablespoons paprika
- 1 tablespoon garlic powder
- 1 tablespoon onion powder

- 1 tablespoon dried oregano
- 2 teaspoons salt
- 1 teaspoon black pepper
- 1 teaspoon cayenne pepper (optional, for heat)

Instructions:

1. Combine all ingredients in a small bowl or jar.
2. Whisk or shake to mix thoroughly.
3. Transfer to an airtight container or jar.
4. Store in a cool, dark place for up to 6 months.
5. Shake before each use to redistribute spices.

How to Use:

For 1 pound of ground meat:
- Add 2-3 tablespoons taco seasoning
- Add 3 tablespoons water
- Cook until water evaporates and meat is well coated

For chicken or pork:
- Rub 1-2 tablespoons directly on meat before cooking

For soups or chili:
- Add 2-3 tablespoons to pot

Tips:

Budget breakdown: Buying bulk spices costs about $2.50 for this batch. Compare to: store-bought packets ($0.50-1.00 each for 1-2 tablespoons) or pre-mixed jars ($4-6 for less seasoning).

Savings: This makes enough seasoning for 5-6 pounds of meat, equivalent to 6-8 store-bought packets. You'll save $3-6 and avoid sugar/fillers.

Why make your own:
- No added sugar (many store brands add sugar or dextrose)
- No fillers (flour, cornstarch, maltodextrin)
- Fresher tasting
- Customizable heat level
- Much cheaper

Storage: Store in a jar with a tight-fitting lid. Keep in a cool, dark place (not above the stove). Spices lose potency after 6-12 months.

Customization:
- **Mild:** Omit cayenne pepper, reduce chili powder to 2 tablespoons
- **Hot:** Increase cayenne to 2 teaspoons or add ½ teaspoon chipotle powder
- **Smoky:** Add 1 teaspoon smoked paprika
- **Earthy:** Increase cumin to 3 tablespoons

Uses:
- Ground beef, turkey, chicken, or pork for tacos
- Taco salad bowls
- Burrito bowls
- Soup or chili
- Roasted vegetables
- Scrambled eggs
- Seasoning for roasted chicken
- Mix into sour cream for a quick dip

Make a big batch: Triple or quadruple this recipe. Put in multiple jars. Give as gifts. Always have it on hand.

CHAPTER 9 SUMMARY

You now have 8 sauces and 1 essential seasoning blend that will transform how you eat. Here's how to use them:

The Sauce System:

Master these 5 sauces:
1. **Garlic butter** - Put on everything. Literally everything.
2. **Ranch dressing** - America's favorite dressing for a reason.
3. **Caesar dressing** - Makes any protein on lettuce exciting.
4. **Sugar-free BBQ sauce** - For when you want summer barbecue flavors.
5. **Taco seasoning** - Ground meat becomes exciting again.

These 5 sauces + basic proteins = 50+ different meals.

My Weekly Sauce Rotation:

Sunday meal prep:
- Make garlic butter (store in fridge, use all week)
- Make ranch dressing (lasts the whole week)
- Refill taco seasoning jar if running low

Throughout the week:
- Monday: Chicken + garlic butter + roasted broccoli
- Tuesday: Taco meat (using taco seasoning) + taco bowl
- Wednesday: Salad with ranch dressing
- Thursday: Chicken + Caesar dressing + romaine
- Friday: Ribs + BBQ sauce

Total sauce prep time: 20 minutes on Sunday. Flavor all week.

Sauce Storage Strategy:

Always in the fridge:
- Garlic butter (2 weeks shelf life)
- Ranch dressing (1 week shelf life)
- Caesar dressing (1 week shelf life)

Make as needed (10 minutes):
- Hollandaise (serve immediately)
- Alfredo (serve immediately or refrigerate 4 days)

Always in the pantry:
- Taco seasoning (6+ months shelf life)

Meal Prep Integration:

Protein + Sauce = Infinite Variety

Same chicken, 8 different meals:
1. Chicken + garlic butter + asparagus
2. Chicken + Caesar dressing + romaine = Caesar salad
3. Chicken + ranch dressing + buffalo sauce = Buffalo chicken
4. Chicken + Alfredo sauce + zucchini noodles
5. Chicken + BBQ sauce + coleslaw
6. Chicken + taco seasoning + cauliflower rice = Mexican bowl
7. Chicken + blue cheese dressing + celery = Buffalo chicken style
8. Chicken + hollandaise + broccoli = Fancy dinner

Cook chicken once on Sunday. Eat 8 different meals.

The Cost Analysis:

Store-bought sauces:
- Good ranch dressing: $4-6 per bottle
- Caesar dressing: $4-6 per bottle
- Sugar-free BBQ sauce: $5-8 per bottle
- Taco seasoning packets: $1 each

Total for one week: $15-20

Homemade sauces (this chapter):
- Ranch dressing: $5.50 (lasts 1-2 weeks)
- Caesar dressing: $4.50 (lasts 1-2 weeks)
- BBQ sauce: $4.50 (lasts 2+ weeks)
- Taco seasoning: $2.50 (lasts months)

Total for several weeks: $17

Savings: $10-20 per month, $120-240 per year

Plus you avoid:
- Added sugars
- Seed oils (soybean, canola)
- Preservatives
- Fillers

Common Mistakes:
1. **Underseasoning everything.** Fat-free, flavor-free eating is why people fail. Use these sauces liberally.
2. **Buying store-bought with added sugar.** Read labels. Many "low-carb" sauces still have hidden sugars.
3. **Not making sauces ahead.** These keep for days or weeks. Make on Sunday, use all week.
4. **Being afraid of fat.** These sauces are high-fat. That's the point. Fat keeps you full and makes food taste good.

5. **Sticking to one sauce.** Rotate your sauces. Variety prevents boredom.

Time Investment:

Per batch:
- Simple sauces (garlic butter, taco seasoning): 5 minutes
- Creamy dressings (ranch, Caesar, blue cheese): 5 minutes
- Cooked sauces (BBQ, Alfredo): 10-25 minutes

Total time to make all sauces: About 90 minutes

How long they last: 1 week to 6 months depending on sauce

Time saved: Never having boring, underseasoned food again. Priceless.

The Complete System:

You've now been through all 9 chapters. You have:
- **Breakfast recipes** (Chapter 1)
- **Quick dinners** (Chapter 2)
- **One-pan meals** (Chapter 3)
- **Budget recipes** (Chapter 4)
- **Make-ahead meals** (Chapter 5)
- **Soups and stews** (Chapter 6)
- **Salads and bowls** (Chapter 7)
- **Sides and snacks** (Chapter 8)
- **Sauces and seasonings** (Chapter 9)

You have everything you need.

You don't need to make every recipe in this book. You need:
- 3-4 breakfasts you can make without thinking
- 5-6 dinners you rotate through
- 2-3 make-ahead meals for busy weeks
- 2-3 soups for comfort food
- 3-4 salads/bowls for lunch
- 3-4 vegetable sides
- 2-3 snacks
- 5 sauces to keep things interesting

That's 25-30 total recipes. Out of 145 in this book.

Find your favorites. Master those. Repeat them. That's how you stick with this long-term.

APPENDIX A: 14-DAY MEAL PLAN

This is where theory meets reality.

You've read through 9 chapters and 145 recipes. Maybe you've tried a few. Maybe you've just been reading, planning to start "when you're ready."

Here's the truth: you'll never feel completely ready. There will always be a birthday party next week, a work event, a vacation coming up, or some reason to delay.

So stop waiting. Start now. This 14-day meal plan shows you exactly how.

What This Meal Plan Is:
- A **practical, realistic** plan using recipes from this book
- Built around **minimal cooking time** (2-3 hours on Sundays, 30 minutes or less on weeknights)
- Designed for **actual humans** with jobs, families, and lives
- **Flexible**—swap meals around based on your schedule and preferences

What This Meal Plan Is NOT:
- A rigid, must-follow-exactly prescription
- Gourmet Instagram-worthy food
- Complicated or time-consuming
- The only way to do this

How to Use This Plan:
Option 1: Follow it exactly If you're brand new and want to remove all decision-making, follow this plan to the letter. Every meal is mapped out. Just execute.

Option 2: Use it as a template If you already have favorite recipes or foods, swap them in. Keep the same structure (meal prep Sunday, easy weeknight meals, leftovers), but use your preferred recipes.

Option 3: Cherry-pick what works Maybe you don't need breakfast planned (you always eat eggs). Maybe you meal prep lunch but cook dinner fresh. Take what helps, ignore the rest.

The Structure:

Sundays: Meal prep day (2-3 hours)
- Cook proteins for the week
- Make 1-2 batch meals (soups, casseroles)
- Prep vegetables
- Hard-boil eggs
- Make 1-2 sauces

Monday-Friday: Use prepped components
- Breakfast: Quick or grab-and-go (5-10 minutes)
- Lunch: Prepped meals or quick assembly (5 minutes)
- Dinner: Quick cooking or reheated prep (15-30 minutes)

Saturdays: Flexible
- Cook something fresh if you want
- Use leftovers
- Eat out
- Experiment with new recipes

Key Principles:
1. **Batch cook proteins** (cook once, eat all week)
2. **Make extra** (intentional leftovers = easy lunches)
3. **Keep it simple** (no recipe needs more than 7 ingredients)
4. **Prep ahead** (Sunday work = easy weeknights)
5. **Stay flexible** (life happens, adjust as needed)

Shopping Strategy:
I've included shopping lists for Week 1 and Week 2. They're organized by store section for efficient shopping.

Before you shop:
- Check your pantry (you may already have spices, oils, etc.)
- Check what's on sale (swap proteins if needed)
- Adjust quantities (this plan serves 1-2 people; multiply as needed)

WEEK 1 MEAL PLAN

WEEK 1 OVERVIEW

Sunday - Meal Prep Day:
- Prep Time: 2.5 hours total
- Cook: Pulled chicken, taco meat, hard-boiled eggs
- Make: Beef chili
- Prep: Vegetables, cauliflower rice
- Make: Ranch dressing, garlic butter

Daily Breakdown:

DAY	BREAKFAST	LUNCH	DINNER
Sunday	Scrambled Eggs 3 Ways	Prep day	Beef Chili (fresh)
Monday	Egg Muffins (prepped)	Beef Chili (leftover)	Garlic Butter Chicken + Broccoli
Tuesday	Egg Muffins	Chicken Bowl (Teriyaki)	Taco Salad Bowl
Wednesday	Greek Yogurt Protein Bowl	Taco Salad Bowl	Chicken Soup (fresh)
Thursday	Bacon & Avocado Plate	Chicken Soup	Sheet Pan Chicken Fajitas
Friday	Egg Muffins	Leftover Fajitas	Chef Salad (quick assembly)
Saturday	Cottage Cheese Pancakes	Chicken Caesar Salad	Whatever you want

Macros Average Per Day:
- Calories: 1,400-1,700
- Protein: 110-140g
- Fat: 90-110g
- Net Carbs: 25-35g

SUNDAY MEAL PREP (Week 1)

Total Time: 2.5 hours **Hands-on Time:** 90 minutes (rest is cooking/cooling)

The Schedule:

9:00 AM - Start
- Preheat oven to 350°F
- Put chicken in slow cooker for Pulled Chicken (Recipe 78)

9:10 AM
- While oven preheats, mix and portion Egg Muffins (Recipe 133)
- Put in oven (20 minutes)

9:30 AM
- Start Beef Chili (Recipe 77) on stovetop
- While chili simmers (45 minutes), move to next tasks

9:40 AM
- Hard-boil 1 dozen eggs (Recipe 81)
- Start water boiling, set timer

9:50 AM
- While eggs cook, chop vegetables:
- Wash and chop lettuce (store in container)
- Dice bell peppers (store in container)
- Dice cucumber (store in container)
- Slice celery (store in container)

10:00 AM
- Eggs done → ice bath → into fridge
- Check egg muffins → should be done → cool on counter

10:15 AM
- Make Ranch Dressing (Recipe 140) - 5 minutes
- Make Garlic Butter (Recipe 138) - 5 minutes
- Store both in fridge

10:30 AM
- Brown ground beef for taco meat (Recipe 86) - 15 minutes
- Add seasoning, cook until done
- Portion into containers

10:45 AM
- Chili should be done → let cool → portion into containers
- Cook 2 batches of Cauliflower Rice (Recipe 124) - 20 minutes
- Store in containers

11:15 AM
- Pulled chicken should be done → shred → portion into containers
- Store with some cooking liquid to keep moist

11:30 AM - Done
- Clean up
- Everything labeled and stored
- Relax, you're done for the week

What You Have:
- Pulled chicken (3-4 cups)
- Taco meat (3-4 cups)
- Hard-boiled eggs (12)
- Egg muffins (12)
- Beef chili (8 servings)
- Prepped vegetables (all week)
- Cauliflower rice (6 servings)
- Ranch dressing (1½ cups)
- Garlic butter (½ cup)

DAILY MEALS - WEEK 1

SUNDAY

Breakfast: Classic Scrambled Eggs (Recipe 1)
- Time: 7 minutes
- While you're cooking anyway, might as well have fresh eggs

Lunch: Light/skip (you've been cooking all morning)

Dinner: Beef Chili (Recipe 77)
- Time: 0 minutes (already made)
- Just heat and serve
- Top with cheese, sour cream, avocado
- Macros: 380 cal, 32g protein, 8g net carbs

MONDAY

Breakfast: Egg Muffins (Recipe 133)
- Time: 1 minute

- Grab 2 muffins from fridge
- Microwave 45 seconds
- Eat in car or at desk
- Macros: 190 cal, 14g protein, 2g net carbs

Lunch: Beef Chili
- Time: 2 minutes
- Heat and eat
- Macros: 380 cal, 32g protein, 8g net carbs

Dinner: Garlic Butter Chicken + Roasted Broccoli
- Use fresh chicken or prepped pulled chicken
- Chicken + garlic butter (Recipe 138)
- Broccoli (Recipe 118)
- Time: 25 minutes
- Macros: 535 cal, 44g protein, 4g net carbs

Daily Total: 1,105 cal, 90g protein, 14g net carbs

TUESDAY

Breakfast: Egg Muffins
- Time: 1 minute
- Macros: 190 cal, 14g protein, 2g net carbs

Lunch: Meal Prep Chicken Bowl - Teriyaki (Recipe 76)
- Use pulled chicken from Sunday
- Cauliflower rice (prepped)
- Broccoli, carrots
- Store-bought teriyaki sauce (check carbs) or soy sauce
- Time: 5 minutes assembly
- Macros: 395 cal, 38g protein, 7g net carbs

Dinner: Taco Salad Bowl (Recipe 104)
- Use taco meat from Sunday
- Prepped lettuce, tomatoes, cucumber
- Top with cheese, sour cream, avocado, salsa
- Time: 5 minutes assembly
- Macros: 495 cal, 36g protein, 8g net carbs

Daily Total: 1,080 cal, 88g protein, 17g net carbs

WEDNESDAY

Breakfast: Greek Yogurt Protein Bowl (Recipe 6)
- Time: 3 minutes
- Fresh berries, nuts, flaxseed

- Macros: 385 cal, 28g protein, 9g net carbs

Lunch: Taco Salad Bowl
- Use remaining taco meat
- Fresh assembly
- Time: 5 minutes
- Macros: 495 cal, 36g protein, 8g net carbs

Dinner: Chicken Soup (Recipe 91)
- Make fresh tonight (45 min) or use canned chicken + broth + vegetables (15 min quick version)
- Make extra for Thursday lunch
- Time: 15-45 minutes depending on method
- Macros: 245 cal, 28g protein, 6g net carbs

Daily Total: 1,125 cal, 92g protein, 23g net carbs

THURSDAY

Breakfast: Bacon & Avocado Plate (Recipe 4)
- Cook bacon and eggs fresh (10 min) or use precooked bacon (2 min)
- Time: 2-10 minutes
- Macros: 465 cal, 28g protein, 3g net carbs

Lunch: Chicken Soup
- Leftover from Wednesday
- Time: 2 minutes
- Macros: 245 cal, 28g protein, 6g net carbs

Dinner: Sheet Pan Chicken Fajitas (Recipe 41)
- Fresh cooking tonight
- Chicken, peppers, onions, spices
- No tortillas, just eat the filling
- Top with sour cream, cheese, avocado
- Time: 30 minutes
- Make extra for Friday lunch
- Macros: 340 cal, 38g protein, 7g net carbs

Daily Total: 1,050 cal, 94g protein, 16g net carbs

FRIDAY

Breakfast: Egg Muffins
- Last 2 from Sunday batch
- Time: 1 minute
- Macros: 190 cal, 14g protein, 2g net carbs

Lunch: Leftover Fajitas
- From Thursday dinner
- Time: 2 minutes
- Macros: 340 cal, 38g protein, 7g net carbs

Dinner: Chef Salad (Recipe 110)
- Use deli meat, hard-boiled eggs, cheese
- Prepped lettuce and vegetables
- Ranch dressing (made Sunday)
- Time: 10 minutes assembly
- Macros: 465 cal, 35g protein, 6g net carbs

Daily Total: 995 cal, 87g protein, 15g net carbs

SATURDAY - FLEX DAY

Breakfast: Cottage Cheese Pancakes (Recipe 10)
- Time: 13 minutes
- A treat for making it through the week
- Macros: 320 cal, 28g protein, 8g net carbs

Lunch: Chicken Caesar Salad (Recipe 106)
- Use remaining pulled chicken
- Fresh romaine
- Caesar dressing (make fresh or use store-bought)
- Time: 15 minutes
- Macros: 515 cal, 42g protein, 4g net carbs

Dinner: Your Choice
- Cook something fresh from the book
- Go out to eat
- Order in (be smart about choices)
- Or just have leftovers if available

Optional: Use Saturday afternoon to do some prep for Week 2 if you want to get ahead

WEEK 1 SHOPPING LIST

PROTEINS:
- 4 lbs boneless, skinless chicken thighs (for pulled chicken)
- 2.5 lbs ground beef (for chili and taco meat)
- 2 lbs chicken breasts or thighs (for Monday dinner and fajitas)
- 18 large eggs (for various meals)
- 1 package bacon (8-12 strips)

- 1 lb deli turkey and ham (for Chef Salad)
- 1 container full-fat Greek yogurt (32 oz)
- 1 container cottage cheese (16 oz)

VEGETABLES:
- 3 heads romaine lettuce
- 3 heads broccoli
- 6 bell peppers (mix of colors)
- 3 onions
- 2 cucumbers
- 4 medium tomatoes (or 2 pints cherry tomatoes)
- 4 celery stalks
- 3 avocados
- 2 large heads cauliflower (or 4 bags frozen cauliflower rice)
- 1 bag fresh spinach
- 3 medium carrots

DAIRY:
- 2 lbs butter (4 sticks)
- 1 quart heavy cream
- 16 oz sour cream
- 16 oz cream cheese
- 2 lbs shredded cheddar cheese
- 8 oz shredded mozzarella
- 8 oz Parmesan cheese (block, not pre-grated)
- 1 cup cottage cheese
- Buttermilk (1 cup - for Ranch dressing)

PANTRY/STAPLES:
(Check your pantry first - you may already have these)
- Olive oil
- Coconut oil or avocado oil
- Mayonnaise (1 jar)
- Dijon mustard
- Hot sauce (Frank's RedHot)
- Soy sauce or coconut aminos
- Apple cider vinegar
- Chicken broth (6 cups)
- Beef broth (6 cups)
- Canned diced tomatoes (28 oz can for chili)
- Tomato paste (6 oz can)
- Salsa (1 jar, sugar-free)
- Almond flour (1 bag)

SPICES: *(If not already in pantry)*
- Salt and black pepper
- Garlic powder
- Onion powder
- Paprika
- Chili powder
- Cumin
- Italian seasoning
- Dried thyme
- Dried oregano
- Dried parsley
- Cayenne pepper

FRESH HERBS:
- Fresh parsley (1 bunch)
- Fresh dill (1 small bunch)
- Fresh chives (1 small bunch)
- Fresh cilantro (1 bunch)

OPTIONAL:
- Berries (for yogurt bowl)
- Nuts (almonds, walnuts - for snacking and yogurt)
- Pork rinds (chip substitute)

Estimated Cost: $120-150 for one person for the week, depending on location and what you already have in the pantry

WEEK 2 MEAL PLAN

WEEK 2 OVERVIEW

Sunday - Meal Prep Day:
- Prep Time: 2.5 hours
- Cook: Pork shoulder (slow cooker), marinated chicken thighs, turkey meatballs
- Make: Zuppa Toscana soup
- Prep: Vegetables, cauliflower rice
- Make: Caesar dressing, garlic butter (refill)

Daily Breakdown:

DAY	BREAKFAST	LUNCH	DINNER
Sunday	Denver Omelet	Prep day	Zuppa Toscana (fresh)
Monday	Breakfast Burrito Bowl	Zuppa Toscana	Marinated Chicken + Green Beans
Tuesday	Spinach & Feta Egg Cups	Greek Chicken Bowl	Turkey Meatballs + Marinara + Zoodles
Wednesday	Smoked Salmon Roll-Ups	Pulled Pork Bowl	Steak Salad (fresh)
Thursday	Egg Roll in a Bowl	Steak Salad (leftover)	Beef & Broccoli Stir-Fry
Friday	Spinach & Feta Egg Cups	Turkey Meatballs	Shrimp Avocado Salad
Saturday	Protein Coffee Smoothie	Buffalo Chicken Salad	Whatever you want

Macros Average Per Day:
- Calories: 1,450-1,750
- Protein: 115-145g
- Fat: 95-115g
- Net Carbs: 25-40g

SUNDAY MEAL PREP (Week 2)

Total Time: 2.5 hours **Hands-on Time:** 90 minutes

The Schedule:

9:00 AM - Start
- Preheat oven to 400°F
- Season and sear pork shoulder, put in slow cooker (Recipe 70) - takes 10 min

9:10 AM
- Mix and portion Turkey Meatballs (Recipe 83) - 15 min
- Put in oven (20 minutes)
- While meatballs bake, move to next tasks

9:25 AM
- Marinate Chicken Thighs (Recipe 87) - 10 min
- Set aside to marinate (will cook later)

9:35 AM
- Start Zuppa Toscana (Recipe 101) on stovetop - 45 min simmer

9:40 AM
- While soup simmers, mix Spinach & Feta Egg Cups (Recipe 12)
- Bake when meatballs come out (20 minutes at 350°F)

9:50 AM
- Prep vegetables while soup simmers:
- Wash and chop lettuce
- Spiralize zucchini or buy pre-spiralized
- Dice cucumbers, tomatoes, peppers
- Prep salad ingredients
- Store all in containers

10:20 AM
- Meatballs done → cool → store in containers
- Put egg cups in oven (20 minutes)

10:30 AM
- Make Caesar Dressing (Recipe 141) - 5 min
- Refill or make new Garlic Butter (Recipe 138) - 5 min

10:40 AM
- Egg cups done → cool → store
- Cook 2 batches Cauliflower Rice (Recipe 124) - 20 min
- Store in containers

11:00 AM
- Soup done → cool → portion into containers
- Grill or bake Marinated Chicken Thighs - 25 min
- While chicken cooks, finish vegetable prep

11:30 AM
- Chicken done → cool → store
- Pork should be done or nearly done (8 hours from start, so will be done by dinner)
- Clean up

What You Have:
- Pulled pork (starts in slow cooker, done by evening)
- Marinated chicken thighs (cooked)
- Turkey meatballs (32 meatballs)
- Spinach & feta egg cups (12 cups)
- Zuppa Toscana (8 servings)
- Prepped vegetables (all week)
- Cauliflower rice (6 servings)
- Caesar dressing (1 cup)
- Garlic butter (½ cup)

DAILY MEALS - WEEK 2

SUNDAY

Breakfast: Denver Omelet (Recipe 2)
- Time: 13 minutes
- Fresh cooked Sunday morning
- Macros: 420 cal, 32g protein, 5g net carbs

Lunch: Light/skip (prep day)

Dinner: Zuppa Toscana (Recipe 101)
- Time: 0 minutes (already made)
- Just heat and serve
- Top with extra Parmesan
- Macros: 385 cal, 22g protein, 6g net carbs

MONDAY

Breakfast: Breakfast Burrito Bowl (Recipe 7)
- Time: 10 minutes
- Scramble eggs, add ground beef or sausage
- Top with cheese, avocado, salsa, sour cream
- Macros: 520 cal, 35g protein, 7g net carbs

Lunch: Zuppa Toscana
- Leftover from Sunday
- Time: 2 minutes
- Macros: 385 cal, 22g protein, 6g net carbs

Dinner: Marinated Chicken Thighs + Garlic Green Beans
- Chicken from Sunday prep
- Make Green Beans (Recipe 119) fresh - 15 min
- Time: 15 minutes total
- Macros: 505 cal, 46g protein, 8g net carbs

Daily Total: 1,410 cal, 103g protein, 21g net carbs

TUESDAY

Breakfast: Spinach & Feta Egg Cups
- From Sunday prep
- Time: 1 minute
- 2 cups, microwave 45-60 seconds
- Macros: 220 cal, 16g protein, 2g net carbs

Lunch: Greek Chicken Bowl (Recipe 105)
- Use marinated chicken from Sunday
- Prepped vegetables, cauliflower rice
- Feta, olives, cucumber, tomatoes
- Greek vinaigrette (make quick or use lemon and olive oil)
- Time: 5 minutes assembly
- Macros: 465 cal, 40g protein, 8g net carbs

Dinner: Turkey Meatballs + Marinara + Zucchini Noodles
- Meatballs from Sunday (4-5 meatballs)
- Store-bought marinara or make simple sauce
- Zucchini noodles (Recipe 123) - cook fresh, 10 min
- Time: 15 minutes
- Macros: 465 cal, 36g protein, 9g net carbs

Daily Total: 1,150 cal, 92g protein, 19g net carbs

WEDNESDAY

Breakfast: Smoked Salmon Roll-Ups (Recipe 5)
- Time: 5 minutes
- Quick and elegant
- Macros: 380 cal, 28g protein, 4g net carbs

Lunch: Pulled Pork Bowl
- Pulled pork from Sunday (should be done by now)
- Cauliflower rice (prepped)
- Coleslaw (Recipe 127, make quick version or use bagged mix)
- Sugar-free BBQ sauce
- Time: 5 minutes assembly
- Macros: 465 cal, 34g protein, 8g net carbs

Dinner: Steak Salad with Blue Cheese (Recipe 107)
- Cook steak fresh tonight - 12 min
- Prepped salad greens and vegetables
- Blue cheese dressing (make fresh or use Recipe 139 from Week 1)
- Time: 22 minutes
- Make extra steak for Thursday lunch
- Macros: 545 cal, 42g protein, 6g net carbs

Daily Total: 1,390 cal, 104g protein, 18g net carbs

THURSDAY

Breakfast: Egg Roll in a Bowl - Breakfast Version (Recipe 15)
- Time: 17 minutes
- Ground pork, cabbage, eggs, Asian seasonings
- Macros: 420 cal, 28g protein, 6g net carbs

Lunch: Steak Salad
- Leftover steak from Wednesday
- Fresh greens
- Time: 5 minutes assembly
- Macros: 545 cal, 42g protein, 6g net carbs

Dinner: Beef & Broccoli Stir-Fry (Recipe 26)
- Fresh cooking tonight
- Sirloin, broccoli, stir-fry sauce
- Serve over cauliflower rice (prepped Sunday)
- Time: 22 minutes

- Macros: 380 cal, 34g protein, 8g net carbs

Daily Total: 1,345 cal, 104g protein, 20g net carbs

FRIDAY

Breakfast: Spinach & Feta Egg Cups
- Last 2 from Sunday batch
- Time: 1 minute
- Macros: 220 cal, 16g protein, 2g net carbs

Lunch: Turkey Meatballs
- Remaining meatballs from Sunday
- Heat with marinara
- Serve over zucchini noodles or eat plain
- Time: 5 minutes
- Macros: 465 cal, 36g protein, 9g net carbs

Dinner: Shrimp Avocado Salad (Recipe 109)
- Fresh cooking tonight (it's quick)
- Shrimp, avocado, greens, cilantro-lime dressing
- Time: 20 minutes
- Macros: 425 cal, 32g protein, 7g net carbs

Daily Total: 1,110 cal, 84g protein, 18g net carbs

SATURDAY - FLEX DAY

Breakfast: Protein Coffee Smoothie (Recipe 11)
- Time: 3 minutes
- Cold brew, protein powder, heavy cream, almond butter
- Macros: 285 cal, 30g protein, 5g net carbs

Lunch: Buffalo Chicken Salad (Recipe 112)
- Use remaining pulled pork or chicken
- Toss with buffalo sauce
- Serve on greens with ranch or blue cheese
- Time: 10 minutes
- Macros: 485 cal, 40g protein, 6g net carbs

Dinner: Your Choice
- Cook something new
- Go out
- Leftovers if any remain
- Rest and prepare for Week 3

WEEK 2 SHOPPING LIST

PROTEINS:
- 4 lbs pork shoulder (for pulled pork)
- 3 lbs boneless, skinless chicken thighs (for marinated chicken)
- 2 lbs ground turkey (for meatballs)
- 1½ lbs Italian sausage (for Zuppa Toscana)
- 12 oz sirloin or flank steak (for steak salad)
- 1½ lbs beef (sirloin or flank) for stir-fry
- 12 oz large shrimp (for salad)
- 1 lb ground pork (for egg roll bowl)
- 24 large eggs
- 8 oz smoked salmon
- 2 lbs ground turkey (for meatballs)

VEGETABLES:
- 3 heads romaine or mixed greens
- 3 heads broccoli
- 3 lbs green beans
- 6 medium zucchini
- 8 cups cabbage (or 1 bag coleslaw mix)
- 4 bell peppers
- 3 onions
- 3 cucumbers
- 3 tomatoes (or 2 pints cherry tomatoes)
- 3 avocados
- 2 large heads cauliflower (or 4 bags frozen cauliflower rice)
- 1 lb fresh spinach
- 1 lb Brussels sprouts (for Zuppa Toscana)
- 3 medium carrots
- 1 head kale
- Fresh ginger root

DAIRY:
- 2 lbs butter (4 sticks)
- 1 quart heavy cream
- 16 oz sour cream
- 8 oz cream cheese
- 2 lbs shredded cheddar cheese
- 1 lb shredded mozzarella
- 8 oz Parmesan cheese
- 8 oz feta cheese
- 6 strips bacon (for Zuppa Toscana)

PANTRY/STAPLES:
- Olive oil
- Sesame oil
- Mayonnaise
- Soy sauce or coconut aminos
- Rice vinegar
- Lemon juice (or 3-4 fresh lemons)
- Lime juice (or 2-3 fresh limes)
- Chicken broth (6 cups)
- Beef broth (2 cups)
- Marinara sauce (2 cups, sugar-free)
- Sugar-free BBQ sauce
- Hot sauce (Frank's RedHot)
- Almond flour
- Worcestershire sauce
- Apple cider vinegar

SPICES: *(Refill if running low)*
- Salt and black pepper
- Garlic powder
- Onion powder
- Paprika (regular and smoked)
- Italian seasoning
- Oregano
- Thyme
- Cumin
- Chili powder
- Red pepper flakes

FRESH HERBS:
- Fresh parsley
- Fresh cilantro
- Fresh dill
- Fresh basil

OPTIONAL:
- Kalamata olives
- Blue cheese (for salad)
- Protein powder (for smoothie)
- Almond butter (for smoothie)
- Cold brew coffee (for smoothie)

Estimated Cost: $130-160 for one person for the week

TIPS FOR SUCCESS

Meal Prep Strategies:

1. **Don't make every recipe from scratch every time**
   - » Use rotisserie chicken instead of cooking chicken
   - » Buy pre-spiralized zucchini
   - » Use frozen cauliflower rice
   - » Buy pre-washed salad greens

2. **Batch your tasks**
   - » Cook all proteins at once
   - » Prep all vegetables at once
   - » Make all sauces at once

3. **Use your time wisely**
   - » While something cooks, prep vegetables
   - » While something marinates, clean up
   - » Multitask when possible

4. **Label everything**
   - » Date your containers
   - » Label what it is
   - » Note what meal it's for

5. **Store strategically**
   - » Put Monday's meals in front
   - » Keep frequently used items accessible
   - » Stack containers efficiently

BEYOND THE 14 DAYS

Week 3 and Beyond:
You don't need a new meal plan every week. Here's what to do:

Option 1: Repeat
- Repeat Week 1 or Week 2
- By the third time through, you'll have it memorized

Option 2: Mix and Match
- Take favorite meals from Week 1 and Week 2
- Create your own weekly rotation
- Stick to meals you actually enjoy

Option 3: Create Your Own
- Use the structure from these two weeks
- Plug in your favorite recipes from the book
- Keep the Sunday prep concept

The Real Goal:
The goal isn't to follow meal plans forever. The goal is to develop a system that works for you:
- 5-7 dinners you rotate through
- 3-4 breakfasts you can make without thinking
- 2-3 lunch options you actually enjoy
- A Sunday prep routine that makes weeknights easy

Once you have that system, you don't need meal plans anymore. You just cook.

APPENDIX B: QUICK REFERENCE GUIDES

You don't need to reread entire chapters when you're standing in the kitchen trying to remember "how long do I cook chicken breasts again?" or "what temperature for roasting vegetables?"

That's what this appendix is for.

These are the cheat sheets, quick references, and at-a-glance guides that you'll actually use. Print these pages. Tape them inside your cabinet. Save photos on your phone. Whatever makes them accessible when you need them.

No fluff. Just the information you need, fast.

1. PROTEIN COOKING GUIDE

CHICKEN

Chicken Breasts (6-8 oz each):
- **Pan-sear:** 6-7 minutes per side, medium-high heat
- **Grill:** 6-7 minutes per side, medium-high heat
- **Bake:** 25-30 minutes at 425°F
- **Internal temp:** 165°F
- **Rest:** 5 minutes

Chicken Thighs (boneless, skinless, 4-5 oz each):
- **Pan-sear:** 5-6 minutes per side, medium-high heat
- **Grill:** 5-6 minutes per side, medium-high heat
- **Bake:** 30-35 minutes at 400°F
- **Internal temp:** 165°F (but can go higher, stays moist)
- **Rest:** 5 minutes

Chicken Thighs (bone-in, skin-on):
- **Pan-sear then bake:** Sear skin-side down 5 minutes, flip, bake 25-30 minutes at 400°F
- **Grill:** 8-10 minutes per side, medium heat
- **Internal temp:** 165°F
- **Rest:** 5 minutes

Ground Chicken/Turkey:
- **Stovetop:** 8-10 minutes, medium-high heat, breaking up as it cooks
- **Done when:** No pink remains, 165°F internal temp

BEEF

Ground Beef:
- **Stovetop:** 8-10 minutes, medium-high heat, breaking up as it cooks
- **Done when:** Browned throughout, 160°F internal temp

Steak (1-inch thick):

DONENESS	INTERNAL TEMP	TIME PER SIDE (HIGH HEAT)
Rare	120-125°F	3-4 minutes
Medium-rare	130-135°F	4-5 minutes
Medium	135-145°F	5-6 minutes
Medium-well	145-155°F	6-7 minutes
Well done	160°F+	8+ minutes (don't do this)
Rest: 5-10 minutes (crucial for steaks)		

Stew Meat (1-inch cubes):
- **Stovetop/braise:** 1.5-2 hours, low simmer
- **Slow cooker:** 6-8 hours low, 3-4 hours high
- **Instant Pot:** 35 minutes high pressure + natural release

PORK

Pork Chops (1-inch thick):
- **Pan-sear:** 4-5 minutes per side, medium-high heat
- **Grill:** 5-6 minutes per side, medium-high heat
- **Bake:** 20-25 minutes at 400°F
- **Internal temp:** 145°F
- **Rest:** 3 minutes

Pork Tenderloin (1-1.5 lbs):
Roast: 20-25 minutes at 425°F
Grill: 15-20 minutes total, turning frequently
Internal temp: 145°F
Rest: 10 minutes

Pork Shoulder (3-5 lbs):
- **Slow cooker:** 8-10 hours low, 4-6 hours high
- **Oven:** 6-8 hours at 275°F
- **Instant Pot:** 60-80 minutes high pressure + natural release
- **Done when:** Falls apart easily, 195-205°F

Ground Pork:
- **Stovetop:** 8-10 minutes, medium-high heat
- **Done when:** No pink remains, 160°F internal temp

SEAFOOD

Salmon Fillets (6 oz):
- **Pan-sear:** 4-5 minutes skin-side down, 2-3 minutes flesh-side
- **Bake:** 12-15 minutes at 400°F
- **Grill:** 4-5 minutes per side, medium heat
- **Internal temp:** 145°F (or when it flakes easily)

White Fish (cod, halibut, mahi-mahi):
- **Pan-sear:** 3-4 minutes per side
- **Bake:** 10-12 minutes at 425°F
- **Internal temp:** 145°F

Shrimp (large, 16-20 count):
- **Pan-sear:** 2-3 minutes per side, high heat
- **Boil:** 2-3 minutes total
- **Done when:** Pink and opaque, curled into "C" shape
- **Warning:** Overcooks fast—watch carefully

2. AT-A-GLANCE MACROS

PROTEINS (per 4 oz cooked)

ITEM	CALORIES	PROTEIN	FAT	CARBS
Chicken breast	185	35g	4g	0g
Chicken thigh	210	26g	11g	0g
Ground beef (80/20)	285	24g	20g	0g
Ground beef (90/10)	215	28g	11g	0g
Ground turkey (93/7)	170	28g	6g	0g
Sirloin steak	200	32g	7g	0g
Ribeye steak	310	28g	22g	0g
Pork chop	200	28g	9g	0g
Ground pork	300	24g	22g	0g
Salmon	235	25g	14g	0g
Shrimp	120	23g	2g	1g
Cod/white fish	120	26g	1g	0g
Eggs (2 large)	140	12g	10g	1g

DAIRY (per serving)

ITEM	SERVING	CALORIES	PROTEIN	FAT	CARBS
Heavy cream	1 tbsp	50	0g	5g	0g
Sour cream	2 tbsp	60	1g	6g	1g
Cream cheese	2 tbsp	100	2g	10g	2g
Cheddar cheese	1 oz	115	7g	9g	1g
Mozzarella	1 oz	85	6g	6g	1g
Parmesan	1 oz	110	10g	7g	1g
Feta	1 oz	75	4g	6g	1g
Greek yogurt (full-fat)	½ cup	120	10g	5g	5g
Cottage cheese	½ cup	110	14g	5g	4g
Butter	1 tbsp	100	0g	11g	0g

VEGETABLES (per 1 cup raw or ½ cup cooked)

VEGETABLE	CALORIES	PROTEIN	FAT	NET CARBS
Spinach	7	1g	0g	0g
Lettuce	5	0g	0g	1g
Broccoli	30	3g	0g	4g
Cauliflower	25	2g	0g	3g
Zucchini	20	1g	0g	3g
Bell pepper	30	1g	0g	4g
Cucumber	15	1g	0g	3g
Tomato	30	1g	0g	5g
Green beans	35	2g	0g	5g
Asparagus	25	3g	0g	3g
Brussels sprouts	40	3g	0g	6g
Cabbage	25	1g	0g	4g
Mushrooms	20	3g	0g	2g
Avocado	240	3g	22g	3g

NUTS & SEEDS (per ¼ cup)

ITEM	CALORIES	PROTEIN	FAT	NET CARBS
Almonds	210	8g	18g	4g
Walnuts	200	5g	20g	2g
Pecans	195	3g	20g	1g
Macadamias	240	3g	25g	2g
Sunflower seeds	190	6g	16g	3g
Pumpkin seeds	180	9g	15g	2g
Chia seeds	195	7g	12g	2g
Flaxseed (ground)	150	5g	12g	0g

Note: Easy to overeat. Pre-portion into ¼ cup servings.

OILS & FATS (per 1 tablespoon)

ITEM	CALORIES	FAT	ITEM	CALORIES	FAT
Olive oil	120	14g	Ghee	120	14g
Coconut oil	120	14g	MCT oil	115	14g
Avocado oil	120	14g	Bacon grease	115	13g
Butter	100	11g	Mayonnaise	90	10g

3. SEASONING RATIOS

BASIC SEASONING FORMULA

For 1 pound of protein:
- 1 teaspoon salt
- ½ teaspoon black pepper
- ½-1 teaspoon garlic powder
- ½-1 teaspoon onion powder
- Optional: ½-1 teaspoon of main spice (paprika, cumin, Italian seasoning, etc.)

QUICK SEASONING BLENDS

Italian Seasoning (3 tablespoons total):
- 1 tbsp dried basil
- 1 tbsp dried oregano
- ½ tbsp dried thyme
- ½ tbsp dried rosemary

Cajun Seasoning (¼ cup total):
- 2 tbsp paprika
- 1 tbsp garlic powder
- 1 tbsp onion powder
- 1 tbsp dried oregano
- 1 tsp cayenne pepper
- 1 tsp black pepper
- 1 tsp salt

Greek Seasoning (3 tablespoons total):
- 1 tbsp dried oregano
- 1 tbsp dried dill
- 1 tsp garlic powder
- 1 tsp onion powder
- 1 tsp lemon zest powder (or use fresh lemon with the blend)
- ½ tsp salt
- ½ tsp black pepper

Ranch Seasoning (¼ cup total):
- 2 tbsp dried parsley
- 1 tbsp dried dill
- 1 tbsp garlic powder
- 1 tbsp onion powder
- 1 tsp salt
- 1 tsp black pepper

Everything Bagel Seasoning (¼ cup total):
- 2 tbsp sesame seeds
- 1 tbsp poppy seeds
- 1 tbsp dried minced garlic
- 1 tbsp dried minced onion
- 2 tsp coarse salt

4. SAUCE RATIOS

BASIC VINAIGRETTE

3 parts oil : 1 part acid

Example (makes ½ cup):
- 6 tablespoons olive oil
- 2 tablespoons vinegar or lemon juice
- 1 teaspoon Dijon mustard (emulsifier)
- Salt and pepper to taste

Variations:
- Balsamic: Use balsamic vinegar
- Lemon-herb: Use lemon juice + fresh herbs
- Asian: Use sesame oil + rice vinegar + soy sauce

BASIC CREAM SAUCE

1 part cream : ¼ part cheese : butter and seasonings

Example (makes 1 cup):
- 1 cup heavy cream
- ¼ cup grated Parmesan
- 2 tablespoons butter
- 2 cloves garlic, minced
- Salt, pepper, nutmeg

Simmer until thickened, 5-8 minutes

COMPOUND BUTTER

1 stick butter : 2-3 tablespoons mix-ins

Example:
- ½ cup (1 stick) softened butter
- 3 cloves garlic, minced
- 2 tablespoons fresh herbs
- ¼ teaspoon salt

Mix, roll into log, refrigerate or freeze

5. COMMON SUBSTITUTIONS

INGREDIENT SWAPS

IF RECIPE CALLS FOR	USE INSTEAD
Bread crumbs	Crushed pork rinds, almond flour, or Parmesan
Flour (for thickening)	Xanthan gum (use ⅛ the amount), or reduce by simmering
Sugar	Erythritol, monk fruit, or allulose (1:1 ratio)
Pasta	Zucchini noodles, shirataki noodles, or spaghetti squash
Rice	Cauliflower rice
Potatoes (mashed)	Cauliflower mash
Potatoes (in soup)	Cauliflower, radishes, or turnips
Tortillas	Lettuce wraps, cheese wraps, or low-carb tortillas
Pizza crust	Cauliflower crust, fathead dough, or chicken crust
Milk	Heavy cream diluted with water, almond milk, or coconut milk
Soy sauce	Coconut aminos (slightly sweeter, gluten-free)
Cornstarch	Xanthan gum (use much less)

PROTEIN SWAPS

Most proteins can be swapped within their category:

Poultry:
- Chicken breasts ↔ Chicken thighs
- Chicken ↔ Turkey
- Ground chicken ↔ Ground turkey

Beef:
- Ground beef ↔ Ground pork
- Sirloin ↔ Ribeye ↔ Strip steak
- Chuck roast ↔ Beef stew meat

Pork:
- Pork chops ↔ Pork tenderloin (adjust cooking time)
- Ground pork ↔ Italian sausage (remove casing)

Seafood:
- Salmon ↔ Other fatty fish (trout, mackerel)
- Cod ↔ Halibut ↔ Mahi-mahi ↔ Tilapia
- Shrimp ↔ Scallops (adjust cooking time)

6. STORAGE TIMES

REFRIGERATOR (40°F or below)

ITEM	STORAGE TIME	ITEM	STORAGE TIME
Raw chicken/turkey	1-2 days	Soups/stews	3-4 days
Raw ground meat	1-2 days	Creamy soups	3-4 days
Raw beef/pork (whole cuts)	3-5 days	Cooked vegetables	3-4 days
Raw fish	1-2 days	Fresh salad greens (washed)	3-5 days
Cooked chicken/turkey	3-4 days	Cut raw vegetables	3-4 days
Cooked beef/pork	3-4 days	Sauces (vinaigrette)	1-2 weeks
Cooked fish	2-3 days	Sauces (creamy)	5-7 days
Hard-boiled eggs	1 week	Compound butter	2 weeks
Egg muffins/cups	5 days		

FREEZER (0°F or below)

ITEM	STORAGE TIME	ITEM	STORAGE TIME
Raw chicken	9-12 months	Cooked fish	2-3 months
Raw ground meat	3-4 months	Soups/stews (no cream)	2-3 months
Raw beef/pork (whole)	4-12 months	Cooked ground meat	2-3 months
Raw fish (fatty)	2-3 months	Bacon	1 month
Raw fish (lean)	6-8 months	Butter	6-9 months
Cooked chicken/turkey	2-6 months	Compound butter	3-4 months
Cooked beef/pork	2-3 months		

Note: Cream-based soups can separate when frozen. Still safe but texture suffers.

7. MEASUREMENT CONVERSIONS

VOLUME

MEASUREMENT	EQUALS	MEASUREMENT	EQUALS
1 tablespoon	3 teaspoons	1 cup	8 fluid ounces
¼ cup	4 tablespoons	1 pint	2 cups
⅓ cup	5 tablespoons + 1 teaspoon	1 quart	4 cups
½ cup	8 tablespoons	1 gallon	4 quarts
1 cup	16 tablespoons		

WEIGHT

MEASUREMENT	EQUALS	MEASUREMENT	EQUALS
1 ounce	28 grams	12 ounces	¾ pound (340 grams)
4 ounces	¼ pound (113 grams)	16 ounces	1 pound (454 grams)
8 ounces	½ pound (227 grams)		

BUTTER

MEASUREMENT	EQUALS
1 stick	½ cup = 8 tablespoons = 4 ounces
2 sticks	1 cup = 16 tablespoons = 8 ounces
4 sticks	2 cups = 1 pound

8. COMMON RECIPE ABBREVIATIONS

ABBREVIATION	MEANS	ABBREVIATION	MEANS
tsp	teaspoon	qt	quart
tbsp	tablespoon	pt	pint
c	cup	gal	gallon
oz	ounce	pkg	package
lb	pound	doz	dozen

9. QUICK TROUBLESHOOTING

COMMON PROBLEMS & FIXES

Problem: Chicken is dry
- **Cause:** Overcooked
- **Fix:** Use a meat thermometer. Pull at 165°F, not higher.
- **Prevention:** Use thighs instead of breasts (more forgiving)

Problem: Steak is tough
- **Cause:** Didn't rest or wrong cut
- **Fix:** Always rest 5-10 minutes. Slice against the grain.
- **Prevention:** Use tender cuts or marinate tough cuts

Problem: Vegetables are mushy
- **Cause:** Overcooked or crowded pan
- **Fix:** Cook less time. Roast in single layer.
- **Prevention:** Check vegetables 5 minutes before recipe says

Problem: Sauce is too thin
- **Cause:** Not enough reduction or thickener
- **Fix:** Simmer longer uncovered, or add tiny amount of xanthan gum
- **Prevention:** Be patient with reduction

Problem: Sauce is too thick
- **Cause:** Over-reduced or too much thickener
- **Fix:** Add liquid (broth, cream, water) 1 tablespoon at a time
- **Prevention:** Add thickeners slowly

Problem: Food is bland
- **Cause:** Not enough salt, fat, or acid
- **Fix:** Add salt first. Then butter or oil. Then acid (lemon, vinegar).
- **Prevention:** Season in layers while cooking, not just at the end

Problem: Eggs are rubbery
- **Cause:** Too high heat
- **Fix:** Lower heat, add fat (butter/cream), don't overcook
- **Prevention:** Cook eggs on medium-low heat with patience

Problem: Ground meat is greasy
- **Cause:** High-fat content
- **Fix:** Drain excess fat after browning (save for cooking)
- **Prevention:** Use leaner ground meat or plan to drain

Problem: Salad is soggy
- **Cause:** Pre-dressed too early
- **Fix:** Can't fix. Make fresh.
- **Prevention:** Always dress right before eating

Problem: Meal prep got boring
- **Cause:** Same meals every week
- **Fix:** Change the sauce/seasoning on the same protein
- **Prevention:** Rotate through 3-4 different sauces weekly

FINAL THOUGHTS

The most common question I get: "Is this realistic long-term?"

My answer: **It becomes your new normal.**

First 2 weeks: Feels hard. You're breaking sugar addiction and changing habits.

Weeks 3-6: Gets easier. Cravings diminish. Energy improves. You start seeing results.

Months 2-4: Feels normal. You know what to eat. You don't think about it constantly.

Month 6+: It's just how you eat. Not a diet. A lifestyle.

You'll know you've made it when:
- You don't crave sugar anymore
- You feel satisfied after meals
- You have consistent energy
- You don't think about food constantly
- You make good choices without effort
- Your default is protein and vegetables

This isn't about perfection.

It's about progress.
Some weeks will be better than others. Some meals will be off-plan. Life will happen.

The difference between success and failure isn't never messing up.

It's getting right back on track when you do.

You've got this.

Now stop reading and go cook something.